P. F. BELL

*Total Intravenous Anaesthesia*

# *Monographs in Anaesthesiology*

VOLUME 21

*Editor-in-Chief*
T.E.J. HEALY

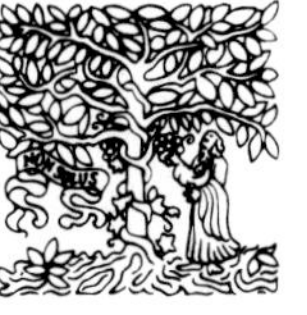

Elsevier · Amsterdam · New York · Oxford

# *Total Intravenous Anaesthesia*

*Edited by*
B. KAY

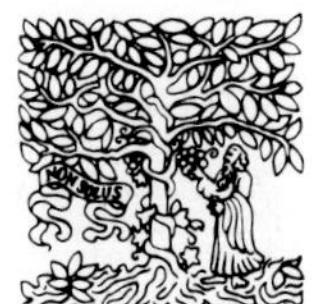

1991
Elsevier · Amsterdam · New York · Oxford

*1st edition © 1974, Excerpta Medica*
*The 1st edition was originally published as Volume 3 in the series.*



ISBN 0-444-81198-2 (volume)
ISBN 0-444-80023-9 (series)

*This book is printed on acid-free paper.*

Published by:
Elsevier Science Publishers B.V.
P.O. Box 211, 1000 AE Amsterdam
The Netherlands

Sole distributors for the USA and Canada:
Elsevier Science Publishing Company, Inc.
655 Avenue of the Americas
New York, NY 10010, USA

Printed in Ireland

# *Contents*

# *List of Contributors*

B. Auty, C.Eng., M.I.E.E.
*University of Bath, Bath Institute of Medical Engineering, Wolfson Centre, Royal United Hospital, Bath, BA1 3NG, UK*

J.G. Bovill, M.D., PhD., F.F.A.R.C.S.I.
*Department of Anaesthesiology, University Hospital Leiden, P.O. Box 9600, 2300 RC Leiden, The Netherlands*

F. Camu, M.D.
*Chairman and Professor of Anaesthesiology, Department of Anaesthesiology, Flemish Free University of Brussels Medical Center, B-1090, Brussels, Belgium*

G.M. Cooper, M.B., Ch.B., F.F.A.R.C.S.
*Senior Lecturer in Anaesthesia, University of Birmingham, Birmingham Maternity Hospital, Queen Elizabeth Medical Centre, Edgbaston, Birmingham, B15 2TG, UK*

H.L. Edmonds, Jr., Ph.D.
*Department of Anesthesiology, University of Louisville School of Medicine, Louisville, KY 40292, USA*

C.S. Goodchild, M.A., M.B., B.Chir., Ph.D., F.C.Anaesth.
*24 Hyde Terrace, Leeds, LS2 9LN, UK*

B. Kay, D.Med.Sci., M.B., Ch.B., F.F.A.R.C.S., D.A.
*Department of Anaesthesia, Victoria University of Manchester, Manchester, UK*

N. Mackenzie, M.B., Ch.B., F.F.A.R.C.S
*Department of Anaesthetics, Ninewells Teaching Hospital, Dundee, Scotland, UK*

E. Moss, M.B. F.C.Anaes.
*Department of Anaesthetics, The General Infirmary at Leeds, Great George Street, Leeds, LS1 3EX, UK*

A. Nilsson, M.D., Ph.D.
*Department of Anaesthesiology, Central Hospital, S-721 Västerås, Sweden*

M.P.J. Paloheimo, M.D.
*Department of Anaesthesiology, University of Helsinki, Helsinki, Finland*

B.J. Pollard, B.Pharm., M.B., Ch.B., F.F.A.R.C.S.
*University Department of Anaesthesia, Manchester Royal Infirmary, Manchester M13 9WL, UK*

M. Rucquoi, M.D.
*Associate Professor, Department of Anaesthesiology, Flemish Free University of Brussels Medical Center, B-1090, Brussels, Belgium*

G.N. Russell, M.B., Ch.B., F.F.A.R.C.S.(E.)
*Regional Adult Cardiothoracic Centre, Broadgreen Hospital, Thomas Drive, Liverpool, UK*

J.W. Sear, M.A., B.Sc., Ph.D., F.F.A.R.C.S.
*Clinical Reader in Anaesthetics, University of Oxford, John Radcliffe Hospital, Headington, Oxford, OX3 9DU, UK*

J. Van Hemelrijck, M.D.
*Department of Anesthesiology, Washington University School of Medicine, St. Louis, MO 63110, USA*

P.F. White, Ph.D., M.D.
*Department of Anesthesiology, Washington University School of Medicine, St. Louis, MO 63110, USA*

# *Preface*

Total Intravenous Anaesthesia (TIVA) is a practical technique that can confer positive benefits not only on the patient but also on the medical and nursing staff who work in the operating theatre and recovery room. Unfortunately it is practised by only a minority of anaesthetists. Why is this?

There are many reasons. The main one may well be that most anaesthetists fear that if they attempt to use what is to them this new technique they will fail to deliver to the patient and the surgeon their usual high standard of anaesthesia. This fear is completely understandable. In many of the early publications about TIVA (including some of the Editor's) reference is made to the abandonment of the technique in favour of inhalational anaesthesia due to technical failure. Far more of the papers written and talks given about TIVA mention that the patient moved during surgery, which is virtually unacceptable to both surgeon and anaesthetist, on whom it casts a doubt about competence. Even worse is the assumption made in the minds of almost all the rest of the operating room staff that the patient is aware of the surgery that is going on and that the anaesthetist has failed in the most basic of his duties. To expose themselves to this sort of risk and even ridicule, anaesthetists must be not only convinced that their attempts to use TIVA will result in all the benefits that exponents of the technique predict but also that they have a very great chance of carrying through their use of TIVA without significant difficulties and, above all, without the risk that the patient will experience the pain of surgery.

The purpose of this book is to help those who wish to practise TIVA competently. This is by no means the first or last book with this aim, but the last major book written primarily with this intention (Editor, Sear, J., 1984) is now more than 6 years old and during this time enormous advances have been made in technique and in the pharmacopoea and equipment available to apply it successfully. In addition, during these six years TIVA has been used far more extensively, by a far greater number of anaesthetists who have not only contributed their accumulated knowledge and experience to the literature but who are also available to teach the best use of the available techniques to those who wish to benefit by them.

This edition is not, however, an anaesthetic recipe book. All the authors believe that good practice can only come about as a result of a thorough understanding of the problems and principles involved and all are aware that whatever drugs and dosages, or methods of application are recommended, trained anaesthetic specialists will adapt these to their patients and the circumstances of their practice. What we hope is that we may offer also an overview and a framework of techniques and, above all, an insight into our experience that we trust will give intending practitioners confidence that they can conduct TIVA competently from the start.

Nevertheless, instant and continued success is not guaranteed. Just as anaesthetists made mistakes and errors of judgement during their training in inhalational anaesthesia it will inevitably take some time and above all practice to ensure the best use of TIVA. Should that statement deter would-be practitioners it should be remembered that the same can be said in regard to the introduction of every new drug and technique in anaesthesia and surely no anaesthetist would wish to halt completely his progress in his profession. One must also remember that continuous success with the practice of long-standing and well-practiced anaesthetic techniques is also not guaranteed; individual patient variability ensures that. So it is not uncommon to see movement in response to surgery in a patient breathing a volatile anaesthetic, embarrassing hiccups, delayed recovery, etc. and, fortunately more rarely, awareness and memory of the pain of surgery, serious anaesthetic-induced complications and even death.

An important point during the initial phase of practice of TIVA is to ensure that all who benefit from the advantages to be gained are able to appreciate them from the start, so that they are immediately more tolerant of any imperfections that may also be apparent. Thus, a surgeon is less likely to complain of slight movement of a patient undergoing a minor surgical procedure if the anaesthesia induction time has been cut to a minute and the patient thanks him personally after waking on the operating table. Nurses in both the operating room and the recovery room will appreciate the fast recovery and rapid turnover that use of TIVA can offer and will also appreciate an explanation that the patient who moves or even phonates during surgery is indeed unconscious, again best reinforced by the patient's own reassurance before leaving the area.

There are also practical difficulties facing the anaesthetist wishing to practice TIVA. Perhaps the greatest and most immediate will be the lack of suitable apparatus. Whilst one of the features of TIVA is that it may be conducted with a minimum of apparatus compared with inhalational anaesthesia, it does demand some pieces that may not be immediately available to every anaesthetist, who must therefore initially spend some of his valuable time in selecting and accumulating appropriate apparatus before embarking on the new venture. Lest this deter, the essential requirements do not include dedicated administration apparatus or special monitoring facilities and particularly not a computer! As reference to the text will indicate, TIVA may be simply applied. What is required is a capacity to deliver an air and oxygen mixture to the patient, although the editor believes that the dangers of giving a patient pure oxygen to breathe for a relatively short time are often greatly exaggerated and are virtually non-existent. For patients breathing spontaneously, it is usually very easy to adapt the connection of an oxygen mask such as is used in the recovery room to fit the outlet of the anaesthetic machine, rather than importing an additional oxygen cylinder in to the operating room, without hazarding the immediate availability of means of ventilating the patient with oxygen manually. For artificial ventilation of a paralysed patient not all ventilators found in operating rooms are capable of delivering an air/oxygen mix and it may be necessary to import an additional one from intensive care or store. Alternatively one may use oxygen, or compromise with a nitrous oxide/oxygen mix.

The latter solution is one favoured by many initially embarking on the use of TIVA in paralysed patients which one would not personally discourage, whilst pointing out the advantages of omitting the gas. Although its use offers some protection against the possibility of awareness in the paralysed patient, it is no guarantee, and the author suggests that the principles described in Chapter 5 are more appropriate.

The problem of potential awareness in paralysed patients leads many anaesthetists into gaining their initial experience of TIVA in unparalysed, spontaneously ventilating patients. Yet these offer the greatest challenge. It is difficult to prevent reflex movement in response to even minor surgical stimulation by using TIVA without inducing an important degree of respiratory depression, impossible if a skin incision is required. The anaesthetist may well not wish to have to support ventilation in an unparalysed patient, however, as this may involve some difficulty, particularly in the case of opioid-induced apnoea. To give the drugs in such a way that significant respiratory depression is avoided, making use of the stimulus of surgery, requires experience not only of the technique but also of the surgeon's practice. Yet the results can be outstanding.

On the other hand the practice of TIVA in paralysed patients will almost invariably be successful from the start. Here the great problem is of overdosage in response to fear of patient awareness. Again, this problem is mainly overcome by experience in the detection of potential awareness and incipient overdose. Whilst use of some of the new, shorter-acting drugs may help to limit the effects of the latter, there is no doubt that the use of appropriate monitoring equipment is the way to obtain the best results.

The Editor has been very fortunate in obtaining some of the best international authorities as authors for this book, including Dr. John Sear, Editor of the last major book on the subject. Not only were these authors prepared to contribute but they also kept to an early, uniform deadline for submission of their Chapters so that the book could be published before their material became out of date in what is a rapidly changing field of anaesthesia. Having said that, it seems very unlikely that any new drugs useful for TIVA will be marketed in the near future. What is certain is that there will be a continued expansion in the practice and experience of TIVA.

*Manchester (U.K.)* B. KAY

*B. Kay (ed.) Total Intravenous Anaesthesia*



# 1

# *Why total intravenous anaesthesia (TIVA)?*

Frederic Camu and Brian Kay

## INTRODUCTION

In order to achieve adequate surgical anaesthesia, the choice of drugs to be used will be determined not only by the pathological condition of the patient but also by the objectives of the anaesthetist. The primary functions of the anaesthetic are to render the patient pain-free throughout surgery by causing unconsciousness or providing adequate analgesia and also to provide the surgeon with a patient who is accessible for surgery, sufficiently immobile and in some circumstances with reduced muscle tone. However, the anaesthetist may have many other objectives. High on the anaesthetist's list of requirements for the effects of any anaesthetic will be the reduction of the effects of surgery (and also anaesthesia itself) on the physiological, pathological and metabolic state of the patient. In its simplest form this usually implies a suppression to some extent of the reflex responses, both somatic and autonomic, to the severe stimulation generally associated with surgery and often with anaesthesia. Many other objectives will spring to the minds of different anaesthetists because these aims will be determined not only by the condition of the patient and the purpose of the surgery but also by the circumstances of anaesthesia and above all by the skill, knowledge and experience of the anaesthetist. Even then, objectives may vary between anaesthetics and anaesthetists as priorities are chosen where aims conflict and the individual preferences of patient, surgeon and anaesthetist are considered.

Not surprisingly, no anaesthetic agent will provide all the requirements that exist, or even, except in rare circumstances, the requirements for a single anaesthetic. Considering only the primary objectives, the volatile anaesthetics will fulfil these aims in the majority of cases whereas TIVA will only occasionally do so; but no patient or anaesthetist is nowadays satisfied with the simple achievement of basic objectives. Thus, although TIVA almost inevitably leads to the occurrence of multiple interactions between different drugs, the use of volatile anaesthetics is in practice never free from such problems. Any comparison between the different modes of anaesthetic administration, i.v. or via the respiratory system, must take into account the whole spectrum of pharmacological and technical problems, these being mainly the pharmacological effects, complications and side-effects, but they also include difficulties of administration, drug interactions and also adequate definition and control of the objectives of the anaesthetic.

Nevertheless, there is a clear difference in the basic concept of achieving the desired objectives by use of TIVA or by volatile anaesthetics. It is the use of individual drugs to obtain specific effects rather than a single drug to do everything. In a majority of circumstances this issue is already resolved in favour of specificity of action, despite the inevitability of inducing complex drug interactions. Anaesthesia is rarely induced by inhalation, which is difficult for the anaesthetist and detested by the patient. Considerable muscle relaxation is infrequently obtained by volatile anaesthetics; neuro-muscular blocking agents are usually used despite the technical and pharmacological problems that they cause. The question is, how practical is it to aim to use drugs that achieve all the objectives of anaesthesia as specifically as possible, which implies TIVA, rather than using the volatile anaesthetics which are relatively unspecific in their effects? Also, will the resulting anaesthesia be any better for its increased specificity?

There is without doubt a theoretical attraction to the concept of being able to tailor the extent of any (specific) pharmacological effect exactly to that required in the circumstances rather than having to increase or decrease a range of effects caused by a volatile anaesthetic; but this is not done simply. Not only are there considerable gaps in the pharmacopoea that would be required but also gaps in the understanding of how the drugs we have work, interact and are eliminated that hopefully will be reduced as experience with TIVA increases. On the grounds of experience alone very few anaesthetists can compare TIVA and volatile anaesthesia in a balanced way.

In the final reckoning, it is the comparative safety and incidence of complications that TIVA and volatile anaesthetics cause in their own hands, in particular circumstances, that will lead to anaesthetists choosing one or the other.

TIVA may have additional theoretical advantages. Many of the drugs used are specific because they act at receptor sites rather than having the more widespread cellular effects that appear to be caused by volatile anaesthetics. Drugs that act at receptor sites have limited effects. Their log•dose-response relations are predictable and usually linear in the region of clinically used dosage. Other drugs acting at the same receptors are frequently available not only giving options of speed of onset and duration of effect but also of competitive antagonists, partial agonists with a reduced maximum efficacy and agonist/antagonists which may find particular application. Understanding of the chemistry of the receptor can also help to produce drugs with greater specificity and more potency and, therefore, fewer side-effects. Many therapeutic advances may be expected and the aims of such developments are clear. Additionally, many receptor sites are complexes or are complex in their structure or function, thus allowing multiple or sophisticated approaches to inhibiting (or enhancing) transmission of impulses. The neuromuscular junction is a case in point, where drugs have been developed to block, competitively, the acetylcholine receptor and also to inhibit, pre-synaptically, the release of acetyl-choline. Thus, combinations of different 'relaxants' may be used to produce not only additive but also synergistic effects, allowing a significant reduction in the dosage and therefore the side-effects (which may be dissimilar) of the drugs used in the combination. One may reasonably expect the development of more of such fortuitous and useful interactions in other areas where drugs acting at receptors are employed, and such developments will be hastened by the more extensive use of TIVA. Perhaps also we may look forward to future advances of this type being based on knowledge and understanding rather than on serendipity.

'Polypharmacy' is a much derided term, with some reason if a multiplicity of drugs are being used in an attempt to ensure that at least one of them has the desired effect; but to use multiple agents each to produce their specific, required effect not only makes sense but is the basis of the concept of 'balanced anaesthesia' that has been one of the major advances in the specialty in the last century. However, as more drugs are required the problems of how they will interact in mulitiple combination, and even of how to study such complex interactions, becomes more difficult. As drugs become more specific, 'cleaner', these problems should be reduced. Computerized predictions of multiple interactions may help us.

For the moment, it is apparent that some anaesthetists use TIVA in some cases because it provides their patients with better anaesthesia than inhaled anaesthetics. In addition to this clear indication for the use of TIVA there are surely two more indications in particular circumstances. One is to study TIVA; to ascertain not only the feasibility of various and new techniques and the suitability of various and new drugs but also to assess these and compare with established inhalation and TIVA techniques. The other is to practice TIVA techniques. For those only trained and experienced in inhalation methods initial ventures into the use of TIVA may be disappointing but results improve remarkably with experience and it would be wrong to reject the new methods, which have now been found to be advantageous in some circumstances by many good anaesthetists, on the grounds of initial difficulties.

## UNCONSCIOUSNESS

### History and development

In the induction of a state of unconsciousness the preference for the i.v. route was rapidly established as soon as fast-acting barbiturates became available more than 50 years ago. Shortly afterwards infusions of the so-called short-acting thiopentone were used (alone) also to maintain anaesthesia, in a 'more or less' manner similar to the almost routine use of ether at the time. Not surprisingly, the results were poor although many anaesthesiologists in the U.S.A. practised the technique extensively and probably developed it to its maximum effectiveness. In the absence of muscle relaxants the need to suppress movement of the patient led to very high doses being given with consequent marked respiratory depression and very prolonged recovery times. The experiences of Pearl Harbour ended extensive use of the technique; it must be remembered that most of the deaths there caused by thiopentone were due to the use of doses intended not to remove consciousness minimally but to induce surgical anaesthesia.

Subsequent reference to Lundy's (1926) original concept of 'balanced anaesthesia' led to the realization that the appropriate use for the barbiturates, which have a selective effect on the cerebral cortex rather than the more uniform central nervous system depression caused by the volatile anaesthetics, was to produce unconsciousness rather than to suppress the reflex motor responses to surgical stimulation which may occur down to spinal cord level. They came to be recognized as hypnotics in practice, although like most hypnotics they have a narcotic effect if given in sufficient dosage. First attempts to substitute an opioid, pethidine, for the (truly awful) ether in a balanced anaesthetic technique failed (see below), so a volatile anaesthetic remained an essential component of most anaesthetics and the maintenance of unconsciousness by drugs given i.v. remained unnecessary and uninvestigated. This situation was reinforced when the modern generation of volatile anaesthetics became available in the middle '50s and ether was replaced. It was also reinforced when the pharmacokinetics of thiopentone were better evaluated and supported experience in suggesting that infusion of the drug was a poor method of maintaining unconsciousness.

A temporary resurgence in the use of TIVA occurred when ketamine was introduced, a drug capable of maintaining unconsciousness and preventing motor responses to surgical stimulation without significant respiratory or cardiovascular depression when used alone. However, the unfortunate side-effects of ketamine soon reduced its frequency of use and relegated it to a small but important area of practice.

A further resurgence came shortly afterwards, however, as new and less persistent i.v. anaesthetics were developed. In the case of methohexitone its use for TIVA was mostly for short anaesthetics, given alone but often after an opioid premedication. Like thiopentone, it often provided unsatisfactory anaesthesia when used in this way but at least recovery was faster. The introduction of Althesin also acted as a spur although the drug used alone was hardly more effective than methohexitone. However, its availability initiated the present resurgence in TIVA techniques when Savege published his results of Althesin/pethidine anaesthesia in 1975. That this technique was not consistently effective was probably due to the drugs used and better results were obtained by Kay (1977a,b,c) using the safer and more effective drugs, etomidate and fentanyl, which became the basis of the subsequent development of TIVA.

The efficacy and safety of fentanyl also allowed the development of opioid anaesthesia by De Castro and Viars (1968), Bovill (1978) and others. The use of morphine by Lowenstein et al. (1971) was less satisfactory as the very high dosage required was less safe. The concept of using the hypnotic effect of opioids to maintain unconsciousness throughout anaesthesia was perhaps not novel but the method was unreliably effective and unsafe until the highly potent and selective fentanyl was developed. Even so, the specificity of effect of fentanyl is for opioid receptors and it is not, like the i.v. anaesthetics, selectively acting at the cerebral cortex so opioid anaesthesia is generally only applied to cases where the other opioid effects are required long after consciousness has been recovered. The subsequent development of other opioids safe enough to use for opioid anaesthesia, e.g. sufentanil and alfentanil, has offered increased flexibility of use but has not changed the basic position, although alfentanil has significantly extended the use of TIVA by its use as the opioid component (see below).

The other new drug that has extended the use of TIVA is propofol. The use of etomidate for long anaesthetics declined due to its capacity to cause extensive myoclonia continuing even after recovery of consciousness (Kay, 1977c) and depression of the adreno-cortical response to stress (Ledingham, 1983). Propofol has few if any qualities that make it unsuitable for TIVA and, being cleared faster than any other i.v. anaesthetic, is probably the drug most frequently used for this purpose.

All the i.v. anaesthetics discussed above, except the opioids, have generalized narcotic cellular effects on the central nervous system, rather like those of the volatile anaesthetics but acting more selectively on the cerebral cortex. There are, however, highly specific hypnotics acting on cortical receptors which maintain consciousness, the benzodiazepines. Naturally, such drugs fit better into the concept of the basis of TIVA than non-specific drugs. Their specificity is reflected in greater safety (i.e., less capacity to kill by respiratory or cardiovascular depression) and fewer side-effects than the i.v. anaesthetics. Thus they have completely replaced the barbiturates as hypnotics for domestic use. A competitive antagonist has also been developed. But, up to the present time, the pharmacokinetic and pharmacodynamic attributes of this group of drugs have not proved to be suitable for wide-spread use to induce and maintain unconsciousness during anaesthesia. The main problems are a relatively slow and uncertain onset of effect and a generally prolonged recovery time. The dose required to induce unconsciousness also varies widely and the slow onset of effect makes titration of dose to effect unacceptably time-consuming on most occasions. Their intensity of hypnotic effect is also more difficult to monitor than that of the i.v. anaesthetics, so that the point of recovery of conscious awareness may be difficult, although essential, to ascertain. However, they do have the often invaluable attribute of being able reliably to induce amnesia in a majority of cases. One may look forward to the development of drugs of this type more suitable for anaesthetic practice. At present a small benzodiazepine effect is widely used as a component of TIVA, the drug being given as premedication to reduce apprehension but also contributing its hypnotic and amnesic effects to the induction and maintenance of unconsciousness throughout anaesthesia, thereby allowing a reduction in the dose of i.v. anaesthetic required.

# COMPARISONS

When seeking to justify the use of TIVA it is necessary to explore not only the range of drugs available and their effects but also the areas of use in order to determine which uses of what drugs may provide better anaesthesia than conventional inhalation anaesthesia. Thus the problems incurred by the use of TIVA are as important as the advantages gained in assessing where the technique is most likely to prove valuable.

## Control of unconsciousness

Consideration of the drugs most often used to induce and maintain unconsciousness during TIVA suggests that they have one outstanding advantage over inhaled anaesthetics; the i.v. route offers the opportunity to induce or deepen the level of unconsciousness very rapidly. With these lipophilic drugs the dynamic equilibrium between concentrations in the plasma and at the effector site is rapid so that the intensity of effect becomes proportional to the plasma concentration. A rise in plasma concentration is rapidly achieved but a fall, leading to a diminution of effect, may not be so readily obtained. Although the i.v. anaesthetics usually used for TIVA have been selected at least partly because of their rapid elimination from the body in general and the plasma in particular, the rate of change may vary greatly even within the individual, the pharmacokinetics depending not only on some of the pharmacodynamic effects but also the effects of surgery. In addition the rate of change of the plasma concentration will also depend on the previous rate of administration and dose of drug given. However, the same limitations of decline in effector site concentrations apply also to the volatile anaesthetics, where a diminution is never fast.

The rapidity with which plasma concentrations of i.v. anaesthetics may change does produce a problem which is less marked when the slower-acting volatile anaesthetics are used, that of maintaining a therapeutic concentration at the effector site. The problems are multiple. During i.v. infusion the plasma concentration at steady state is the ratio of the zero-order infusion rate to the plasma clearance of the drug; but as we have seen the latter may vary for a number of reasons and, being primarily dependent on hepatic function, may decrease profoundly during the course of surgery, leading to an increasing effect of the drug. Volatile agents are much less susceptible to such an effect. Drug clearance may also be affected by other drugs used by the anaesthetist, e.g. propofol and fentanyl.

A second problem is the maintenance of a therapeutic concentration of i.v. anaesthetic after an initial injection usually given to obtain a fast induction of unconsciousness. One may calculate a pattern of infusion by using patient-related parameters and mean pharmacokinetic data but such calculations can only be crude approximations due to the large individual pharmacokinetic variability seen with all these drugs, compounded by pre-existing pathology or age. The usual technique used, in order to obtain the desired fast induction, leads to an 'overshoot' above the minimum concentration required to maintain unconsciousness; but then this is the usual pattern of induction with volatile anaesthetics, so why is it more important in TIVA? One reason is the rate at which the overshoot is approached, inevitably slow with volatile anaesthetics and faster with i.v. agents, readily leading to a greater temporary overdosage. This argument may be more theoretical than real as all anaesthetists become adept at giving the induction dose of their i.v. anaesthetic at a rate appropriate to the patient's condition and requirements in order to minimize the overshoot and its effects, whilst few users of volatile agents are looking closely to prevent overshoot and usually only react to indications of overdosage.

This is because of the second reason why overshoot may be more important in TIVA than inhalation anaesthesia, that the i.v. agents mostly used have a small therapeutic index compared with the volatile agents, opioids or benzodiazepines. However, this index is based on animal toxicology which does not allow for the maintenance of ventilation normal in anaesthetic practice. Nevertheless the concept embodies a sensible way of thinking about dosage and in order to avoid the main consequences of overshoot overdosage, respiratory and cardiovascular depression, the practitioner of TIVA must take steps to minimize the possibility, mainly by slowing the rate of initial administration and close observation so that the rate may be further reduced to an appropriate level as soon as the initial objective of loss of consciousness is achieved.

This is one reason why predetermined dosage on a mg/kg basis should not be used to initiate TIVA. The second and more important reason is that individual variation between plasma concentration and effect is very great with all the drugs used. Thus although an optimal therapeutic plasma concentration exists, it cannot be predicted for the individual from mean statistics. Indeed, it may change greatly during the course of anaesthesia as the degree of stimulation and the effects of interacting drugs vary. If this variability of pharmacodynamic response is added to individual pharmacokinetic variability it may be seen that the prediction of dose requirement and patterns of infusion based on mean pharmacokinetics and dynamics can only be a crude guide. But does the situation differ when volatile anaesthetics are used? Only in degree. It appears from experience and the little data available that individual variation in pharmacokinetics and pharmacodynamic response is less with volatile anaesthetics than with i.v. anaesthetics, so that administration of inhalation anaesthesia is in some ways easier than TIVA. However, the rate of administration must always be controlled by patient responses and if the monitoring of such responses has to be closer when TIVA is being used the patient is all the safer.

One area where the smaller therapeutic index and greater individual pharmacokinetic and pharmacodynamic response variation of i.v. anaesthetics is of most concern is in the maintenance of unconsciousness in paralysed patients. With volatile anaesthetics one may usually give a small 'overdose' in terms of optimum concentrations to maintain unconsciousness (although these are not well studied or defined and may not even be directly related to minimum alveolar concentration (MAC) values) and rely on a patient being unconscious throughout anaesthesia. The assessment of the extent of effect of the volatile agent is also usually readily and reliably made by observation of its cardiovascular effects and other indications such as pupil size. To have such confidence in a given dosage regimen of an i.v. anaesthetic one would have to give a dose that would constitute a significant overdose for many and a severe overdose for some. The assessment of the narcotic effect of the drug is also more difficult as it is not reliably related to its cardiovascular and other effects, which in any case may be far more inconsistent and volatile. Some method of monitoring conscious awareness is essential, yet there is no simple, cheap and utterly reliable method. This problem has proved to be the single most important reason why TIVA has not been more extensively used in paralysed patients. Yet it may be avoided, rather than overcome, by allowing the patient a sufficient degree of neuro-muscular transmission to alert the anaesthetist to impending consciousness and by diminishing muscle tone and response by the use of an adequate dose of opioid, which will also diminish autonomic responses, add to the hypnotic effect of the i.v. anaesthetic and ensure that the patient is at least pain-free should consciousness occur. Many anaesthetists will consider that this is simply giving a better anaesthetic. Unrecognized consciousness should not occur in unparalysed patients so this is not a problem in these cases. See also Chapter 10.

This discussion has so far only elicited one aspect where TIVA has a significant advantage over inhalation anaesthesia but faster induction of anaesthesia may also be accompanied by faster recovery from anaesthesia if advantage is taken of the flexibility of manipulation of plasma concentration levels referred to above (e.g. Ledderose et al., 1987). It is not surprising that faster recovery has mainly been demonstrated after short anaesthetics. Redistribution of the drug to below levels at which consciousness will return is likely to be faster if only small amounts of the drug have been given and concentrations in the sites to which distribution occurs are low. Also in most of the short anaesthetics where faster recovery has been demonstrated the patients have not been paralysed so that excessive plasma concentrations have not been maintained to ensure unconsciousness. Indeed, the plasma concentrations in these cases have mostly been decreased towards the end of anaesthesia by reducing or stopping administration of the drug, with the knowledge that unconsciousness could be deepened within seconds should imminent awareness be apparent.

The use of nitrous oxide to maintain unconsciousness must be considered separately. As the original anaesthetic agent used there is no doubt that it is capable of inducing and maintaining unconsciousness despite the most intense surgical stimulation, although its highly selective effect on the cerebral cortex affords little or no suppression of reflex responses, so that even MAC is in effect unattainable. It is also very rapidly eliminated from the brain and the body so that recovery, like onset of effect, is very fast. Yet its use for this purpose has almost disappeared from anaesthetic practice, although it is considered to have a supplementary effect to that of the volatile anaesthetic so often carried with it. This disappearance was due to the realization that some patients required concentrations of nitrous oxide to ensure unconsciousness that were so high that the patient became hypoxic, and that some paralysed patients given nitrous oxide to maintain unconsciousness had been consciously aware during surgery. The situation was exacerbated when an (inappropriate) instruction to use a minimum concentration of 35% oxygen was generally accepted and the use of nitrous oxide as the sole hypnotic was forbidden. The use of an accurate oximeter can avoid the problem of hypoxia and nitrous oxide may again be used to maintain unconsciousness during anaesthesia, with some advantages. But the problem of assessment of its effect in a paralysed patient is even greater and more critical than that when an i.v. agent is used, as the margin of tolerance between an effective concentration and one leading to hypoxia is so small. Also the drug is by no means short of side-effects and in particular recovery may well be marred by an increased incidence of nausea and vomiting compared with TIVA.

So nitrous oxide is likely to remain an adjuvant to other hypnotic or narcotic drugs, including those used for TIVA. It has a particular role in relation to TIVA in that many anaesthetists wishing to practise TIVA may find that initially the use of nitrous oxide and oxygen in addition to their TIVA technique will help their confidence in the application of the new method and allow its development and also facilitate their acquisition of technical expertise without concern for potentially disastrous failure. In assessing results, however, the deleterious effects of nitrous oxide must always be remembered.

**Cardiovascular effects**

These are generally similar in extent during TIVA and inhalational anaesthesia, although cardiovascular stability is considered by many to be better during TIVA. The risk of dysrhythmias is reduced by TIVA and negative cardiac inotropy is not an inevitable consequence, as it is when volatile anaesthetics are used. TIVA may also avoid the problem of obliteration of the pulmonary vascular response to hypoxia. Cardiovascular effects are considered more fully in Chapter 8.

**Respiratory effects**

Most anaesthetics depress breathing. Their depressant action on the central nervous system does not selectively exclude the respiratory centre and only nitrous oxide has a sufficiently selective action to cause negligible respiratory depression, although respiratory arrest occurs more rapidly during inhalation of nitrous oxide alone than during inhalation of nitrogen.

When muscle paralysis and artificial ventilation is used as a part of the anaesthetic technique, respiratory depression is only of consequence if it persists after the end of anaesthesia. With both the intravenous and volatile anaesthetics some depression will persist after recovery of consciousness, but as recovery is usually faster after the use of the modern i.v. agents persistent respiratory depression is less evident. Perhaps more important in relation to these two groups of drugs is a persistance of poor airway control with a liability to obstruction, which is usually of far greater frequency and importance after the use of a volatile anaesthetic than after an i.v. anaesthetic, where recovery is usually characterized by clear-headed responsiveness and good control of the larynx and pharynx.

The use of an opioid in a TIVA technique with artificial ventilation is potentially far more dangerous, however. A dose of opioid that is effective in reducing reflex responses through to the end of surgery will usually cause significant respiratory depression in the post-operative period, although this may be avoided by the use of alfentanil. Opioid-induced post-operative respiratory depression is all the more likely when the analgesic effect of the opioid is required for pain control. However, this is inherent in the treatment of pain by opioids, and in this respect TIVA has an advantage over inhalation anaesthesia, where the persistent respiratory depression caused by the volatile anaesthetic, which contributes nothing to analgesia, adds to the opioid-induced depression. It is obvious that when an opioid is used in a TIVA technique the persistance of its effects into the post-operative period must be carefully controlled by the choice of drug used and by the dose and time of administration, or by the use of an antagonist or partial antagonist (agonist/antagonist). See Chapter 5.

A further respiratory complication of the use of an opioid with artificial ventilation in TIVA or otherwise is the problem of controlling ventilation to produce an acceptable $PaCO_2$ when spontaneous ventilation is required after anaesthesia. The effect of the opioid on respiratory centre sensitivity to $CO_2$ means that a higher $PaCO_2$ than normal is required for return of adequate ventilation. Intentional or inadvertent artificial hyperventilation may therefore prevent the resumption of spontaneous ventilation or, even more dangerously, result in periodic ventilation with apnoeic periods in which the patient could suffer hypoxia. The use of a capnograph is obviously appropriate.

It is in spontaneously ventilating patients that TIVA is at a significant disadvantage compared with inhalational anaesthesia. The relatively unselective volatile anaesthetics may readily be used to prevent movement in response to surgery, whilst retaining adequate, although depressed, spontaneous ventilation. Whilst this is possible by using TIVA in some cases such as dental surgery or minor urological or gynaecological surgery, if the surgical stimulation is severe (and this includes incision of the skin) the dose of drugs required to prevent movement will almost invariably cause apnoea, unless ketamine is used. Otherwise the choice of i.v. anaesthetic is unimportant. The simultaneous use of an opioid will reduce the extent of the problem, without eliminating it; indeed, if a large dose of opioid is used in an attempt to prevent movement in response to severe surgical stimulation not only may apnoea result but it may also be accompanied by muscle rigidity making artificial ventilation difficult.

Another significant respiratory effect seen during inhalational anaesthesia but less significant during TIVA is due to the effects of the volatile anaesthetics on the muscles and neuro-muscular junction. Not only do these agents reduce neuromuscular transmission, muscle tone and movement but they alter the pattern of respiration in a manner that may reduce ventilation to some areas of the lung, tending to induce a mismatch of ventilation and perfusion, and also interact with muscle relaxants, making them particularly dangerous to use in patients with myasthenia gravis. Some agents used in TIVA may also affect the relative contributions of the rib cage, diaphragm and abdominal muscles to ventilation of the lungs (Hedenstierna et al., 1981; Rigg and Rondi, 1981).

The response of the brain stem respiratory control centres to hypercapnia and hypoxia is also affected by most anaesthetics. These adaptive mechanisms are of importance to the anaesthetised patient, especially during spontaneous breathing and during recovery. If all agents impair $CO_2$ sensitivity, the opioids have the greatest influence. Most agents impair $O_2$ chemosensitivity but this is maintained during administration of barbiturates (but not halothane) (Duffin et al., 1976) and etomidate (but not propofol) (Ponte and Sadler, 1989).

Inhibition of ciliary movement by volatile anaesthetics may be of clinical importance in affecting the incidence of post-operative chest infection, as may be the use of dry anaesthetic gases, oxygen/air mixes as used in TIVA containing water vapour or being more readily humidified. The nitrogen in an oxygen/air mix also helps to prevent alveolar collapse.

## Recovery from anaesthesia

This is generally better and faster after TIVA than after inhalational anaesthesia. See Chapter 9.

## Renal effects

Volatile anaesthetics decrease renal blood flow (RBF) and glomerular filtration rate (GFR) with a consequent reduction in urine output. At equipotent concentrations, isoflurane seems to have the most dramatic effect, reducing urine output by about 66% (Mazze et al., 1974). The mechanism of this effect is mainly haemodynamic and mediated through the autonomic nervous system. Influences on the renin-angiotensin system and ADH secretion could also be involved, especially during periods of hypotension (Ishihara et al., 1978). The renal effects of volatile anaesthetics are not only dose-related but are also dependent on the existence of pre-operative dehydration (Deutsch et al., 1966). Inorganic fluoride ion toxicity may occur after the use of some volatile anaesthetics.

A similar reduction in urine output may occur during $N_2O$-relaxant-opioid anaesthesia despite the absence of haemodynamic effects (Deutsch et al., 1969).In this study RBF was reduced by 36% and GFR by 27%, changes attributed to an increase in ADH levels; what relevance this study has to TIVA using relatively larger doses of modern opioids is, however, debatable.

## Hepatic effects

During anaesthesia hepatic blood flow (HBF) usually decreases by 20—25%, mainly through a reduction in perfusion pressure and changes in splanchnic vascular resistance. If cardiac output is maintained, this decrease in HBF is probably mediated by orthosympathetic nervous system stimulation and by hypocarbia resulting from controlled ventilation. Drug specific effects on liver perfusion are more likely to occur after volatile anaesthetics than after i.v. agents. Volatile anaesthetics have a propensity to induce hypotension by peripheral vasodilatation and a reduced myocardial inotropy, which will directly reduce hepatic perfusion pressure. Halothane, enflurane and isoflurane produced a similar dose-dependent reduction in HBF but, due to splanchnic vasodilatation, no change in hepatic oxygen consumption (Hughes et al., 1980; Price et al., 1966; Thomson et al., 1983).

Hepatotoxicity to volatile anaesthetics is a well-known but rare event. An immune response to a trifluoroacetic hapten is more likely to occur in patients who are obese and female, and also under conditions of hypoxaemia, enzyme induction or repeated halothane anaesthesia. Althogh the incidence of this phenomenon is much less after isoflurane or enflurane, all volatile anaesthetics should be regarded as potential hepatotoxins.

## Cerebral effects

Volatile anaesthetics increase cerebral blood flow and intracranial pressure and may be particularly dangerous in patients with unsuspected head injury or intracranial haemorrhage. TIVA will generally reduce brain metabolism and therefore intracranial pressure and may be specifically designed to maximize these effects.

## Other effects

Other reasons that have been given for the use of TIVA in preference to inhalational anaesthesia include fewer side-effects, particularly nausea and vomiting and the avoidance of atmospheric pollution with its possible and potential effects on the health and performance of personel in the operating room environment. TIVA is also capable of being administered using small and simple apparatus and may therefore be used in conditions where direct continuous access to the patient's airway is not available, or where conventional anaesthetic apparatus is not available or may not be used.

Volatile anaesthetics induce stress-related metabolic changes and usually cause some degree of disturbance to acid-base balance. TIVA avoids both these problems and may be designed to minimize hormonal responses to surgical stress.

TIVA avoids the use of nitrous oxide with its effects on $B_{12}$ metabolism, it also avoids the occurrence of diffusion hypoxia. By using air and oxygen instead of nitrous oxide and oxygen, which may be entirely absorbed from the alveoli, TIVA helps to prevent alveolar collapse. It does not involve the use of explosive or flammable gases. In may allow anaesthesia to be given safely to patients liable to malignant hyperpyrexia, whereas all volatile anaesthetics may trigger this often fatal condition.

See also Chapters 2 and 5 for further reasons for the choice of TIVA.

## CONCLUSIONS

As may be seen from the above discussion, whilst the toxic and side-effects of TIVA and inhalational anaesthesia vary, on overall balance there is little to choose between the two methods in regard to danger to the patient. In the minds of most anaesthetists who do not regularly practise TIVA two questions remain; is TIVA practicable and is it preferable?

These may be to some extent answered by the experience of one of the authors (B.K.), who in 1976 conducted virtually all of his practice using TIVA and who subsequently used it for over 60% of his anaesthetics. The reasons for his choice were simple, that it allowed faster induction of and recovery from anaesthesia, thus pleasing both surgeons and also operating room and recovery room nurses, and that the rapid, clear-headed recovery with pain control and virtual absence of nausea and vomiting pleased the patients. Such attributes do not inevitably follow the use of TIVA, but they are obtainable in the majority of cases (if monitoring facilities are good enough) after sufficient experience with the various techniques.

## REFERENCES

De Castro, J. and Viars, P. (1968) Utilisation pratique des analgesiques centraux en anesthesie et reanimation. *Ars Med.* 23, No. special Juin, 1—228.

Deutsch, S., Goldberg, M., Stephen, G.M. and Wu, W.H. (1966) Effects of halothane on renal function in normal man. *Anesthesiology* 27, 793—804.

Deutsch, S., Bastron, R.D., Pierce, E.C. and Vandam, L.D. (1969) The effect of anesthesia with thiopentone, nitrous oxide and neuromuscular blocking drugs on renal function in normal man. *Br. J. Anaesth.* 41, 807—815.

Duffin, J., Triscott, A. and Whitwam, J.G. (1976) The effect of halothane and thiopentone on ventilatory responses mediated by the peripheral chemoreceptors in man. *Br. J. Anaesth.* 48, 975—980.

Hedenstierna, G., Lofstrom, B. and Lundh, R. (1981) Thoracic gas volume and chest-abdomen dimensions during anaesthesia and muscle paralysis. *Anesthesiology* 55, 499—506.

Hughes, R.L., Campbell, D. and Fitch, W. (1980) Effects of halothane and enflurane on liver blood flow and oxygen consumption in the greyhound. *Br. J. Anaesth.* 52, 1079—1086.

Ishihara, H., Ishida, K., Oyama, T., Kudo, T. and Kudo, M. (1978) Effects of general anaesthesia and surgery on renal function and plasma ADH levels. *Can. Anaesth. Soc. J.* 25, 312—318.

Kay, B. (1977a) Total intravenous anaesthesia with etomidate 1. A trial in children. *Acta Anaesthesiol. Belg.* 28, 107—113.

Kay, B. (1977b) Total intravenous anaesthesia with etomidate 2. Evaluation of a practical technique for children. *Acta Anaesthesiol. Belg.* 28, 115—121.

Kay, B. (1977c) Total intravenous anaesthesia with etomidate 3. Experience with adults. *Acta Anaesthesiol. Belg.* 28, 157—164.

Ledderose, H., Rester, P. and Carlsson, P. (1987) Comparison of recovery time and side-effects after propofol infusion or isoflurane in ENT patients with regional block. In: *Update on Propofol p.A17*, ICI Pharmaceuticals, Macclesfield, U.K.

Ledingham, I.M. and Watt, I. (1983) Influence of sedation on mortality in critically ill multiple trauma patients. *Lancet* 1, 1270.

Lowenstein, E. (1971) Morphine "anesthesia" — a perspective. *Anesthesiology* 35, 563—566.

Lundy, J.S. (1926) Balanced anaesthesia. *Minn. Med.* 9, 399.

Mazze, R.I., Cousins, M.J. and Barr, G.A. (1974) Renal effects and metabolism of isoflurane in man. *Anesthesiology* 40, 536—542.

Ponte, J. and Sadler, C.L. (1989) Effect of thiopentone, etomidate and propofol on carotid body chemoreceptor activity in the rabbit and the cat. *Br. J. Anaesth.* 62, 41—45.

Price, H.L., Deutsch, S., Davidson, I.A., Clement, A.J., Behar, M.G. and Epstein, R.M. (1986) Can general anaesthetics produce splanchnic visceral hypoxia by reducing regional blood flow? *Anesthesiology* 69, 72—83.

Rigg, J.R.A. and Rondi, P. (1981) Changes to rib cage and diaphragm contribution to ventilation after morphine. *Anesthesiology* 55, 507—514.

Savege, T.M., Ramsay, M.A.E., Curran, J.P.J., Cotter, J., Walling, P.T. and Simpson, B.R. (1975) Intravenous anaesthesia by infusion *Anaesthesia* 30, 757—761.

Thomson, I.A., Fitch, W., Hughes, R.L. and Campbell, D. (1983) Effects of increased concentrations of carbon dioxide during halothane anaesthesia on liver blood flow and hepatic oxygen consumption. *Br. J. Anaesth.* 55, 1231—1237.

B. Kay (ed.) Total Intravenous Anaesthesia



# 2

# Continuous infusions of hypnotic agents for maintenance of anaesthesia

J.W. Sear

## INTRODUCTION

It is now over 50 years since the introduction of thiopentone into clinical practice. This is still judged by many to be the archetypal agent for induction of anaesthesia — and therefore the standard against which newer drugs are evaluated.

Over the past 15—20 years, there has been a renewed interest in the use of intravenous agents for either techniques of total intravenous anaesthesia (TIVA), or as supplements to nitrous oxide — thereby replacing the volatile agents as the hypnotic component of the balanced anaesthetic technique. During this time, a number of drugs have been investigated — some are no longer in clinical practice (hydroxydione, propanidid, the Althesin steroids) others have not progressed beyond the early clinical trials stage of their development (minaxolone citrate, fluoretomidate), and there is still debate over the efficacy of etomidate when given by continuous infusion for sedation or the maintenance of anaesthesia. At the same time, there have been preliminary reports of the efficacy of several interesting new agents, such as zolpidem, 3α- hydroxy, 5β- pregnane-20-one and 3α-hydroxy, 5α-pregnane-20-one (Arbilla et al., 1985; Durand et al., 1986; Hogskilde et al., 1987a,b; Norberg et al., 1987; Larsson-Backstrom et al., 1988; Tatti et al., 1989).

Why has there been a resurgence in this interest? This stems, I believe, from several different factors. Firstly there are concerns over the effects of the volatile and inhalational agents in causing tissue and organ toxicity. Repeated administration of halothane has been associated with hepatic damage, and there are now reports in the literature of liver toxicity appearing after enflurane and isoflurane anaesthesia. In addition, the recent papers from Christ and colleagues (1988a,b) have suggested possible cross-sensitivity between the three halogenated volatile agents by way of acetylating intermediates that bind covalently to liver proteins rendering them immunogenic (Hubbard et al., 1988).

Dose-related renal damage from methoxyflurane led to its withdrawal from clinical practice, and increased free fluoride concentrations (the causative factor) may also be found after use of enflurane in patients with impaired renal function, and in patients in the intensive care unit receiving isoflurane for sedation. Some of the complications of the potent inhalational agents can also be avoided by TIVA — ventricular arrhythmogenicity, myocardial depression, and incompatibility with catecholamines. Other adverse effects include the epileptogenic potential of enflurane, and the possible 'coronary steal phenomenon' associated with use of isoflurane in the patient with coronary artery occlusive disease (Bindslev, 1988).

Of the new volatile agents, sevoflurane has been demonstrated to undergo degradation in contact with soda-lime (although not with Baralyme); while I-653 (Desflurane) has physiochemical characteristics (low boiling point, high MAC, high volatility) that will make its delivery both a challenge and, in all likelihood, a great expense. Furthermore, the concern over the haematological effects of nitrous oxide has made several authorities, including Eger, question the role of this adjunctive agent as part of a volatile or balanced anaesthetic.

There is also still debate over the effects of prolonged exposure of operating personnel to the trace concentrations of anaesthetic gases present in that environment. Early studies showed a clear relationship between exposure and the incidence of spontaneous abortions and foetal abnormalities in the pregnant female, a reduction in the immune response to infection, an increased incidence of tissue and blood malignancies, as well as a reduction in mental capacity and judgement (Knill-Jones et al., 1972 Spence, 1987).

## INDICATIONS FOR INTRAVENOUS ANAESTHESIA

The properties of the ideal drug for use during continuous infusion anaesthesia may be summarised as follows (Morgan, 1983):

(i) soluble in water such that use of an additional solvent is avoided;

(ii) stable in solution, and on exposure to light for prolonged periods of time;

(iii) no adsorption onto plastic tubing or giving sets;

(iv) no venous damage (pain on injection, venous phlebitis or thrombosis) or tissue damage when administered either extravascularly or intra-arterially;

(v) sleep in one arm-brain circulation time;

(vi) short duration of action, and inactivation by metabolism in either the liver, blood or other organs of the vessel-rich group of tissues;

(vii) inactive, non-toxic, water soluble metabolites;

(viii) minimal cardiovascular and respiratory side-effects.

It will be instantly appreciated that *none* of the present hypnotic agents fulfills all of these criteria, but that some are more suitable than others under different circumstances.

What are the indications for i.v. anaesthesia?

(1) By infusion as an alternative to volatile agents as a supplement to nitrous oxide in oxygen anaesthesia (Sear and Prys-Roberts, 1979; Sear et al., 1981; Prys-Roberts et al., 1983a,b; Monk et al., 1987; Coates et al., 1987; Korttila et al., 1990b).

(2) To provide sedation during local or regional anaesthetic techniques (Jessop et al., 1985; Wilson et al., 1990b).

(3) For ambulatory surgery; where the speed and completeness of recovery are important (Mackenzie and Grant, 1985; Korttila et al., 1988; Sanders et al., 1989; Marais et al., 1989).

(4) For situations where conventional anaesthetics may be difficult to administer: due to the non-availability of resources such as nitrous oxide; at sites of military or non-military trauma, and anaesthesia at increased ambient pressure.

(5) In circumstances where nitrous oxide may be either undesirable (e.g., due to the need for high inspired oxygen concentrations) or contraindicated (e.g., one-lung ventilation, middle ear surgery, some aspects of neuroanaesthesia, prolonged abdominal surgery, relief of cardiac tamponade, bronchoscopy, laryngoscopy and broncho-tracheal surgery) (Magnusson et al., 1986; Rees and Howell, 1986).

(6) Prevention of awareness during cardio-pulmonary bypass; cerebral protection during episodes of potential brain ischaemia (Cottrell et al., 1982; Shapiro, 1985; Katz et al., 1987; Russell et al., 1989; Van Hemelriyck et al, 1989).

The choice of agent for each of these areas of clinical usage will obviously vary according to the pharmacological profiles of the different drugs. Although many authors have advocated or described the clinical usage of TIVA (i.e., i.v. hypnotics and opioids without either an associated volatile agent or nitrous oxide) (Lees, 1983; Versichelen et al., 1983; Raeder et al., 1987; Schuttler et al., 1988; Nilsson et al., 1988a), this approach is not without some important disadvantages:

(i) difficulties over assessment of adequacy of anaesthesia especially in the paralysed patient, so leading to the possibility of awareness;

(ii) the likelihood of postoperative respiratory depression due to persistent effects of concurrently administered narcotic agents;

(iii) the requirement of a separate, dedicated i.v. access site;

(iv) appropriate infusion pumps and appropriate administration regimens;

(v) depth of anaesthesia may not be as controllable as with the volatile agents.

Against this background, newer intravenous agents have become available to the clinical anaesthetist. These drugs all show dynamic profiles closer to the ideal agents than do previous agents, and most have kinetic properties which make them suitable for continuous administration. In the present chapter, only true hypnotic agents will be discussed, except where there is need to compare hypnotic agents with other drugs; or the combination of hypnotic and opioid.

## BASIC PHARMACOKINETICS

When drugs are given by the intravenous route, their distribution around and elimination from the body depends on a number of inter-related physiological and pharmacological processes. Pharmacokinetics describes the mathematics of these processes and their associated rates of drug movement from the site of administration into the body; their distribution to various target organs, tissue binding sites or storage sites; and their metabolism and elimination. Once these concepts are known for any drug, then administration regimens can be designed to achieve desired goals — namely those blood or plasma concentrations associated with therapeutic effects.

The behaviour of drugs can be described in terms of physiologically based, mathematically based (compartmental), and non-compartmental models.

## 1. Mathematical modelling

When a single dose of an i.v. agent is given, the decline in the plasma drug concentration with time will be the result of both drug distribution and elimination. If we consider the body as a single compartment (q.v.), the plasma concentration ($C_0$) immediately after administration will be the dose ($M_0$) divided by the apparent volume of distribution ($V_d$). However, the drug concentration does not remain constant — the decline occurring in an exponential manner, so that at time $t$, the concentration of drug remaining in the body will be $C_t$,

where: $C_t = M_t/Vd$

($M_t$ being the amount of drug present at this time point).

As the rate of elimination ($dM/dt$) for most drugs is a first order rate process (i.e. a constant fraction of that drug remaining in the body is eliminated per unit time),

$dM/dt = -k\ [M]_t$; $k$ being the elimination rate constant.

However, the rate of drug elimination is also proportional to clearance ($Cl$), as well as the drug concentration at that time.

thus: $dM/dt = Cl \cdot C_t$

by re-arrangement: $Cl \cdot C_t = -k\ [M]_t$

but: $[M]_t = C_t \cdot Vd$

therefore: $Cl = -k \cdot Vd$ (1)

Clearance may be defined as the volume of a body compartment (usually plasma or body fluids) from which a drug is completely removed per unit time; it is therefore independent of the drug concentration. The main site of drug clearance is the liver, but other tissues (kidneys, lungs, plasma, gut mucosal cells) may also contribute. A second kinetic parameter of importance is the *half-life* — the time taken for the drug concentration to decrease to 50% of its initial value. After four or five half-lives, the plasma drug concentration will therefore have fallen to about 6% of the initial value. The numerical value of the half-life may be calculated from the relationship between drug concentration and elimination rate constant:

$dM/dt = -k\ [M]_t$

By integration: $M_t = M_0 e^{-kt}$

As the mass (dose) of the drug is the product of plasma (blood) concentration and volume of distribution, the above equation can be rewritten as:

$$C_t = C_0 e^{-kt}$$

Thus, if the drug concentration declines from $C$ to $C/2$, then

$$k = \frac{\ln C - \ln C/2}{t_{1/2}}$$

but: $\ln C - \ln C/2 = \ln 2 = 0.693$
therefore: $k = 0.693/t_{1/2}$ (2)

By substitution of Eqn. (1) into Eqn. (2), we can derive the relationship between half-life, clearance and volume of distribution:

$$Cl = \frac{0.693 \cdot Vd}{t_{1/2}} \qquad (3)$$

However, most drugs do not follow simple mono-exponential kinetics; rather the decline in the plasma drug concentration is the summation of a number of different exponential equations:

$$C_t = A_{1-n} e^{-k_{1-n}t}$$

where $A_{1-n}$ are the equation constants, and $-k_{1-n}$ are the elimination rate constants of the different exponential terms. The various compartments represented by the different elimination rate constants have no strict anatomical confines, nor do they necessarily comprise only one type of tissue. The faster exponential terms of the polyexponential equation describe the distribution phases, where drug movement from the blood to the peripheral tissues predominates over elimination. The slower exponential(s) describe mainly elimination of drug from the body.

For many drugs, the decline in the plasma drug concentration can be adequately modelled by a bi-exponential equation:

$$C_t = Ae^{-\alpha t} + Be^{-\beta t}$$

where: $\alpha$ and $\beta$ are the rate constants, and $A$ and $B$ the intercept constants. From these constants, various volumes of distribution (q.v.) as well as clearance can be determined, together with the inter-compartmental transfer rate constants.

*Volumes of distribution*

These are measures of the extent of drug dispersion within the body. A number of different volumes may be determined ($V_1$, $V_2$, $Vd_{ss}$, $V_\beta$); where $V_1$ is the volume of the central kinetic department, $V_2$ the volume of the peripheral compartment, $Vd_{ss}$ the overall apparent volume of distribution of steady state (equals the sum of the other two volumes), and $V_\beta$ the apparent volume of distribution during the elimination phase. $V_1$ reflects the distribution space of drug within the vessel-rich group of tissues, and the associated rate constant ($\alpha$) will be influenced by its magnitude. $Vd_{ss}$ is that volume at a state of pseudo-equilibrium between blood and all the various tissue concentrations. This assumes that the partition coefficient between the tissues and blood is unity. This is a necessary assumption as only blood concentrations can be assayed. For many drugs, especially those with high liposolubility, $Vd_{ss}$ will be extremely large and in excess of the total body mass. This implies that there are anatomical areas within the body where tissue concentrations are greater than those in the plasma and hence most of a given dose of the drug will be in the peripheral kinetic compartment(s).

By reference to Eqn. (3), we can define the terminal half life in terms of the apparent volume of distribution at steady state and clearance. Thus, as the distribution volume increases, so the terminal half life becomes longer; similarly as clearance increases, so the half life will become shorter.

## 2. Physiological modelling

As an alternative to mathematical equations to describe drug behaviour within the body, some authors have derived 'perfusion models' — where drug disposition is considered in terms of drug: tissue partition coefficients, tissue masses, and tissue blood flows. Tissues with similar partition coefficients and blood flow can then be grouped together as 'physiological compartments'. By definition, these models have a number of major limitations, as they incorporate many assumptions, such as averaged tissue masses, and averaged organ blood flows. They also ignore the inter-individual variability that exists between healthy subjects, as well as those alterations occurring due to co-existing disease states, or through concurrent administration of other drugs or anaesthetics.

Nevertheless, some of the earliest work on the modelling of the thiobarbiturates was carried out using this approach. Initial clinical observations with thiopentone led to the concept that the short duration of effect of a single bolus dose was attributable to rapid metabolism. However, Brodie et al. (1950) first demonstrated that the elimination half life of the barbiturate was between 4 and 5 h. These same investigators later showed that the rapid rate of cerebral uptake was dependent on the high cerebral blood flow, and the drug's high lipid solubility. Recovery occurred by redistribution of drug away from the brain to other lipid tissues including muscle.

In 1960, Price described a physiological model for the behaviour of thiopentone; the model predicting that the lean tissues (muscle and skin) were of greater importance than the fat tissues in the initial phase of redistribution of drug from the central nervous system (Price et al., 1960). Thus, although the blood/muscle partition coefficient for thiopentone was less than that for blood/fat, muscle bulk constituted about 55% total body mass, compared with the 20% for the fatty tissues. However, this model ignored the contribution of hepatic metabolism.

Later studies by Saidman and Eger (1966) showed that hepatic degradation of thiopentone was also important in the termination of its effect. Further elaboration of the physiological model by Bischoff and Dedrick (1968) involved inclusion of the influences of hepatic metabolism, regional blood flows, and tissue and plasma protein binding in the kinetics and dynamics of thiopentone. Although the binding data have been questioned by Shen and Gibaldi (1974), Gillis and colleagues (1976) were able to delineate a plausible physiological model for the action of both thiopentone and methohexitone.

### 3. Statistical moment analysis

In 1978, Yamaoka and colleagues introduced non-compartmental modelling into kinetics, where the disposition of drugs is considered in terms of two main parameters — the area under the concentration-time curve (AUC) (= zero moment), and its first statistical moment (MRT, mean residence time). The latter is that time taken for the elimination of 62.3% of an injected dose from the body. From these two estimates, we can determine two other kinetic descriptors — clearance and apparent volume of distribution at steady state ($Cl$ and $Vd_{ss}$) (Yamaoka et al., 1978; Chan et al., 1982).

Of these two derived parameters, only clearance is 'truly model independent' in so much that it is not influenced by the nature of the 'drug exit site' (i.e. whether the drug is exclusively eliminated from the central kinetic compartment, or also from the peripheral tissues as well). This latter concept is clearly of importance in the parameter estimation for drugs such as atracurium, morphine (and perhaps propofol) where clearance may be from both central and peripheral compartments (Ward et al., 1983; Mazoit et al., 1990; Lange et al., 1990).

The relationships between AUC, AUMC (area under the product of concentration and time versus time curve) and the other derived parameters are shown below:

$$\mathrm{AUC} = \int_0^{\infty} C\,\mathrm{d}t$$

$$\mathrm{AUMC} = \int_0^{\infty} t \cdot C\,\mathrm{d}t$$

$$Cl = \mathrm{Dose/AUC}$$

$$\mathrm{MRT} = \mathrm{AUMC/AUC}$$

$$Vd_{ss} = \mathrm{Dose} \cdot \mathrm{AUMC/AUC}^2;\ \text{or MRT} \cdot Cl$$

All these calculations for an i.v. bolus dose require an extrapolation for AUC and AUMC from the first measured drug concentration back to the $t = 0$ intercept to determine $C_t = 0$; and similarly from the last data point to infinity. For calculation in those cases where drugs are not solely eliminated from the central compartment, the reader should refer to the review by Nakashima and Benet (1988).

From the known or calculated values for a drug's kinetic profile (half-life, clearance, volumes of distribution), it is usually possible to predict whether the agent may be useful and/or suitable for administration by multiple increments or continuous infusion for the maintenance of anaesthesia. The most appropriate drugs will have: a high clearance, a short terminal (elimination) half-life, non-saturable metabolic pathways, no active metabolites, and a lack of solvent toxicity if water-insoluble.

## KINETICS OF THE CONTINUOUS INFUSION

For i.v. hypnotic drugs given either as multiple incremental doses or by continuous infusion, the relationship between the infusion rate and the efficacy (in terms of quality of anaesthesia) will depend on the drug concentration not in the blood or plasma, but in the so-called 'effect compartment' or biophase. This concept was suggested by Hull and colleagues (1978), and has been successfully applied to the kinetic-dynamic modelling of the muscle relaxants pancuronium and *d*-tubocurarine (Sheiner et al., 1979). There is not necessarily a unique one-to-one relationship between the plasma concentration and that in the biophase. Scott et al. (1985) describe a finite lag period between the change in the plasma fentanyl concentration, and the dynamic effect (when measured in terms of the spectral edge frequency). Thus, for any plasma drug concentration, there may be a wide range of biophase concentrations, and vice versa. The finite delay in changes in drug concentrations in the one compared to the other is termed the 'hysteresis effect'. The magnitude of this delay varies for different hypnotic and analgesic agents (Table 2.1). The speed of equilibration between plasma and biophase will be related to the physiochemical properties of the individual agents (e.g. p$K_a$, lipophilicity etc.). Thus, although high lipophilicity and low ionisation may facilitate drug transfer across the blood-brain barrier, it may also confer slow receptor kinetics.

When a constant stable drug concentration is required for clinical anaesthesia, it is clear, therefore, that there is need to achieve a constant biophase concentration, and hence a continuous input of drug into the system. However, the elegant studies of Ausems and colleagues using the analgesic agent alfentanil (Ausems and Hug, 1983; Ausems et al., 1983; Ausems et al., 1986), and the clinical intuition of the anaesthetist based on the normal practice with the volatile agents, have clearly demonstrated that the magnitude of the stress of surgery will vary with a number of different, yet well definable factors: patient age, sex, operator technique, operation site, and the phase of the operation, e.g. incision, gut traction or skin closure, etc. Thus, the clinical anaesthetist wishing to pursue intravenous anaesthesia must

TABLE 2.1

Half-time for blood/brain equilibration for hypnotic and other i.v. agents

Pharmacokinetic-dynamic modelling has been carried out, correlating blood concentrations of the various anaesthetic agents to the parameters of the power spectral analysis of the EEG. Brain sensitivity is shown as the magnitude of the maximal slowing of the spectral edge ($E_{max}$), and the plasma drug concentration that causes 50% of the maximal EEG slowing ($IC_{50}$). Data are shown as mean (S.D.).

| | Sampling site | $t_{1/2}k_{eo}$ [a] (min) | $E_{max}$ (Hz) | $IC_{50}$ ($\mu$g/ml) | Reference |
|---|---|---|---|---|---|
| Thiopentone | A[b] | 1.2 (0.3) | 16.6 (6.7) | 19.2 (6.3) | Stanski et al., 1984 |
| Etomidate | A | 1.6 (0.5) | 7.2 (1.2) | 0.39 (0.14) | Arden et al., 1986 |
| Ketamine | A | | 7.9 (1.7) | 2.0 (0.5) | Schuttler et al., 1987 |
| Diazepam | A | 5.4 (0.8) | — | 0.19 (0.11) | Buhrer et al., 1988 |
| Midazolam | A | 1.6 (0.5) | — | 1.0 (0.21) | Buhrer et al., 1988 |
| Propofol | A | 2.9 (2.2) | 8.6 (1.5) | 2.3 (0.8) | Schuttler et al., 1986 |
| Fentanyl | A | 4.7 (1.5) | 13.0 (2.7) | 7.8 (2.6)[c] | Scott and Stanski, 1987 |
| Alfentanil | A | 0.9 (0.3) | 13.5 (4.1) | 479 (271)[c] | Scott and Stanski, 1987 |
| Sufentanil | A | 6.2 (2.8) | — | 0.68 (0.31)[c] | Scott et al., 1991 |

[a] $t_{1/2}k_{eo}$: equilibration half life between blood and brain (biophase).
[b] A: arterial sampling.
[c] ng/ml.

learn to adopt the same approach as with the volatile agents — namely vary the input (inspired concentration or infusion rate) according to the patient's individual requirements. Changes in drug infusion rate, and therefore in drug concentration in the plasma and hence in the biophase, should be conducted so as to minimise the marked dynamic effects of inadequate or excessive anaesthesia (viz. patient movement in the spontaneously ventilating subject, increases in heart rate or blood pressure, or awareness in the paralysed subject, cardiorespiratory depression).

The design of appropriate infusion regimens depends on two factors: knowledge of those concentrations associated with clinical efficacy, and the basic kinetic profile of a given drug under a given set of conditions. If a drug is administered by incremental dosing at regular intervals, the amount given will be additive with that already persisting in the body. In this way, the total amount of drug in the body will gradually increase until the rate of administration equals the rate of elimination. In general, if the incremental period is less than twice the elimination half-life for a particular agent, accumulation of drug will occur. If the same drug is given by continuous fixed rate infusion for a long period of time, then there will be a progressive increase in the plasma drug concentration until so-called 'steady-

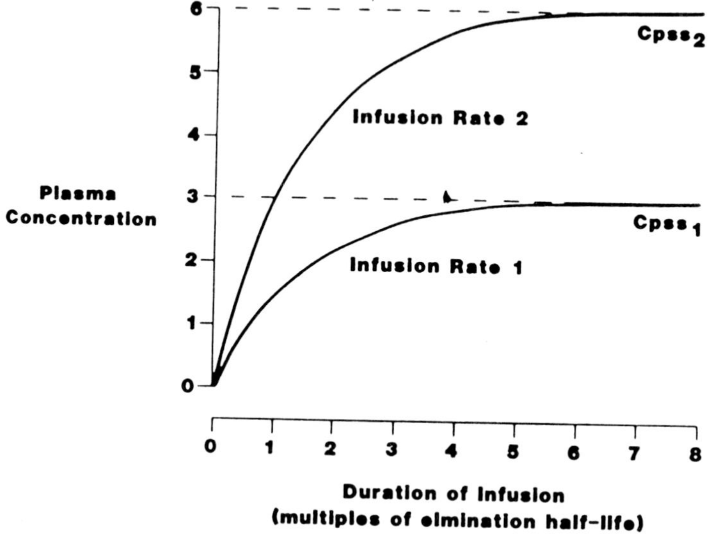


Fig. 2.1. Plasma drug concentration versus time after starting a fixed rate infusion. Three to four multiples of the elimination half life are needed to achieve steady-state conditions; shown as $Cp_{ss1}$. Doubling the infusion rate only doubles the steady-state concentration ($Cp_{ss2}$); the time taken to achieve the higher steady-state concentration is unaltered.

state' concentrations are reached. At the point, the rate of input and rate of output must be equal. There is a defined relationship between the steady state concentration and the infusion rate:

$$C_{ss} = Q/Cl$$

where $C_{ss}$ is the required steady drug concentration, $Q$ the infusion rate, and $Cl$ systemic clearance.

The time to reach steady state concentrations will vary from drug to drug, being dependent only on the terminal half life and volume of distribution. Increasing the infusion rate does not alter the time to achieving steady state, rather it will result in a greater eventual steady state drug concentration (Fig. 2.1). There are a number of different approaches to the attainment of steady state drug concentrations.

(1) A fixed rate (zero-order) infusion will cause the blood drug concentration to increase exponentially. Unless the drug has a very short elimination half-life, it will not be feasible to use this infusion alone to provide stable concentrations, as this would require an infusion of duration 3—4 times the elimination half life. The use of a higher infusion rate may allow the drug concentration at the time of incision to be adequate for clinical anaesthesia, but the concentration will then continue to increase until the steady state is achieved. Such an approach may cause both cardiovascular depression by the high drug concentration, and delayed recovery.

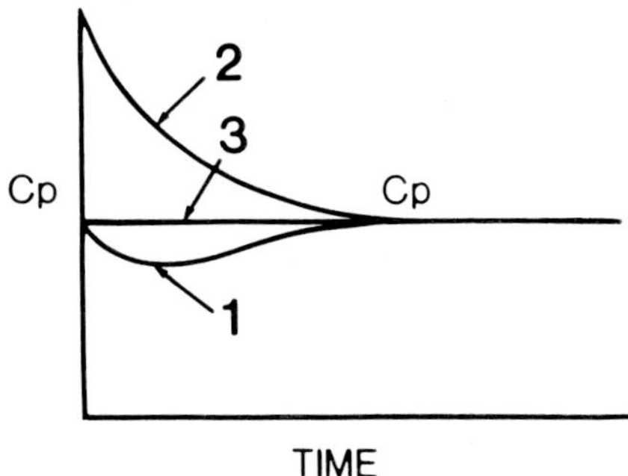


Fig. 2.2. Plasma concentration against time profile for two different infusion regimens aimed at attaining the same steady-state concentration (3). For curve 1, the loading dose was determined as the product of the initial volume of distribution ($V_1$) and the steady-state concentration; for curve 2, as the product of the apparent volume of distribution at steady-state ($Vd_{ss}$) and the steady-state concentration.

(2) Combination of a loading dose plus a zero-order infusion, as described by Boyes et al. (1971) and Mitenko and Ogilvie (1972). The size of the loading dose may be based on either the initial volume of distribution of the agent ($V_1$), the apparent volume of distribution at steady state ($Vd_{ss}$), or the apparent volume of distribution during the elimination phase ($V_\beta$). In each case, the loading dose will be the product of the volume of distribution and the target steady state drug concentration ($B = Vd \cdot C_{ss}$). If the latter two volumes of distribution are used, the initial drug concentration will exceed the target concentration, and the area under the target concentration line will be minimised (Fig. 2.2). When $V_1$ is employed, there will be a greater area under this target concentration line, and therefore a longer period when the patient is inadequately anaesthetised. The size of the loading dose may, however, be limited for some drugs with narrow therapeutic concentration ranges by the toxic or adverse effects associated with supra-therapeutic concentrations.

(3) A double infusion regimen, based on the calculation of Wagner (1976). In place of the bolus loading dose, which may result in marked dynamic adverse effects (e.g. hypotension, bradycardia), two different infusion rates may be employed — the first (a rapid infusion, $Q_1$) takes the place of the bolus loading dose, while the second ($Q_2$, the maintenance rate) is calculated to achieve the target steady-state concentration. Thus, the concentration-time profile will initially overshoot the projected steady-state concentration, and then gradually decline back towards it. The magnitude of the overshoot may be limited by extending the duration of the rapid infusion.

(4) Combination of a single bolus dose and two or more constant rate infusions. This approach was initially proposed by Kruger-Thiemer (1968) and subsequently developed by Vaughan and Tucker (1976), Rigg and Wong (1981) and Schwilden et al. (1986). The regimen is made up of three components:

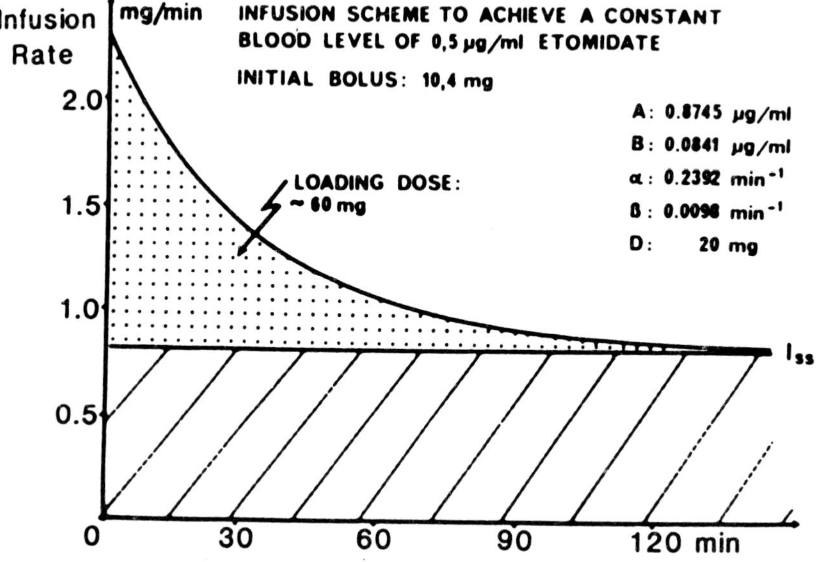


Fig. 2.3. BET (Bolus-elimination-transfer) infusion scheme for etomidate, with those data necessary to achieve a constant plasma drug concentration of 0.5 μg/ml. The initial bolus dose is 10.4 mg, together with a constant rate infusion replacing drug lost by elimination (metabolic clearance, 0.8 mg/min.), and an exponentially declining infusion rate to compensate for drug transfer to the peripheral tissues (a total dose of approximately 60 mg over 170 min). The bolus dose and different infusion rates for this scheme have been derived from kinetic data obtained from blood sampling following a bolus dose of 20 mg etomidate (D). The parameters A, B, $\alpha$ and $\beta$ are the ordinates and hybrid rate constants of the bi-exponential equation describing the decline of the plasma etomidate concentration with time. (Produced with kind permission of Dr H. Schwilden, and Georg Thieme Verlag, Stuttgart; from *Quantitation, Modelling and Control in Anaesthesia,* ed. H. Stoeckel.)

(i) the bolus dose ($B$) to achieve target concentration ($C_{ss}$); $B = C_{ss} \cdot V_1$;

(ii) the maintenance infusion rate ($E$) to replace drug lost from the body by elimination or metabolism; $E = C_{ss} \cdot Cl_p$;

(iii) an exponentially declining infusion rate ($T$) to compensate for drug transfer from the central compartment to the peripheral tissues; $T = C_{ss} \cdot k_{12} \cdot e^{-k_{21}t \cdot V_1}$ (Fig. 2.3).

To provide these three consecutively occurring modes of drug input, it is normally appropriate to use computer control, as typified by the work of Alvis and colleagues (1985a,b). Other examples of similar schema can be seen in the models of Schuttler and colleagues for etomidate (Schwilden et al., 1983; Schuttler et al., 1985). However, this technology is clearly outside the remit of most clinical anaesthetists, and thus Roberts and colleagues (1988) have recently described a manual version of this model by approximating the various phases to a loading dose and three fixed rate infusions.

(5) Another novel approach to the attainment of constant plasma drug concentrations without resource to complex computerisation has been described by Riddell and colleagues (1984). An exponentially decreasing drug delivery rate can be achieved by removing solution from a container at a constant rate, at the same time replacing it with solvent at the same rate. Riddell described its use for infusions of lignocaine; McMurray et al. (1986) have used the same method for infusing methohexitone for maintenance of anaesthesia.

**Fixed rate versus variable rate infusion regimens**

Kinetically designed infusion regimens aim to achieve predesignated drug concentrations. However, as shown by Ausems et al. (1986), Glass and colleagues (1989), Shafer and colleagues (1988), and Sear et al. (1988a) for alfentanil and propofol respectively, the same drug concentration will not necessarily be associated with adequate anaesthesia in all patients and at all phases of surgery. In addition, there is the very real problem of inter-individuality of drug disposition and dynamic sensitivity. The data of Tackley et al. (1988) illustrate this well; an infusion regimen for propofol designed to give a steady-state concentration of 3 μg/ml resulted in drug concentrations between 1.5 and 5 μg/ml in the eight patients studied. Besides these usual factors which may influence drug disposition (physiological, pharmacological, pathological, chronological, and perhaps gender), it is essential that derived pharmacokinetic parameters incorporated into computer programmes are determined under similar anaesthetic conditions to those being investigated. Thus, the application of bolus dose kinetics to the design of infusion regimens may be an appropriate method for drugs having no haemodynamic effects; but is clearly inappropriate for the i.v. anaesthetic agents and will therefore account for some of the reported failures to achieve or maintain the desired drug concentrations. Drug kinetics will also be altered by the presence of hypovolaemia or shock (haemorrhagic, septic, cardiogenic) and by the use of cardiopulmonary bypass. For further consideration of those factors affecting drug disposition, the reader should refer to Sear (1987a,b; 1989).

There are increasing numbers of researchers who, realising this variability, have chosen to investigate the administration of i.v. hypnotic drugs by variable rate infusion to supplement either an infusion of alfentanil or 70% nitrous oxide in the spontaneously breathing patients and those receiving controlled ventilation (White, 1984; Doze et al., 1986; Shafer et al., 1988; Sear et al., 1988b). In none were there any episodes of awareness or recall — despite the occasional patient moving due to inadequate anaesthesia. The average maintenance rate for outpatients was greater than the $ED_{50}$ infusion rates derived from the dose-response studies of the Bristol group (Spelina et al., 1986), with values being closely to their $ED_{95}$ rates. To date, there are no published data comparing the quality of anaesthesia and post-anaesthetic recovery for comparable groups of patients receiving either a variable infusion regimen or a fixed protocol. These are clearly needed — one would expect the former to be the more appropriate!

Because fixed rate regimens are usually based on average kinetic parameters, it will be clear that 50% of the patients should be overdosed, and 50% have episodes of light anaesthesia. Thus, the rationale for variable rate administration should be obvious. Whether the regimen depends on minute-by-minute changes of the infusion rate, or the use of a background infusion (based, say, on the $EC_{25}$ concentration) topped up according to the individual patients own needs, is uncertain. This latter approach has been further developed in the case of propofol, where it forms the basis of the 'Ohmeda' pump adminsitration system.

## BARBITURATES

Infusions of the barbiturates (especially thiopentone and methohexitone) have been used by several authors for the maintenance of anaesthesia.

### Thiopentone

Early studies of the properties of thiopentone by Lundy in Rochester, and Waters in Madison, Wisconsin, indicated the safety of this first thiobarbiturate (Lundy and Tovell, 1934; Platt et al., 1936). However, the subsequent experience, especially in the context of anaesthesia for the traumatised patient following Pearl Harbour, led Halford (1943) to describe the use of thiopentone in the presence of shock and hypovolaemia as 'an ideal form of euthanasia'. This disaster led to the realization that reduced doses of the barbiturate were indicated under such circumstances, and that oxygen was an important adjunct to thiopentone anaesthesia, particularly in those patients with hypovolaemic shock.

Despite the passage of over 55 years since its introduction into clinical practice, there have been few studies critically evaluating the concentration-effect relationships in either healthy or infirm patients when thiopentone is administered either as a sole agent, or as an agent to supplement nitrous oxide, or to supplement an infusion or incremental dosing of an opioid. When used in conjection with either of the latter, infusion rates of the order of 150—300 μg/kg per min are required (Hunter, 1972a, Blunnie et al., 1981; White, 1984). These will produce plasma drug concentrations of between 15 and 25 μg/ml (Crankshaw et al, 1985, 1987; Crankshaw and Karasawa, 1989) and are in general agreement with White and colleagues (1983) who found the mean plasma thiopentone concentration, in conjunction with nitrous oxide, necessary to allow gynaecological surgery in the spontaneously breathing patient to be 13.7 μg/ml. In a separate study, Becker (1978) reported the plasma concentration associated with abolition of the response to squeezing the trapezius muscle (equitable with the initial surgical stimulus) to be 42.2 μg/ml in the absence of nitrous oxide. These concentrations compare with peak concentrations in excess of 150 μg/ml following the induction of anaesthesia with 4—6 mg/kg. Crankshaw et al. (1989) have recently reported EEG burst suppression (in the absence of nitrous oxide) in 12 patients at mean thiopentone concentrations of 37 (S.D. 11) μg/ml; similar to the 51 μg/ml reported by Todd et al. in 1985.

There has been considerable debate as to whether acquired tolerance may be seen with thiopentone. This implies that exposure of the brain to an initial dose of the hypnotic renders it less sensitive to a subsequent dose.

Brodie et al. (1951), Dundee et al. (1956) and Toner et al. (1980) have reported that the larger the dose of thiopentone administered, the higher the concentration in the plasma at awakening. However, their data have been questioned by at least two other sets of results. Hudson and colleagues (1983), using power spectral analysis of the EEG to assess the brain effect of the barbiturate, showed that after three sequential infusions of thiopentone 20—25 min apart, burst suppression occurred after similar total doses (9.6, 5.6 and 5.2 mg/kg). Using the spectral edge frequency as the marker, the thiopentone concentration needed to produce a 50% of maximal shift (termed the $IC_{50}$ concentration) was also similar after each infusion (13.9, 13.9 and 16.0 μg/ml). This indicates that acute tolerance does not occur after repeated infusions.

The second set of data from Crankshaw and colleagues in Melbourne (1985) showed that after doses of thiopentone up to 10 times normal, there was little difference in the plasma drug concentration at awakening. Why then do these two papers appear to differ from the earlier results? The concentration appears to vary according to the sampling site. Stanski et al. (1984) demonstrated that during thiopentone infusion, there was a lag period between the arterial and venous concentrations reaching the same level, and that after cessation of the infusion, this difference remained (although its magnitude was reduced). This importance in sampling site is also emphasized by the kinetic modelling of Barrett et al. (1984a,b).

One argument against the use of thiopentone is that with continuous infusions there is saturation of the peripheral tissue storage sites, and recovery may be slow. This is due to the low hepatic clearance rate for thiopentone — the major factor in the decline of the plasma drug concentration being redistribution to peripheral tissues rather than elimination. Change in drug kinetics to zero-order elimination is not seen below concentrations of the order of 50—60 μg/ml. If the concentrations are retained in the range 15—25 μg/ml, then a prompt decline occurs in the drug concentration over the first 15 or so minutes after cessation of the infusion, and the patient awakens (Crankshaw et al., 1985, 1987). This can be explained on a kinetic basis. The clearance rate of thiopentone from the central compartment (volume: 5 l) is about 200 ml/min; thus the initial fall in the plasma drug concentration (30—50%) will bring the brain concentration below that associated with hypnosis.

At infusion rates greater than about 300 μg/kg per min, thiopentone concentrations will increase exponentially as the peripheral stores become saturated. Under these circumstances, use of the drug is associated with a prolonged recovery. This accumulation of drug is the result of two separate processes — a change in the kinetics to zero-order elimination (as outlined above), and the metabolic breakdown of thiopentone to pentobarbitone, an active metabolite. After 2-h infusion, about 20% of the total drug dose will be present as pentobarbitone (Chan et al.,1985). The elimination half life of this barbiturate is longer than that of thiopentone —

so resulting in persistent drowsiness into the immediate post-operative period (Table 2.2).

There are also other disadvantages with use of infusions of thiopentone: a low therapeutic index, porphyrinogenicity, and in large doses, possible hepatotoxicity (Dundee, 1955); although this latter aspect has been questioned by the studies of other authors including Blunnie et al. (1981). However, there are some potential pluses: minimal cardiovascular depression (Todd et al., 1985) and an effectiveness in offering brain protection during episodes of cerebral ischaemia (Shapiro, 1985).

### Methohexitone

The use of methohexitone either as a sole agent, or as a supplement to nitrous oxide or opioids has been described for body surface, intra-abdominal and neurosurgical operations (Hunter, 1972b; Prys-Roberts et al., 1983; Sear et al., 1983a, 1984a; White, 1984; Doze et al., 1986).

There are, however, few data on the kinetics of methohexitone when given by continuous infusion. In a study in volunteers, Breimer (1976) infused the barbiturate at a dose of 3 mg/kg over 60 min, and calculated the following mean disposition parameters: elimination half-life 97 min, and clearance 826 ml/min. However, these estimates are probably an underestimate of the half-life, based on bolus dose kinetics described by Hudson et al. (1983). A more recent infusion kinetic study has been made by le Normand et al. (1988) where methohexitone was infused at 60 and 90 $\mu$g/kg per min to patients for 14 h, and the post-infusion decay followed for a further 12 h. The derived mean kinetic estimates were similar to those of Hudson and colleagues; namely half-life 420—460 minutes, volume of distribution at steady state 4.5—4.7 l/kg, and clearance 9.6—9.8 ml/kg per min (Table 2.2).

When compared with thiopentone, methohexitone is associated with faster and more complete initial recovery — and recovery of psychomotor skills over the first 2—4 h after anaesthesia (Mackenzie and Grant, 1985). However, the later recovery profile is similar for the two barbiturates (Korttila et al., 1975). Residual effects following single bolus dosing of methohexitone may be demonstrated for at least 8 h. The main metabolite of the methoxybarbiturate in most species, including man, is 4-hydroxy methohexitone (Welles et al., 1963; Heusler et al., 1981). A recent study by Korttila and colleagues (1990a) has examined whether the prolonged action of methohexitone might be due to this metabolite. Effects following its administration i.p. to mice were assessed using the 'rotarod test'. The $ED_{50}$ values for the metabolite were about 10-fold greater than those for the parent drug; and since, after acute administration of methohexitone to children, Engelhardt et al. (1986) found metabolite concentrations to be only about 50% those of the parent drug, it would seem unlikely that, during normal clinical anaesthesia, the metabolite contributes significantly to central nervous system impairment.

Dynamic concentration-effect relationship data are scarce for methohexitone. In volunteers, Lauven et al. (1987) found the venous drug threshold concentrations for sleeping to be 3.4 $\mu$g/ml, for loss of the eyelash reflex 4.4—6.5 $\mu$g/ml and

TABLE 2.2

Disposition of thiopentone and methohexitone when given by continuous infusion

Data shown as mean (S.D.) or mean and range.

| Source | $n$ | Sampling site | Duration of infusion (min) | Duration of sampling (h) | Model[a] | $V\beta$ (l) | $Vd_{ss}$ (l) | $Cl$ (ml/min) | $t_{1/2}el$ (h) |
|---|---|---|---|---|---|---|---|---|---|
| **Thiopentone** | | | | | | | | | |
| Christensen et al., 1983 | 8P[b] | v[c] | 50—130 | 24 | — | 161 (60—254) | — | 180 (120—240) | 14.2 (8.4—22.2) |
| Crankshaw et al., 1985 | 12P | a/v | 40—300 | up to 70 | — | — | 146 (63) | 162 (53) | 15.0 (7.2) |
| Turcant et al., 1985 | 62P | a/v | 4—8 days | 72 | 1C | — | — | 108[d] (47) | 10.2[e] (5.7) |
| Stanski et al., 1980 | 5P | a/v | 42—89 h | 175 | 1C | — | — | — | 7.6—30.3[e] |
| **Methohexitone** | | | | | | | | | |
| Breimer et al., 1976 | 4V | v | 60 | 7 | 2C | 1.13[f] (0.19) | — | 12.14[f] (2.28) | 1.6 (0.4) |
| Le Normand et al., 1988 | 16P | a | 14 h | 12 | 3C | 5.21[f] (1.83) | 4.60[f] (1.70) | 9.67[f] (3.77) | 7.3 (3.5) |

[a]Model: number of compartments.
[b]P or V: patients or volunteers.
[c]a or v: arterial or venous sampling.
[d]Estimated steady-state clearance.
[e]Terminal half life following zero-order decay.
[f]Values given as l/kg or ml/kg per min.

10.7 μg/ml for burst suppression — thus indicating a wide therapeutic window. The values were similar in a given individual patient for each of the three input cycles; so confirming the apparent absence of tolerance.

In a series of dose-response studies in patients premedicated with either diazepam or morphine-atropine, Sear et al. (1983a, 1984a) determined the $ED_{50}$ and $ED_{95}$ infusion rates when methohexitone was used to supplement nitrous oxide in patients aged 20—60 years. The values for those rates, when the applied stimulus was the initial surgical incision, were 66.0 and 80.7 μg/kg per min for diazepam premedicated patients, and 48.8 and 75.9 μg/kg per min, respectively, after opioid premedication. There were no reported data relating drug concentration to effect in these patients, although in a separate study, Todd et al. (1984) infused methohexitone at higher infusion rates (400 μg/kg per min) as the sole anaesthetic for neurosurgical anaesthesia. The concentration associated with burst suppression of the EEG varied between 8 and 10 μg/ml, and isoelectric EEGs at concentrations between 9 and 13 μg/ml.

Methohexitone has no active metabolites, and most clinical studies infusing the agent with either nitrous oxide or an opioid infusion use rates between 50 and 120 μg/kg per min. Recovery is prompt unless the total drug dose administered is in excess of 500—600 mg (Prys-Roberts et al., 1983b). However, its use may be accompanied by some unwanted side-effects, such as excitatory movements, pain on injection and a predisposition to convulsions. Indeed, Todd et al. (1984) reported post-operative seizures in three out of the 8 neurosurgical patients receiving infusions of methohexitone, at a mean plasma drug concentration of ≥ 18 μg/ml. This is significantly greater than those concentrations required to maintain anaesthesia with methohexitone and nitrous oxide or an infusion of opioid; but the property may limit the overall usefulness of the barbiturate.

Comparative studies of methohexitone with other i.v. and inhalational agents suggest that recovery is faster after both etomidate and propofol when given by incremental doses or infusion, although the quality of recovery after the initial wake-up period needs to be evaluated further to delineate whether real differences exist between the different agents. There are no reported adverse sequelae following methohexitone with regard to liver function tests or adrenal cortical function (Prys-Roberts et al., 1983b; Crozier et al., 1987) although Bittrich et al. (1963) reported increases in some non-specific liver enzymes when patients received large doses of the hypnotic.

## CHLORMETHIAZOLE

This is a derivative of the thiazole part of vitamin $B_1$. It has sedative, hypnotic and anticonvulsant properties. As a continuous i.v. anaesthetic, it is mainly used to supplement regional or spinal anaesthesia (Schweitzer, 1978; Mather and Cousins, 1980). The drug is eliminated mainly by hepatic metabolism, with < 1% excreted unchanged in the urine (Moore et al., 1975). Its kinetics during continuous infusion have been reported in volunteers by Seow et al. (1981), and show an elimination half-life between 101 and 476 min, clearance between 690 and 2170 ml/min, and a volume of distribution ($Vd_{ss}$) of 114 and 273 l. Amnesia occurred at concentrations between 6.9 and 16.2 $\mu$g/ml, and light sedation between 5.5 and 9.6 $\mu$g/ml. In a series of studies involving use of chlormethiazole as a basal sedative for patients undergoing angiography, Mather et al. (1981) measured liver extraction to be 70—80%, and apparently unrelated to drug concentration. Lung and kidney extraction varied among the seven patients, ranging between 0% and 20%.

In all of these studies, there was a noted ease in rapidly changing the depth of sedation, and the associated cardiovascular effects were minimal (an increase in heart rate, and no change in cardiac output) (Wilson et al., 1969). Modig (1988) has suggested that chlormethiazole may have a protective role in endotoxic shock, through minimising cardiovascular and pulmonary instability.

There are few reports of the use of chlormethiaziole for the maintenance of anaesthesia (Kristoffersen et al., 1982; Christensen et al., 1983). Christensen infused the sedative at a mean rate of 4.7 mg/kg per h to supplement 67% nitrous oxide and increments of pethidine in elderly (60—85 years) female patients. Kinetic data gave an elimination half-life of 5.1 h (range 4 to 6.6), clearance 0.73 l/min (0.41 to 1.01), and $V_{\beta}$ 328 l (142 to 529). Impedance cardiography showed no significant effect on cardiac output, although there was an increase in stroke volume and decrease in heart rate. The plasma chlormethiazole concentration at the abolition of the eyelash reflex was 134 $\mu$mol/l (range 68 to 215); this compares with the 42 $\mu$mol/l required for hypnosis in patients undergoing surgery under epidural blockade (Mather and Cousins, 1980) and 40 $\mu$mol/l for basal sedation in volunteers (Seow et al., 1981).

The drug has, however, a number of disadvantages: its preparation as an 0.8% infusion in 4% glucose results in a large fluid load, which may limit its usefulness, especially in patients with renal failure and those with fluid and electrolyte problems; concentrations $>5\%$ may lead to an increased red cell fragility and haemolysis (Runciman et al., 1981); an absence of any analgesic properties; the need to infuse via a central vein to overcome the high incidence of thrombophlebitis; and nasal irritation and stuffiness. There is also adsorption of the sedative on to the surface of the i.v. giving set. During prolonged infusion, saturation of peripheral tissues may occur, such that recovery is then lengthy, being dependent not on redistribution but rather on hepatic metabolism (Robson et al., 1984). Its use as a sedative agent may be limited by the magnitude of the accompanying tachycardia (up to +50%).

## ETOMIDATE

The carboxylated imidazole etomidate has been in clinical practice in the United Kingdom since 1978, having been introduced into European practice in the early 1970s. It is considered by many anaesthetists to be the ideal agent for the induction and maintenance of anaesthesia in the cardiac-compromised or hypovolaemic patient. It has been formulated in four separate solvents to date (and a fifth, Intralipid, has also recently been studied), but none has significantly resulted in a reduction in the incidence of pain on injection and the accompanying venous sequelae of thrombosis and phlebitis. Other minor side-effects include involuntary muscle movements (especially in the unpremedicated patient) which may occur throughout induction, maintenance and recovery, coughing and hiccups.

Single dose studies investigating the disposition of etomidate revealed a terminal half-life of between 80 and 200 min, and a clearance of 800 to 1600 ml/min (Van Hamme et al., 1978; Schuttler et al., 1980). The drug is biotransformed by enzymes present in both the plasma and the liver, with formation of inactive, water-soluble metabolites (the main one being the corresponding carboxylic acid). This has a longer elimination half-life than the parent compound. Etomidate is bound to plasma proteins (76%: binding to both albumin and alpha$_1$-acid glycoprotein).

When given by continuous infusion, de Ruiter et al. (1981) described the kinetics of etomidate with an elimination half-life of 170 min, volume of distribution at steady state of 310 l, and clearance 1280 ml/min. Similar data have been reported in volunteers by Schuttler and colleagues (1985) (terminal half life 87—126 min; clearance 1175—2550 ml/min), and Hebron et al. (1983) in post-surgical ITU patients (half-life 43—119 min, clearance 1045—2254 ml/min) (Table 2.3). Anaesthesia was associated with concentrations between 300 and 500 ng/ml, with burst suppression of the EEG found at concentrations greater than 1.0 μg/ml.

When given at high infusion rates, etomidate causes a decrease in both cardiac output and liver blood flow, so causing greater plasma drug concentrations than might otherwise have been predicted (Van Lambalgan et al., 1982; Thomson et al., 1984). In addition, Schuttler et al. (1983b) have shown a significant decrease in etomidate clearance in the presence of a steady-state concentration of fentanyl (10 ng/ml). Although they hypothesize this to be due to an alteration in the volume of drug distribution, there is little evidence from other studies to support this. Another interaction involving etomidate has shown greater steady-state etomidate concentrations when the hypnotic was infused by fixed regimen to patients breathing nitrous oxide and oxygen rather than oxygen-enriched air (Sear et al., 1984b). The average plasma etomidate concentration during the maintenance infusion (10 μg/kg per min) was 501 (S.D. 135) ng/ml in the presence of nitrous oxide; and 367 (S.D. 110) ng/ml with oxygen-enriched air. The effect of nitrous oxide of decreasing cardiac output (and hence liver blood flow) has been described by Thomson et al. (1982) in a dog model, and McDermott and Stanley (1977) in man. The decrease in the hepatic extraction of etomidate results not only in a greater etomidate concentration during the maintenance infusion phase, but also an increase in the area under the concentration-time curve (0 to 120 min) (nitrous oxide group: 85.3 μg/ml per min vs. oxygen enriched air group: 64.7 μg/ml per min) (Sear et al., 1984b).

Etomidate has many of the ideal properties of an hypnotic agent: sleep in one arm-brain circulation time, no detectable histamine release, minimal cardiovascular and respiratory depressive effects, reduction in cerebral metabolism, cerebral blood

TABLE 2.3

Disposition of kinetics of etomidate, midazolam, chlormethiazole and propofol when given by continuous infusion

Data shown as mean (S.D.) or range.

| | $n$[a] | Sampling site | Duration of infusion (min) | Duration of sampling (h) | Model[b] | $Vd\beta$ (l) | $Vd_{ss}$ (l) | $Cl$ (ml/min) | $t_{1/2}el$ (h) |
|---|---|---|---|---|---|---|---|---|---|
| **Etomidate** | | | | | | | | | |
| Hebron et al., 1983 | 6P[c] | A[d] | — | 24 | 3C | — | — | 25 (3)[e] | 5.88 (1.22) |
| Fragen et al., 1983 | 11P | V | 30—110 | 4 | 2C | — | 183 (88) | 1.21 (0.3) | 2.9 (1.1) |
| Schuttler et al., 1985 | 6V | — | 120 | — | 2C | 252 (51) | — | 1.69 (0.5) | 1.77 (0.28) |
| Sear et al., 1984b | 12P | V | 120 | — | — | — | — | 24 (9)[e] | — |
| **Midazolam** | | | | | | | | | |
| Persson et al., 1987 | 15P | V | 75—120 | 6 | 2C | 1.9 (0.6)[e] | — | 483 (109) | 3.1 (0.8) |
| **Chlormethiazole** | | | | | | | | | |
| Christensen et al., 1983 | 8P | V | 70—105 | 24 | — | 328 (142—529) | — | 730 (410—1010) | 5.1 (4.0—6.6) |
| **Propofol** | | | | | | | | | |
| Schuttler et al., 1986 | 6V | A | 120 | — | 2C | 153 (21) | — | 1890 (400) | 1.05 (0.27) |
| | 6V | V | 120 | — | 2C | 209 (36) | — | 1880 (360) | 1.38 (0.22) |
| Cockshott et al., 1990 | 8V | V | 120 | — | 3C | 832 (325) | 263 (95) | 1930 (417) | 5.1 (2.2) MIR[f] |
| | | | | | 3C | 996 (652) | 319 (224) | 1540 (360) | 8.5 (7.0) MIR[f] |
| Gepts et al., 1987 | 18P | A/V | 120—240 | 8 | 3C | 860 (432) | 287 (213) | 1770 (320) | 5.9 (3.8) |
| Gepts et al., 1988 | 11P | A | 120—230 | 8 | 3C | 717 (392) | 280 (220) | 1910 (480) | 4.7 (3.1) |
| Shafer et al., 1988 | 50P | V | 100 | 10 | 2C | — | 2.3 (0.8)[e] | 30 (8)[e] | 1.93 (0.57) |
| Vandermeersch et al., 1989 | 20C | V | 60+ | — | — | — | — | 39 (12)[e] | — |
| Albanese et al., 1990 | 9P | A | 3 days | — | NC | — | 166 (756) | 1570 (560) | 31.3 (11.2) |

[a]$n$: number of subjects studied.
[b]Model: number of compartments to which the data has been fitted. NC: non-compartmental modelling.
[c]P, V, C: patients (adult), volunteers (adult), children.
[d]A or V: arterial or venous sampling.
[e]Values given as l/kg or ml/kg per min.
[f]MIR: minimum infusion rate ($ED_{50}$). For propofol, the rates employed in the study reported by Cockshott et al. (1990) were 54 and 108 μg/kg per min.

flow and intracranial pressure, and rapid recovery after single doses and continuous infusions.

There are two problems with etomidate which question its use by continuous infusion for either sedation or maintenance of anaesthesia. The first relates to the solvent, propylene glycol; there being a recommended limit as to the total dose of etomidate given because of the potential haemolytic consequences following large volumes of the solvent. This may be overcome by use of the infusion preparation (125 mg/ml, dissolved in absolute alcohol). When diluted with normal saline or dextrose-saline to a concentration of 1 mg/ml, the resulting pH is about 3.5. This reformulation does not remove the problem of pain on injection.

The second and more important adverse property of etomidate relates to its effects on adrenal and gonadal steroidogenesis. A letter from Ledingham and Watt (1983) in the Lancet reported that use of the drug by infusion for the provision of sedation in the ITU was associated with an increased mortality. Watt and Ledingham (1984) also noted that many of the patients receiving etomidate exhibited low plasma cortisol levels ($<$ 100 nmol/l; normal range 260—550 nmol/l). Their hypothesis; that the increased mortality associated with etomidate by infusion was due, at least in part, to adrenal cortical suppression, was supported by the animal experiments of Preziosi and Vacca (1982) and Preziosi (1983) who demonstrated that 20 $\mu$mol/kg of *d*-etomidate inhibited stress- and drug-induced corticosteroid production in the adrenal gland, as well as inhibiting the ACTH-induced stress response. In the rat, etomidate also inhibited the rise in prolactin, which is similarly part of the neurophysiological response to stress. Some suppression of this response also occurs with deep Althesin (alphaxalone/alphadolone acetate) anaesthesia, but is not caused by hydroxydione or ketamine (Preziosi, 1983). Other in vitro data from Lambert et al. (1985) and Kenyon et al. (1985) have shown etomidate, at normal therapeutic concentrations, to be a more potent inhibitor of steroid synthesis than metyrapone; while other hypnotic agents (e.g., thiopentone and propofol) cause inhibition only at supra-therapeutic concentrations.

Many authors have delineated the mechanisms of the lowered cortisol levels in response to etomidate. Moore et al. (1985) used a standard clinical model — premenopausal patients undergoing abdominal hysterectomy. After premedication with diazepam, patients were randomly allocated to receive either thiopentone and halothane to supplement nitrous oxide and fentanyl (control group) or etomidate 0.3 mg/kg for induction of anaesthesia, and an infusion of 10 $\mu$g/kg per min to supplement nitrous oxide and fentanyl (study group). Blood samples were collected prior to induction of anaesthesia (always at 08.30 h to avoid the diurnal variation in cortical hormone levels), 1 h later, at the end of surgery, and at 4, 10 and 24 h after induction. The responses of both plasma cortisol and aldosterone to the stimulus of surgery were obtunded in those patients receiving an infusion of etomidate.

In order to evaluate whether the reduction in corticosteroid synthesis was due to adrenal gland inhibition, or through inhibition of the anterior pituitary-adrenal axis (as had been suggested by Preziosi (1983) in the rat), ACTH levels were also measured at induction, at the time of the maximum cortisol response in the control group (4 h) and at 24 h. There were large increases in plasma ACTH concentrations, with no differences between the groups, indicating the effect of etomidate to be on the adrenal cortex. Further studies have shown four different sites of enzyme inhibition, with apparent dose dependence: 11$\beta$ hydroxylase, 17$\alpha$ hydroxylase, 18 hydroxylase and probably the cholesterol side chain cleavage enzyme (20,22 lyase) (de Jong et al., 1984; Fry and Griffiths, 1984; de Coster et al., 1985; Moore et al., 1985; Allolio et al., 1985). The main hormonal effects of etomidate are, therefore, to decrease cortisol and aldosterone synthesis and secretion, and increase the plasma concentrations of their precursors, 11-deoxycortisol and 18-deoxycorticosterone.

The effect of etomidate on 11$\beta$ hydroxylation is both dose- and concentration-related. Data from Sear et al. (1983a), Moore et al. (1985) and Sear et al. (1988a) show a decrease in cortisol and aldosterone synthesis with doses of 0.3 mg/kg and a greater effect from 1.2 mg/kg total dose. Crozier and colleagues (1988) found a sigmoidal relationship between the relative inhibition of cortisol in response to ACTH stimulation and the log of the plasma etomidate concentration. The $ED_{50}$ etomidate concentration was 110 nM (20 ng/ml), with suppression negligible at concentrations below 40 nM. On the basis of these data and the known kinetics of the drug, the expected duration of the inhibition will be about 4—8 h, in agreement with data from Fragen et al. (1984), Wagner and White (1984) and Moore et al. (1985).

In vitro studies by Horai et al. (1985) have confirmed this concentration dependence of the inhibition of P-450 metabolism, and especially that of certain drugs (ketamine *N*-demethylation, pethidine *N*-demethylation, *p*-nitroanisole *O*-demethylation, and aniline *p*-hydroxylation). The $IC_{50}$ concentrations were of the order of 10 $\mu$M. The mechanisms of inhibition vary. Other in vivo studies by the same group (Atiba et al., 1988) using ketamine and antipyrine as the marker substrates have shown an infusion of etomidate to increase the elimination half-life of antipyrine, but to cause no significant change in clearance. There was no effect when ketamine was used as the anaesthetic agent. These data suggest etomidate might prolong the elimination of drugs with a low extraction ratio, but not those of the flow-dependent type.

Etomidate is not the only i.v. agent to cause a decrease in plasma cortisol levels. Kapp (1988) in a review article describes studies where the effects on adrenal cortical function of morphine 10 mg/70 kg i.v., morphine 30 mg p.o., and nalbuphine 20 mg/70 kg i.v. were investigated in volunteers in the absence of surgical stimulation. Each opioid caused a decrease in cortisol and ACTH concentrations, but there was no indication as to whether this was a dose-related phenomenon as has been shown for etomidate. Hence the combination of etomidate and an opioid may lead to a compounded effect.

Data for other hypnotics are conflicting. Our own work on midazolam (Dawson and Sear, 1986) and that of Nilsson et al. (1988a) show increased cortisol levels in response to the stimulus of lower abdominal surgery. However, studies from

Crozier and colleagues (1987) have reported different responses. They compared infusions of methohexitone, etomidate and midazolam as supplements to nitrous oxide and fentanyl anaesthesia in patients undergoing body surface orthopaedic surgery. Hormone levels were measured pre-induction, at the end of surgery, at 6 h and then at 20 h post-surgery. In the barbiturate group, there were the expected increases in both cortisol and ACTH levels; in the etomidate group, there was the expected blunting of the cortisol response. However, there was also blunting of the cortisol response to surgery in the midazolam group. The rises of ACTH and beta-endorphin levels in this group were obtunded in comparison to the increases seen at the end of surgery in both the methohexitone and etomidate groups. Thus, although both etomidate and midazolam caused a reduced cortisol response, the mechanisms responsible were different. For etomidate, these decreases are due to enzyme inhibition; for midazolam, there appears to be central inhibition of ACTH release. Glisson et al. (1982) have shown a similar effect from midazolam in dogs subjected to the stress of hypovolaemic hypotension; with decreases in cortisol, ACTH and adrenaline. Data for other i.v. hypnotics (thiopentone, propofol) indicate no effect on the response to surgical stress, although both drugs can result in an initial decrease in the plasma cortisol concentration (Kay et al., 1985; Fragen et al., 1987).

Why should the results of Nilsson and ourselves differ from those of Crozier? It is probable that abdominal surgery offers a greater noxious stimulus to the anaesthetised patient than does body suface surgery; and that with this increased stress, the central inhibition may be overridden. This hypothesis remains to be clarified.

## KETAMINE

Ketamine, a phencyclidine derivative, is the only one of the present hypnotic agents that possesses defined analgesic properties. It is a racemic mixture — the ratio of $R(-)/S(+)$ being 1 : 1 — although the latter isomer has greater anaesthetic and analgesic properties. Ketamine is also water soluble (hence requires no additional solvent), and has a liposolubility more than 10 times that of thiopentone — so resulting in rapid onset of hypnosis and analgesia.

Following i.v. and i.m. bolus administrations, there was a biphasic decline in the plasma drug concentration, due to a combination of both redistribution to the peripheral tissues and hepatic clearance — the latter being flow-dependent. The terminal half-life after i.v. administration was 186 min, and clearance 19.1 ml/kg per min (Clements et al., 1982). Similar values were observed following intramuscular injection, and the bioavailability was estimated at 93%. The metabolic fate of ketamine is complex, but one of the main metabolites (norketamine: metabolite I) is pharmacologically active. Indeed, it has been suggested that this metabolite has an anaesthetic potency of about 33% that of the parent drug, while metabolite II (dehydronorketamine) has about 1% activity. Studies of the urinary excretion of ketamine show about 2.5% appearing as parent drug, 1.6% per 24 h as metabolite I and 16% per 24 h as metabolite II. The remaining 80% is excreted as glucuronide conjugates of ketamine and its metabolites.

There are few kinetic data on the plasma disposition of ketamine when given by continuous infusion; although Idvall et al. (1979) and Clements et al. (1982) have established the concentration-effect relationships in respect of both analgesia and hypnosis. These data indicate an analgesic threshold of about 200 ng/ml; and a concentration required for hypnosis, when ketamine is given as supplement to nitrous oxide, of 1.5—2.5 μg/ml. Idvall and colleagues gave 2 mg/kg as a loading dose and then an infusion of 40 μg/kg per min. The corresponding steady state drug concentration was between 1.7 and 2.4 μg/ml. The mean terminal half-life post-infusion in 31 patients was 79 min. Metabolite I appeared in the plasma by 5 min, and metabolite II by 20 min after the start of the infusion. The concentrations of these metabolites increased still further after the infusion was stopped.

When administered alone, the side-effects of ketamine may limit its usefulness. These include cardiovascular stimulation (resulting from peripheral constriction and an increase in sympathetic tone) which leads to hypertension and a tachycardia; postoperative dreaming and hallucinations; and excessive salivation. Each of these side-effects may be attenuated with benzodiazepine premedication (either diazepam or midazolam). However, it must be noted that pretreatment with the former results in a significant drug interaction, with prolongation of the elimination half-life of ketamine and increased duration of effect (Idvall et al., 1983).

As a sole agent, regimens of a loading dose (0.50—1.0 mg/kg) followed by a maintenance infusion rate of 25—75 μg/kg per min will achieve unconsciousness and provide haemodynamically stable anaesthesia. In the presence of nitrous oxide, the required maintenance rate is reduced to the range 10—30 μg/kg per min. In a study of patients receiving ketamine to supplement nitrous oxide for body surface anaesthesia, White et al. (1983), using a variable rate infusion according to patient response, found the average maintenance infusion rate to be between 2 and 6 mg/min, with the associated drug concentration of 1.1 μg/ml (range: 0.5—1.8). The concentrations of metabolite I varied between 0.2 and 0.8 μg/ml. Lower infusion regiments (1—2 mg/min) will provide sedation and analgesia in patients being ventilated in the ITU post-surgery (Joachimsson et al., 1986).

There is some debate over the effects of ketamine on hepatic function. Zsigmond and colleagues (1980) reported no change of any of the routine enzyme tests of liver function. However, this was in contrast to Dundee et al. (1980) who found significant increases in serum transaminases, when infusions of ketamine were given to supplement either nitrous oxide in oxygen, or oxygen-enriched air. However, the nonspecificity of the enzymes measured may be an important factor in the study, and therefore the significance of these observations needs to be re-examined. In vitro testing of the effects of ketamine in hepatocyte function revealed an $ED_{50}$ dose for inhibition of gluconeogenesis of the order of 300 to 500 μmol/l (Sear and McGivan, 1979).

Other studies from the department in Belfast and our own data have shown none of the other i.v. hypnotic agents (methohexitone, etomidate, midazolam and propofol) to affect liver cell integrity when given by continuous infusion to patients undergoing body surface or abdominal surgery (Dundee and Zacharias, 1979; Blunnie et al., 1981; Kawar et al., 1982; Prys-Roberts et al., 1983b; Sear et al., 1983c; Sear et al., 1984b; Robinson and Patterson, 1985).

## PROPOFOL

A sterically hindered phenol, which is water insoluble, propofol (di-isopropyl phenol) was first administered to volunteers in 1977 by Kay and Rolly; but problems firstly with severe pain on injection, and then with complement mediated adverse reactions to a Cremophor formulation have resulted in three solvents being investigated. The present one, a 1% oil in water emulsion formulation containing 10% soyabean oil, 1.2% egg phosphatide and 2.25% glycerol was first given to human subjects here in Oxford in July 1983 by my colleague Dr Nigel Kay; and the ensuing multicentre study showed the $ED_{95}$ induction dose in unpremedicated ASA I and II patients to be 2.5 mg/kg (Cumming et al., 1984). At this dose, there was a significantly lower incidence of side-effects than had been observed with an equipotent dose of the Cremophor formulation. In a separate study, Kay and colleagues (1985) investigated the clinical properties of the drug when given by increments to supplement nitrous oxide (70%) in oxygen for the maintenance of anaesthesia in opioid premedicated patients undergoing body surface surgery. The mean overall administration rate was 79.7 μg/kg per min (95% limits: 62.6 to 96.8 μg/kg per min; and recovery post-anaesthesia was rapid and complete.

Kinetic data from several different studies where patients were receiving a single dose of propofol (2.5 mg/kg) give mean values for elimination half-life of 226—674 min, clearance of 1.66—1.91 l/min), a central volume of distribution of 13—56 l, and a volume of distribution at steady state of 171—781 l (Cockshott, 1985). The large volume of distribution reflects the high octanol/water partition coefficient (log *P*: 3.7); while the high plasma protein binding (97—99%) may explain the large central volume of distribution. There is, however, considerable variability between individuals, and indeed our own data (based on 8-h sampling in patients undergoing body surface surgery during halothane-nitrous oxide anaesthesia) shows a terminal half-life of 146—592 min; clearance of 1.36—2.78 l $min^{-1}$, and $V_{\gamma}$ of 409—1318 l (Kay et al., 1986).

The metabolic fate of propofol has been reported by both Vree et al. (1987) and Simons et al. (1988). In the volunteer study of Simons, less than 0.3% of the parent drug was excreted unchanged. The major metabolites were propofol glucuronide, and the glucuronide and sulphate conjugates of the hydroxylated derivative, 2,6 di-isopropyl 1,4-quinol. In four patients undergoing body surface surgery, the half-lives of the three metabolites ranged between 7 and 20 h; while the excretion of each was 15.6—33.3%, 0.6—2.4%, and 22.5—50.3%, respectively. None of these metabolites is known to possess significant pharmacological activity.

More recent studies from Campbell and colleagues in Melbourne (1988) have suggested an even greater variability in the various kinetic parameters (terminal half-life 3.6—63 h; clearance 870—2140 ml/min; and volume of distribution ($V_\gamma$) 180—1730 l). These data were obtained after a single dose of propofol 2—3 mg/kg, and a longer sampling period than in all other studies to date (up to 52 h — the duration being limited by the sensitivity of the assay, 2 ng/ml). This terminal half-life is probably representative of the rate of drug efflux from the peripheral lipid tissues. After a single bolus dose, the terminal half-life will not be significant as it does not contribute to the decay profile until the blood drug concentration has fallen below levels associated with clinical anaesthesia or sedation. However, this may not be the case when the drug is administered by prolonged infusion, and this is clearly in need of study.

The high clearance rate for propofol has been commented on by several authors, including ourselves, to be in excess of liver blood flow, so begging the question of whether there are other sites of metabolism of the hindered phenol (e.g. lungs or kidney). Recent data from Lange and colleagues (1990) in Gottingen has proposed that extra-hepatic metabolism may be the primary method of drug elimination. This has been supported by data from Mather and colleagues at Flinders University, Adelaide, who found similar evidence of extra-hepatic clearance using their chronically instrumented sheep model. If, however, the data from Campbell are a truer reflection of the kinetics of this compound, then there is little need to consider extra-hepatic metabolism as being such a major component in drug removal.

Either way, the high clearance characteristics and rapid initial decline in drug concentration in the blood make propofol an ideal agent for administration by continuous infusion either alone, or as supplement to nitrous oxide or an infusion of an opioid. There are a number of data sets for the kinetics of propofol given by infusion; these are summarised in Table 2.3. However, all these parameter estimates have been obtained in ASA I or II patients (or volunteers), and there is urgent need for more data on the influence of ageing, obesity, disease states and intercurrent therapy on the kinetics of propofol.

Kirkpatrick et al. (1988) have shown significant reductions in both total clearance and the volume of distribution ($V_1$) in elderly patients aged 65 to 80 years; while Dundee et al. (1986), Monk et al. (1987) and others have shown the dosage requirements both for induction or maintenance of anaesthesia to be reduced in the elderly patient. Renal disease and compensated hepatic cirrhosis (Child's classification A and B) have been reported to have little effect on the handling of propofol (Morcos and Payne, 1985; Reiter et al., 1989; Servin et al., 1988). There are no data at present (February 1991) on the kinetic interaction of propofol with beta-adrenoceptor blocking agents, and $H_2$ receptor antagonists. Despite the data from Cockshott et al. (1987), the present emulsion formulation shows no kinetic interaction with either fentanyl or alfentanil when given by continuous infusion (Gill et al., 1990; Gepts et al., 1988). However, Gepts et al. (1988) have shown the combination propofol-alfentanil to result in higher than predicted plasma alfentanil concentrations. Again, this needs further investigation.

**Concentration-effect relationships**

Although propofol is a central nervous system depressant drug, there are few data investigating the effects of different infusion rates or drug concentrations on the EEG. Hazeaux et al. (1987) showed that following a bolus dose of 2.5 mg/kg propofol, there was burst suppression of EEG activity. The awake pattern began returning after about 4 min, and was back to normal within 6 min of an induction dose. During maintenance infusions of propofol at 9 mg/kg per h, there were periods of burst suppression. However, a better correlation between EEG pattern and propofol input was seen when comparing the EEG pattern with the blood propofol concentration. An awake-type EEG was seen at drug concentrations up to about 3.74 μg/ml. Loss of consciousness was induced at concentrations of about 6 μg/ml, while surgical anaesthesia required levels of 7 to 10 μg/ml. During the infusion, burst suppression started at concentrations around 8.5 μg/ml; but following cessation of the infusion, similar activity was also observed at lower propofol concentrations. Other studies by Vandesteene and colleagues (1988) found a better correlation between EEG activity and blood propofol concentrations. The usual endpoints of anaesthesia (eyes opening to command, and giving date of birth) have been measured by several authors and found to occur at concentrations of the ranges of 1.0 to 2.9 μg/ml and 0.6 to 1.8 μg/ml, respectively.

Prys-Roberts and his colleagues (Spelina et al., 1986; Turtle et al., 1987; Monk et al., 1987) have conducted a series of experiments designed to determine the $ED_{50}$ and $ED_{95}$ rates, with respect to the intial surgical incision, and their associated drug concentrations ($EC_{50}$ and $EC_{95}$), for infusions of propofol. For ASA I or II patients aged 20—60 years, and premedicated with morphine 0.15 mg/kg, the $ED_{50}$ rate to supplement 70% nitrous oxide was 53.5 μg/kg per min, and the $EC_{50}$, 1.7 μg/ml. Table 2.4 lists the respective values for propofol under a variety of different conditions. There are, however, no data at present for propofol infusions given to patients with intercurrent pathology or receiving medication. In such patients, the adoption of infusion regiments based on the results of the ASA I and II patients may lead to overdose with toxic side-effects, or underdosing with resulting awareness due to either kinetic or dynamic interactions.

Shafer and colleagues (1988) and Glass et al. (1989) have both delineated other aspects of the concentration-effect relationship. In ventilated patients receiving an infusion of propofol to supplement 70% nitrous oxide and incremental doses of pethidine (meperidine), the average blood propofol concentration associated with an obtunding of the autonomic responses was higher during abdominal surgery (4.05 μg/ml) when compared with 2.97 μg/ml during body surface surgery (Shafer et al., 1988). Blood propofol concentrations at which responses to surgery were observed were also greater in the major surgery group (3.46 compared with 2.39 μg/ml).

TABLE 2.4

Dose requirements for continuous infusions of propofol to supplement either 67% nitrous oxide in oxygen, or the combination alfentanil infusion-oxygen enriched air, in patients premedicated with either a benzodiazepine or opioid-vagolytic

Mean (± S.D.) or range of 95% confidence interval.

| Premed | Air/ $N_2O$ | $ED_{50}$[a] | $EC_{50}$[b] | $ED_{95}$[a] | $EC_{95}$[b] | Reference |
|---|---|---|---|---|---|---|
| Morphine 0.15 mg/kg i.m. | $N_2O$ | 53.5 (39.9—63.0) | 1.66 | 112.2 (85.6—306.2) | 3.39 | Spelina et al., 1986 |
| Lorazepam 2—3 mg p.o. | $N_2O$ | 130 (106—167) | 2.5 | 348 (233—1296) | 5.92 | Turtle et al., 1987 |
| Temazepam 20—30 mg p.o. | Air | 49.0 (39.1—56.2) | 1.40 (0.62—1.87) | 83 (68.8—1.87) | 4.05 (2.78—30.5) | Richards et al., 1990[c] |
| Pethidine 1 mg/kg i.v. | $N_2O$ | 8.3 (2.4)[d] | 4.05 (1.01) | Major surgery | | Van Doze et al., 1988; |
| | $N_2O$ | 7.8 (2.8)[d] | 2.97 (1.07) | Non-major surgery | | Shafer et al., 1988 |

[a]$ED_{50}$ and $ED_{95}$: infusion rates for 50% and 95% of population necessary to prevent movement to the initial surgical incision (termed 'minimum infusion rate' for $ED_{50}$; Sear and Prys-Roberts, 1979) (μg/kg per min).
[b]$EC_{50}$ and $EC_{95}$: blood propofol concentrations at the $ED_{50}$ and $ED_{95}$ infusion rates (μg/ml).
[c]Alfentanil infusion: 50 μg/kg loading dose and infusion rate of 50 μg/kg per h.
[d]Rates shown as mg/min.

Similar data, based on propofol-nitrous oxide anaesthesia, have recently been presented by Glass and colleagues (1989). Our own data, obtained from studies in spontaneously breathing patients where a variable rate infusion regimen of propofol was used to supplement 70% nitrous oxide in oxygen, suggest that somatic and/or autonomic response to incision showed wide inter-individual variability in terms of the blood propofol concentration. Inadequate anaesthesia (taken as movement in response to the initial surgical incision or during surgery) was seen in 10 out of 30 patients, at blood propofol concentrations between 3.11 and 8.42 μg/ml at incision, and 2.58 and 5.54 μg/ml during body surface surgery (Sear et al., 1988b) (Figure 2.4).

## MIDAZOLAM

Although not usually considered an hypnotic agent (rather a sedative drug), there has been recent interest in the use of midazolam as supplement to either nitrous

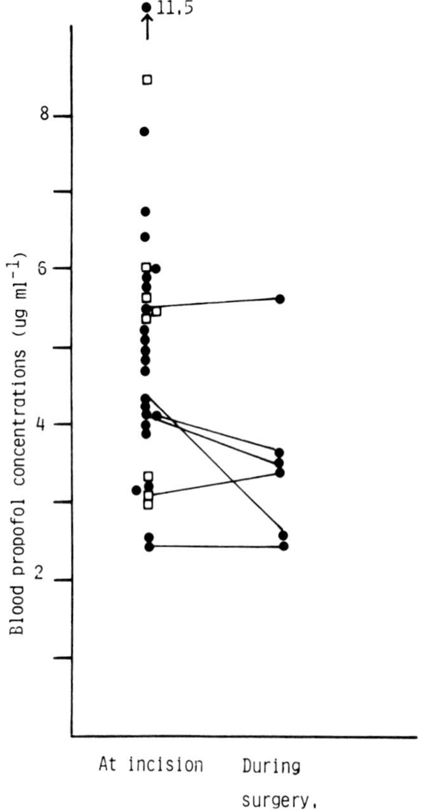


Fig. 2.4. Blood propofol concentrations in patients receiving a variable rate infusion of the drug to supplement 67% nitrous oxide in oxygen anaesthesia, and undergoing body surface surgery. All patients breathed spontaneously. The individual points represent data from 29 patients at the time points shown. Episodes of inadequate intra-operative anaesthesia are linked to the respective concentration at the time of incision. Propofol concentrations: ○ = response; ● = no response.

oxide in oxygen, or oxygen-enriched air plus an opioid for the maintenance of anaesthesia.

As an induction agent, midazolam has a slower onset of action than thiopentone, methohexitone or etomidate, a longer recovery period, and a higher incidence of amnesia (Nilsson et al., 1984). In animal and human studies, midazolam (and diazepam) reduce the MAC for volatile anaesthetic agents (Perisho et al., 1971; Melvin et al., 1982; Hall et al., 1988). Apnoea following induction is less frequent than after thiopentone, except in those patients with chronic obstructive airways disease where midazolam may cause prolonged ventilatory depression. The effects of midazolam on ICP, $CMRO_2$ and CBF are minimal.

In 1986, Nilsson and colleagues first described the use of an infusion of midazolam (0.25 mg/kg per h) to supplement nitrous oxide and increments of fentanyl for lower abdominal surgery. The average plasma midazolam concentration during the maintenance phase was 400 ng/ml, with a range of 298—764 ng/ml. Although the technique provided satisfactory anaesthesia, with cardiovascular stability, there was prolonged recovery, with many of the patients taking over 2 h from the end of the infusion to being able to give their correct names. A modification of the technique, using alfentanil by infusion in place of fentanyl, and a lower maintenance rate of midazolam (0.125 mg/kg per h), was accompanied by improved recovery (Nilsson et al., 1988). There were no adverse effects on the adrenocortical or glucose responses to surgery, when randomly compared with patients receiving thiopentone-nitrous oxide and alfentanil. These data support the earlier findings of Dawson and Sear (1986) following single doses of midazolam (0.3 mg/kg) for the induction of anaesthesia. There have been no reported adverse effects of midazolam on hepatic function (Kawar et al., 1982).

Kinetic studies with infusions of midazolam indicate an elimination half-life of 3—4 h, a clearance of 330—507 ml/min, and the volume of distribution, $V_\beta$ of 1.5—2.0 l/kg (Raeder et al, 1987, Persson et al, 1987). In patients premedicated with pethidine and atropine, Nilsson evaluated the concentration-effect relationship for the combination midazolam-alfentanil (Persson et al., 1988). Adequate anaesthesia for surgery required plasma drug concentrations $>$250—300 ng/ml, while arousal was seen when the concentration fell below 150—200 ng/ml. Sedation was associated with drug concentrations in excess of 75—100 ng/ml.

Recovery may be enhanced by use of the benzodiazepine antagonist, flumazenil in doses of 0.5 to 1 mg (Nilsson et al., 1988a; Raeder et al., 1988). However, the effect of single doses of the antagonist appears to be evanescent, with no differences in recovery from sedation and anxiolysis between treated and placebo control groups at time points greater than 1 h after flumazenil administration.

Disposition studies in the ITU have further highlighted the wide variability with elimination half-lives of 1.5—50 h, and clearance 35—1680 ml/min (Behne et al., 1987; Dirksen et al., 1988; Oldenhof et al., 1988; Michalk et al., 1988); as well as the metabolic ratio of midazolam/1-hydroxy midazolam glucuronide (0.03—15.6) (Dirksen et al., 1988; Oldenhof et al., 1988). 1-Hydroxy midazolam may have pharmacological activity, although this has not been reported for the glucuronide. Whether high blood concentrations of the glucuronide influence the patient's level of consciousness, midazolam hydroxylation or midazolam glucuronidation is not known; and therefore further studies are clearly needed to elucidate the effects of multi-organ failure on rates of metabolism of midazolam and its hydroxy metabolites.

## CONCLUDING REMARKS

Although this volume has been entitled Total Intravenous Anaesthesia, implying the avoidance of all gaseous supplements, the concept of the combined simultaneous administration of an opioid and an hypnotic to provide total surgical anaesthesia is still very alien to most anaesthetists' practice. There are many reasons for this reticence — a lack of familarity with the techniques of i.v. infusions; an absence of appropriate equipment; a more complex drug disposition profile resulting in greater variability in the achieved blood drug concentrations; and greater uncertainty over the assessment of depth of anaesthesia. In addition, there is often lack of data on the relationships between drug infusion rates and plasma drug concentrations, and adequacy of anaesthesia. For these reasons, and because of the many positive qualities of nitrous oxide as an anaesthetic adjunct, many anaesthetists will find it advantageous initially to employ infusions of hypnotics in place of the usual volatile supplements, assessing the required infusion regimens in the spontaneously breathing patient, before proceeding to their use in the paralysed individual. In this way, the risk of under-dosage and awareness should be reduced.

## REFERENCES


Albanese, J., Martin, C., Lacarelle, B., Saux, P., Durand, A. and Gouin, F. (1990) Pharmacokinetics of long-term propofol infusion used for sedation in ICU patients. *Anesthesiology* 73, 214—217.

Allolio, B., Dorr, H., Stuttmann, R., Knorr, D., Engelhardt, D. and Winkelmann, W. (1985) Effect of a single bolus of etomidate upon eight major corticosteroid hormones and plasma ACTH. *Clin. Endocrinol.* 22, 281—286.

Alvis, J.M., Reves, J.G., Govier, A.V., Menkhaus, P.G., Henling, C.E., Spain, J.A. and Bradley, E. (1985a) Computer-assisted continuous infusions of fentanyl during cardiac anesthesia: comparison with a manual method. *Anesthesiology* 63, 41—49.

Alvis, J.M., Reves, J.G., Spain, J.A. and Sheppard, L.C. (1985b) Computer-assisted continuous infusion of the intravenous analgesic fentanyl during general anesthesia — an interactive system. *IEEE: Trans. Biomed. Eng. MBE* 32, 323—329.

Arbilla, S., Depoortere, H., George, P. and Langer, S.Z. (1985) Pharmacological profile of the imidazopyridine zolpidem at benzodiazepine receptors and electrocorticogram in rats. *Naunyn Schmiedeberg's Arch. Pharmacol.* 330, 248—251.

Arden, J.R., Holley, F.O. and Stanski, D.R. (1986) Increased sensitivity to etomidate in the elderly: Initial distribution versus altered brain response. *Anesthesiology* 65, 19—27.

Atiba, J.O., Horai, Y., White, P.E., Trevor, A.J., Blaschke, T.F. and Sung, M.-L. (1988) Effect of etomidate on hepatic drug metabolism in humans. *Anesthesiology* 68, 920—924.

Ausems, M.E. and Hug, C.C., Jr. (1983) Plasma concentrations of alfentanil required to supplement nitrous oxide anaesthesia for lower abdominal surgery. *Br. J. Anaesth.* 55, Suppl. 2, 191s—197s.

Ausems, M.E., Hug, C.C., Jr. and de Lange, S. (1983) Variable rate infusion of alfentanil as a supplement to nitrous oxide anesthesia for general surgery. *Anesth. Analg.* 62, 982—986.

Ausems, M.E., Hug, C.C., Jr., Stanski, D.R. and Burm, A.G.L. (1986) Plasma concentrations of alfentanil required to supplement nitrous oxide anesthesia for general surgery. *Anesthesiology* 65, 362—373.

Barrett, R.L., Graham, G.G. and Torda, T.A. (1984a) The influence of sampling site upon the distribution phase kinetics of thiopentone. *Anaesth. Intensive Care* 12, 5—9.

Barrett, R.L., Graham, G.G. and Torda, T.A. (1984b) Kinetics of thiopentone in relation to the site of sampling. *Br. J. Anaesth.* 56, 1385—1390.

Becker, K.E. (1978) Plasma levels of thiopental necessary for anesthesia. *Anesthesiology* 49, 192—196.

Behne, M., Asskali, F., Steurer, A. and Forster, H. (1987) Continuous infusion of midazolam for sedation of ventilator patients. *Anaesthesist* 36, 228—232.

Bindslev, L. (1988) Inhalation anaesthesia. *Acta Anaesthesiol. Scand.* 32, Suppl. 87, 11—16.

Bischoff, K.B. and Dedrick, R.L. (1968) Thiopental pharmacokinetics. *J. Pharm. Sci.* 57, 1346—1351.

Bittrich, N.M., Kane, A.V. and Mosher, R.F. (1963) Methohexital and its effect on liver function tests: a comparative study. *Anesthesiology* 24, 81—90.

Blunnie, W.P., Zacharias, M., Dundee, J.W., Doggart, J.R., Moore, J. and McIlroy, P.D.A. (1981) Liver enzyme studies with continuous infusion anaesthesia. *Anaesthesia* 36, 152—156.

Boyes, R.N., Scott, D.B., Jebson, P.J., Godman, M.J. and Julian, D.G. (1971) Pharmacokinetics of lidocaine in man. *Clin. Pharmacol. Ther.* 12, 105—115.

Breimer, D.D. (1976) Pharmacokinetics of methohexitone following intravenous infusion in humans. *Br. J. Anaesth.* 48, 643—649.

Brodie, B.B., Mark, L.C., Lief, P.A., Bernstein, E. and Papper, E.M. (1951) Acute tolerance to thiopental. *J. Pharmacol. Exp.* Ther. 102, 215—218.

Buhrer, M., Maitre, P.O., Crevoisier, C., Hung, O. and Stanski, D.R. (1988) Comparative pharmacodynamics of midazolam and diazepam. *Anesthesiology* 69, A 642.

Campbell, G.A., Morgan, D.J., Kumar, K. and Crankshaw, D.P. (1988) Extended blood collection period required to define distribution and elimination kinetics of propofol. *Br. J. Clin. Pharmacol.* 26, 187—190.

Chan, H.N.J., Morgan, D.J., Crankshaw, D.P. and Boyd, M.D. (1985) Pentobarbitone formation during thiopentone infusion. *Anaesthesia* 40, 1155—1159.

Chan, K.K.H. and Gibaldi, M. (1982) Estimation of statistical moments and steady-state volume of distribution for a drug given by intravenous infusion. *Pharmacokinetics Biopharmaceutics* 10, 551—558.

Christ, D.D., Kenna, J.G., Kammerer, W., Satoh, H. and Pohl, L.R. (1988a) Enflurane metabolism produces covalently bound liver adducts recognised by antibodies from patients with halothane hepatitis. *Anesthesiology* 69, 833—838.

Christ, D.D., Satoh, H., Kenna, J.G. and Pohl, L.R. (1988b) Potential metabolic basis for enflurane hepatitis and the apparent cross-sensitization between enflurane and halothane. *Drug Metab. Disposition* 16, 1—6.

Christensen, J.H., Andreasen, F. and Kristoffersen, M.D. (1983) Comparison of the anaesthetic and haemodynamic effects of chlormethiazole and thiopentone. *Br. J. Anaesth.* 55, 391—397.

Clements, A., Nimmo, W.S. and Grant, I.S. (1982) Bioavailability, pharmacokinetics and analgesic activity of ketamine in humans. *J. Pharm. Sci.* 71, 539—541.

Coates, D.P., Monk, C.R., Prys.-Roberts, C. and Turtle, M. (1987) Hemodynamic effects of infusions of the emulsion formulation of propofol during nitrous oxide anesthesia in humans. *Anesth. Analg.* 66, 64—70.

Cockshott, I.D. (1985) Propofol (Diprivan) pharmacokinetics and metabolism — an overview. *Postgrad. Med. J.* 61, Suppl. 3, 45—50.

Cockshott, I.D., Briggs, L.P., Douglas, E.J. and White, M. (1987) Pharmacokinetics of propofol in female patients: studies using single bolus injection. *Br. J. Anaesth.* 59, 1103—1110.

Cockshott, I.D., Doughlas, E.J., Prys-Roberts, C., Turtle, M.J. and Coates, D.P. (1990) Pharmacokinetics of propofol during and after i.v. infusion in man. *Eur. J. Anaesthesiol.* 7, 265—276.

Cooke, J.E. and Scott, J.C. (1986) Do sufentanil and fentanyl have the same pharmacodynamics? *Anesthesiology* 65, A 552.

de Coster, R., Helmers, J.H.J.H. and Noorduin, H. (1985) Effect of etomidate on cortisol biosynthesis: site of action after induction of anaesthesia. *Acta Endocrinol.* 110, 526—531.

Cottrell, J.E., Griffin, J.P., Lim, K., Milhorat, T., Stein, S. and Shwiry, V. (1982) Intracranial pressure, mean arterial pressure and heart rate following midazolam or thiopental in humans with intracranial masses. *Anesthesiology* 57, A 323.

Crankshaw, D.P., Edwards, N.E., Blackman, G.L., Boyd, M.D., Chan, H.N.J. and Morgan, D.J. (1985) Evaluation of infusion regimens for thiopentone as a primary anaesthetic agent. *Eur. J. Clin. Pharmacol.* 28, 543—552.

Crankshaw, D.P., Boyd, M.D., and Bjorksten, A.R. (1987) Plasma drug efflux — a new approach to optimization of drug infusion for constant blood concentration of thiopental and methohexital. *Anesthesiology* 67, 32—41.

Crankshaw, D.P., Boon, L.C., Bjorksten, A.R. and Edward, N.E. (1989) Analysis of the electroencephalogram for burst suppression produced by prolonged infusion of thiopental. *J. Clin. Monit.* 5, 289 (abstract).

Crankshaw, D.P. and Karasawa, F. (1989) A method for implementing programmed infusion of thiopentone and methohexitone with a simple infusion pump. *Anaesth. Intensive Care* 17, 496—499.

Crozier, T.A., Beck, D., Schlaeger, M., Wuttke, W. and Kettler, D. (1987) Endocrinological changes following etomidate, midazolam or methohexital for minor surgery. *Anesthesiology* 66, 628—635.

Crozier, T.A., Beck, D., Wuttke, W. and Kettler, D. (1988) In vivo suppression of steroid synthesis by etomidate is concentration-dependant. *Anaesthesist* 37, 337—339.

Cummings, G.C., Dixon, J., Kay, N.H., Windsor, J.P.W., Major, E., Morgan, M., Sear, J., Spence, A.A. and Stephenson, D.K. (1984) Dose requirements of ICI 35868 (propofol, Diprivan) in a new formulation for induction of anaesthesia. *Anesthesia* 38, 1168—1171.

Dawson, D. and Sear, J.W. (1986) Influence of induction of anaesthesia with midazolam on the neuroendocrine response to surgery. *Anaesthesia* 41, 268—271.

Dirksen, M.S.C., Vree, T.B. and Driessen, J.J. (1987) Clinical pharmacokinetics of long-term infusion of midazolam in critically ill patients — preliminary results. *Anaesth. Intensive Care* 15, 440—444.

Doze, V.A., Shafer, A. and White, P.F. (1988) Propofol-nitrous oxide versus thiopental-isoflurane-nitrous oxide for general anesthesia. *Anesthesiology* 69, 63—71.

Doze, V.A., Westphal, L.M. and White, P.F. (1986) Comparison of propofol with methohexital for outpatient anesthesia. *Anesth. Analg.* 65, 1189—1195.

Dundee, J.W. (1955) Thiopentone as factor in production of liver dysfunction. *Br. J. Anaesth.* 27, 14—23.

Dundee, J.W., Price, H.L. and Dripps, R.D. (1956) Acute tolerance to thiopentone in man. *Br. J. Anaesth.* 28, 344—352.

Dundee, J.W. and Zacharias, M. (1979) Etomidate. In: *Current Topics in Anaesthesia Series 1: Intravenous Anaesthetic Agents.* Editor: J.W. Dundee, Arnold, London, pp. 46—66.

Dundee, J.W., Fee, J.P.H., Moore, J., McIlroy, P.D.A. and Wilson, D.B. (1980) Changes in serum enzyme levels following ketamine infusions. *Anaesthesia* 35, 12—18.

Dundee, J.W., Robinson, F.P., McCollum, J.S.C. and Patterson, C.C. (1986) Sensitivity to propofol in the elderly. *Anaesthesia* 41, 482—485.

Durand, A., Ferrandes, B., Garrigou, D. and Morselli, P. (1986) Plasma and brain kinetics of zolpidem, a new hypnotic, in the rat. *Br. J. Pharmacol.* 87, 730p.

Engelhardt, W., Ebert, W., Rietbrock, I. and Richter, E. (1986) Dosiswirkungsbeziehung und serumkonzentrationen von methohexital und hydroxymethohexital nach rektaler anaestesieeinleitung mit 1% iger und 5% iger methohexitallosung mit kindern.*Anaesthesist* 35, 491—495.

Fragen, R.J., Avram, M.J. and Henthorn, T.K. (1983) A pharmacokinetically designed etomidate infusion regimen for hypnosis. *Anesth. Analg.* 62, 654—660.

Fragen, R.J., Shanks, C.A., Molteni, A. and Avram, M.J. (1984) Effects of etomidate on hormonal responses to surgical stress. *Anesthesiology* 61, 652—656.

Fragen, R.J., Weiss, H.W. and Molteni, A. (1987) The effect of propofol on adrenocortical steroidogenesis: a comparative study with etomidate and thiopental. *Anesthesiology* 66, 839—842.

Fry, D.E. and Griffiths, H. (1984) The inhibition by etomidate of the 11$\beta$ hydroxylation of cortisol. *Clin. Endocrinol.* 20, 625—629.

Gepts, E., Camu, F., Cockshott, I.D. and Douglas, E.J. (1987) Disposition of propofol administered as constant rate intravenous infusions in humans. *Anesth. Analg.* 66, 1256—1263.

Gepts, E., Jonckheer, M., Maes, V., Sonck, W. and Camu, F. (1988) Disposition kinetics of propofol during alfentanil anaesthesia. *Anaesthesia* 43, Suppl., 8—13.

Gillis, P.P., de Angelis, R.J. and Wynn, R.L. (1976) Non-linear pharmacokinetic model of intravenous anesthesia. *J. Pharm. Sci.* 65, 1001—1006.

Gill, S.S., Wright, E.M. and Reilly, C.S. (1990) Pharmacokinetic interation of propofol and fentanyl: single bolus injection study. *Br. J. Anaesth.* 65, 760—765.

Glass, P.S.A., Markham, K., Ginsberg, B. and Hawkins, E.D. (1989) Propofol concentrations required for surgery. *Anesthesiology* 71, A 273.

Glisson, S.N., Haddad, W, Kubak M.A. and Hieber, M.F. (1983) Midazolam action on catecholamine, cortisol and renin responses to surgical stress in dogs. *Anesthesiology* 59, A 239.

Grant, I.S. and MacKenzie, N. (1985) Recovery following propofol (Diprivan) anaesthesia — a review of three different anaesthetic techniques. *Postgrad. Med. J.* 61, Suppl. 3, 133—137.

Halford, F.J. (1943) A critique of intravenous anesthesia in war surgery. *Anesthesiology* 4, 67—69.

Hall, R.I., Schwieger, I.M. and Hug, C.C., Jr. (1988) The anesthetic efficacy of midazolam in the enflurane-anesthetized dog. *Anesthesiology* 68, 862—866.

Hazeaux, C., Tisserant, D., Vespignani, H., Hummer-Sigiel, M., Kwan-Ning, V. and Laxenaire, M.C. (1987) Electroencephalographic changes produced by propofol. *Ann. Fr. Anesth. Reanim.* 6, 261—266.

Hebron, B.S., Edbrooke, D.L., Mather, L.E. and Newby, D.M. (1983) Pharmacokinetics of etomidate associated with a prolonged intravenous infusion. *Br. J. Anaesth.* 55, 281—287.

Heusler, H., Epping, J., Heusler, S., Richter, E., Vermeulen, N.P. and Breimer, D.D. (1981) Simultaneous determination of blood concentrations of methohexital and its hydroxy metabolite by gas chromatography and identification of 4′-hydroxymethohexital by combined gas-liquid chromatography-mass spectrometry. *J. Chromatogr.* 226, 403—412.

Hogskilde, S., Nielsen, J.W., Carl, P. and Bredgaard-Sorensen, M. (1987a) Pregnanolone emulsion. A new steroid preparation for intravenous anaesthesia. *Anaesthesia* 42, 586—590.

Hogskilde, S., Wagner, J., Carl, P. and Bredgaard-Sorensen, M. (1987b) Anaesthetic properties of pregnanolone emulsion. *Anaesthesia* 42, 1045—1050.

Horai, Y., White, P.F. and Trevor, A.J. (1985) The effect of etomidate on rabbit liver microsomal drug metabolism in vitro. *Drug Metab. Dispos.* 13, 364—367.

Hubbard, A.K., Gandolfi, A.J. and Brown, B.R. (1988) Immunological basis of anesthetic-induced hepatotoxicity. *Anesthesiology* 69, 814—817.

Hudson, R.J., Stanski, D.R., Saidman, L.J. and Meathe, E. (1983) A model for studying depth of anesthesia and acute tolerance to thiopental. *Anesthesiology* 59, 301—308.

Hull, C.J., van Beem HBH, McLeod, K. and Watson, M.J. (1978) A pharmacodynamic model for pancuronium. *Br. J. Anaesth.* 50, 1113—1123.

Hunter, A.R., (1972a) Thiopentone supplemented anaesthesia for neurosurgery. *Br. J. Anaesth.* 44, 506—510.

Hunter, A.R. (1972b) Methohexitone as a supplement to nitrous oxide during intracranical surgery. *Br. J. Anaesth.* 44, 1188—1190.

Idvall, J., Ahlgren, I., Aronsen, K.F. and Stenberg, P., (1979) Ketamine infusions: pharmacokinetics and clinical effects. *Br. J. Anaesth.* 51, 1167—1173.

Idvall, J., Aronsen, K.F., Stenberg, P. and Paalzow, L. (1983) Pharmacodynamic and pharmacokinetic interactions between ketamine and diazepam. *Eur. J. Clin. Pharmacol.* 24, 337—343.

Jessop, E., Grounds, R.M., Morgan, M. and Lumley, J. (1985) Comparison of infusions of propofol and methohexitone to provide light general anaesthesia during surgery with general anaesthesia during surgery with regional blockade. *Br. J. Anaesth.* 57, 1173—1177.

Joachimsson, P.-O., Hedstrand, U. and Eklund, A. (1986) Low-dose ketamine infusion for analgesia during postoperative ventilator treatment. *Acta Anaesthesiol. Scand.* 30, 697—702.

de Jong, F.H., Mallios, C., Jansen, C., Scheck, P.A.E. and Lamberts, S.W.J. (1984) Etomidate suppresses adrenocortical function by inhibition of 11$\beta$ hydroxylation. *J. Clin. Endocrinol. Metab.* 59, 1143—1147.

Kapp, W. (1988) Opioids in anaesthesia. *Acta Anaesthesiol. Scand.* 32, Suppl. 87, 33—37.

Katz, R.I., Skeen, J.T., Quartarao, C. and Poppers, P.J. (1987) Varied use of a thiopental infusion. *Anesth. Analg.* 60, 1328—1330.

Kawar, P.K., Briggs, L.P., Bahar, M., McIlroy, P.D.A., Dundee, J.W., Mettett, J.D. and Nesbitt, G.S. (1982) Liver enzyme studies with disoprofol (ICI 35868) and midazolam. *Anaesthesia* 37, 305—308.

Kay, B., and Rolly, G. (1977) ICI 35868, a new intravenous induction agent. *Acta Anaesthesiol. Belg.* 28, 303—316.

Kay, N.H., Uppington, J., Sear, J.W. and Allen, M.C. (1985) Use of an emulsion of ICI 35868 (propofol) for the induction and maintenance of anaesthesia. *Br. J. Anaesth.* 57, 736—742.

Kay, N.H., Sear, J.W., Uppington, J., Douglas, E.J. and Cockshott, I.D. (1986) Disposition of propofol in patients undergoing surgery. A comparison of men and women. *Br. J. Anaesth.* 58, 1075—1079.

Kenyon, C.J., McNeill, L.M. and Fraser, R. (1985) Comparison of the effects of etomidate, thiopentone and propofol on cortisol synthesis. *Br. J. Anaesth.* 57, 509—511.

Kirkpatrick, T., Cockshott, I.D., Doughlas, E.J. and Nimmo, W.S. (1988) The pharmacokinetics of propofol in elderly patients. *Br. J. Anaesth.* 60, 146—150.

Knill-Jones R.D., Rodriques, L.V., Moir, D.D. and Spence, A.A. (1972) Anaesthetic practice and pregnancy. Controlled survey of women anaesthetists in the U.K. *Lancet* i, 1326—1328.

Korttila, K., Linnoila, M., Ertama, P. and Hakkinen, S. (1975) Recovery and simulated driving after intravenous anesthesia with thiopental, methohexital, propanidid or alphadione., *Anesthesiology* 43, 291—299.

Korttila, K., Ostman, P.L., Faure, E., Apfelbaum, J.L., Ekdawi, M. and Roizen, M.F. (1989) Randomized comparison of outcome after propofol-nitrous oxide or enflurane-nitrous oxide anaesthesia in operations of long duration. *Can. J. Anaesth.* 36, 651—657.

Korttila, K., Ghoneim, M., Chiang, C.-K., Nuotto, E and Fischer, L.J. (1990a) Metabolites of methohexitone do not contribute to its prolonged action on the central nervous system. *Acta Anaesthesiol. Scand.* 34, 55—58.

Kortilla, K., Ostman, P., Faure, E., Apfelbaum, J., Prunskis, J., Ekdawi, M. and Roizen, M. (1990b) Randomized comparison of recovery after propofol-nitrous oxide versus thiopentone-isoflurane-nitrous oxide anesthesia in patients undergoing ambulatory surgery. *Acta Anaesthesiol. Scand.* 34, 400—403.

Kristoffersen, M.B., Kjaer Hansen, E., Jostell, K.-G. and Stockman, O. (1982) Chlormethiazole and nitrous oxide as compared to halothane for general anaesthesia. *Acta Anaesthesiol. Scand.* 26, 337—343.

Kruger-Thiemer, E. (1968) Continuous intravenous infusion and multicompartmental accumulation. *Eur. J. Pharmacol.* 4, 317—324.

Lambert, A., Mitchell, R. and Robertson, W.R. (1985) Effect of propofol, thiopentone and etomidate on adrenal steroidogenesis in vitro. *Br. J. Anaesth.* 57, 505—508.

Lange, H., Stephan, H., Rieke, H., Kellerman, M., Sonntag, H. and Bircher, J. (1990) Hepatic and extrahepatic disposition of propofol in patients undergoing coronary by-pass surgery. *Br. J. Anaesth.* 64, 563—570.

Larsson-Backstrom, C., Lustig, L.L., Eklund, A. and Thorstensson, M. (1988) Anaesthetic potency of pregnanolone in mice in an emulsion preparation for intravenous administration: a comparison with thiopentone. *Pharmacol. Toxicol.* 63, 143—149.

Lauven, P.M., Schwilden, H. and Stoeckel, H. (1987) Threshold hypnotic concentration of methohexitone. *Eur. J. Clin. Pharmacol.* 33, 261—265.

Ledingham, I.M.cA. and Watt, I. (1983) Influence of sedation on mortality in critically ill multiple trauma patients. *Lancet* i, 1270.

Lees, N. (1983) Experience with etomidate as part of a total intravenous anaesthetic technique. *Anaesthesia* 38, Suppl., 70—73.

Lundy, J.S. and Tovell, R.M. (1934) Some of the newer local and general anesthetic agents. Methods of their administration. *Northwest Med.* (Seattle) 33, 308—311.

Mackenzie, N. and Grant, I.S. (1985) Comparison of the new emulsion formulation of propofol with methohexitone and thiopentone for induction of anaesthesia in day cases. *Br. J. Anaesth.* 57, 725—731.

Magnusson, H., Ponten H. and Sonander, H.G. (1986) Methohexitone anaesthesia for microlaryngoscopy: circulatory modulation with metoprolol and dihydralazine. *Br. J. Anaesth.* 58, 976—982.

Marais, M.L., Maher, M.W., Wetchler, B.V., Korttila, K. and Apfelbaum, J.L. (1989) Reduced demands on recovery room resources with propofol (Diprivan) compared to thiopental-isoflurane. *Anesthesiology Rev.* 16, 29—40.

Mather, L.E. and Cousins, M.J. (1980) Low dose chlormethiazole infusion as a supplement to central neural blockade: blood concentrations and clinical effects. *Anaesth. Intensive Care* 8, 421—425.

Mather, L.E., Runciman, W.B., Ilsley, A.H., Thomson, K. and Goldin, A. (1981) direct measurement of chlormethiazole extraction by liver, lung and kidney in man. *Br. J. Clin. Pharmacol.* 12, 319—325.

Mazoit, J.X., Sandouk, P., Schermann, J.-H. and Roche. A. (1990) Extrahepatic metabolism of morphine occurs in humans. *Clin. Pharmacol. Ther.* 48, 613—618.

McDermott, R.W. and Stanley, T.H. (1974) The cardiovascular effects of low concentrations of nitrous oxide during morphine anesthesia. *Anesthesiology* 41, 89—91.

McMurray, T.J., Robinson, F.P., Dundee, J.W. and McClean, E. (1986) A new method for producing constant plasma drug levels: application to methohexitone. *Br. J. Anaesth.* 57, 1085—1090.

Melvin, M.A., Johnson, H.B. and Quasha, A.L. (1982) Induction of anesthesia with midazolam decreases halothane MAC in humans. *Anesthesiology* 57, 238—241.

Michalk, S., Moncorge, C., Fichelle, A., Huot, O., Servin, F., Farinotti, R. and Desmonts, J.M. (1988) Midazolam infusion for basal sedation in intensive care: absence of accumulation. *Intensive Care Med.* 15, 37—41.

Mitenko, P.A. and Ogilvie, R.I. (1972) Rapidly achieved plasma concentration plateaus with observations on theophylline kinetics. *Clin. Pharmacol. Ther.* 13, 329—335.

Modig, J. (1988) Indications of chlormethiazole as a protective agent in experimental endotoxinaemia. *Eur. Surg. Res.* 20, 195—204.

Monk, C.R., Coates, D.P., Prys-Roberts, C., Turtle, M.J. and Spelina, K.R. (1987) Haemodynamic effects of prolonged infusion of propofol as a supplement to nitrous oxide anaesthesia. Studies in association with peripheral arterial surgery. *Br. J. Anaesth.* 59, 954—960.

Moore, R.A., Allen, M.C., Wood, P.J., Rees, L.H. and Sear, J.W. (1985) Perioperative endocrine effects of etomidate. *Anaesthesia* 40, 124—130.

Moore, R.G., Robertson, A.V., Smyth, M.P., Thomas, J. and Vine, J. (1975) Metabolism and urinary excretion of chlormethiazole in humans. *Xenobiotica* 5, 687—696.

Morcos, W.E. and Payne, J.P. (1985) The induction of anaesthesia with propofol (Diprivan) compared in normal and renal failture patients. *Postgrad. Med. J.* 61, Suppl. 3, 62—63.

Morgan, M. (1983) Total intravenous anaesthesia. *Anaesthesia* 38, Suppl., 1—9.

Nakashima, E. and Benet, L.Z. (1988) General treatment of mean residence time, clearance and volume parameters in linear mammillary models with elimination from any compartment. *J. Pharmacokinet. Biopharm.* 16, 475—492.

Nilsson, A., Lee, P. and Revenas, B. (1984) Midazolam as induction agent prior to inhalational anaesthesia: a comparison with thiopentone. *Acta Anaesthesiol. Scand.* 28, 249—251.

Nilsson, A., Tamsen, A. and Persson, P. (1986) Midazolam-fentanyl anaesthesia for major surgery. Plasma levels of midazolam during prolonged total intravenous anesthesia. *Acta Anaesthesiol. Scand.* 30, 66—69.

Nilsson, A., Persson, M.P., Hartvig, P. and Wide, L. (1988a) Effect of total intravenous anaesthesia with midazolam/alfentanil on the adrenocortical and hyperglycaemic response to abdominal surgery. *Acta Anaesthesiol Scand.* 32, 379—382.

Nilsson, A., Persson, M.P. and Hartvig, P. (1988b) Effects of the benzodiazepine antagonist flumazenil on postoperative performance following total intravenous anaesthesia with midazolam and alfentanil. *Acta Anaesthesiol. Scand.* 32, 441—446.

Norberg, L., Wahlstrom, G. and Backstrom, T. (1987) The anaesthetic potency of $3\alpha$ hydroxy $5\alpha$ pregnan-20-one and $3\alpha$ hydroxy $5\beta$ pregnan-20-one determined with an intravenous EEG-threshold method in male rats. *Pharmacol. Toxicol.* 61, 42—47.

Le Normand, Y., de Villepoix, C., Pinaud, M., Bernard, J.M., Fraboul, J.P., Athouel, A., Ribeyrol, M., Beneroso, N. and Larousse, C. (1988) Pharmacokinetics and haemodynamic effects of prolonged methohexitone infusion. *Br. J. Clin. Pharmacol.* 26, 589—594.

Obermaier, M. (1985) Effect of etomidate on human adrenal $11\beta$ hydroxylase and 18 hydroxylase activity. *Acta Endocrinol.* 108, Suppl. 267, 26.

Oldenhof, H., de Jong, M., Steenhoek, A. and Janknegt, R. (1988) Clinical pharmacokinetics of midazolam in intensive care patients, a wide interpatient variability? *Clin. Pharmacol. Ther.* 43, 263—269.

Perisho, J.A., Buechel, D.R. and Miller, R.D. (1971) The effect of diazepam (Valium) on minimum alveolar anaesthetic requirement (MAC) in man. *Can. Anaesth. Soc. J.* 18, 536—540.

Persson, M.P., Nilsson, A., Hartvig, P. and Tamsen, A. (1987) Pharmacokinetics of midazolam during total intravenous anaesthesia. *Br. J. Anaesth.* 59, 548—556.

Persson, M.P., Nilsson, A. and Hartvig, P. (1988) Relation of sedation and amnesia to plasma concentrations of midazolam in surgical patients. *Clin. Pharmacol. Ther.* 43, 324—331.

Platt, T.W., Tatum, A.L., Hathaway, H.R. and Waters, R.M. (1936) Sodium ethyl (1-methyl butyl) thiobarbiturate: preliminary experimental and clinical study. *Am. J. Surg.* 31, 464—466.

Preziosi, P. (1983) Etomidate, sedative and neuroendocrine changes. *Lancet* ii, 276.

Preziosi, P. and Vacca, M. (1982) Etomidate and the corticotrophic axis. *Arch. Int. Pharmacodyn. Ther.* 256, 308—310.

Price, H.L., Kovnat, P.J., Safer, J.N., Conner, E.H. and Price, M.L. (1960) The uptake of thiopental by body tissues and its relation to duration of narcosis. *Clin. Pharmacol. Ther.* 1, 16—22.

Prys-Roberts, C., Davies, J.R., Calverley, R.K. and Goodman, N.W. (1983a) Haemodynamic effects of infusions of di-isopropyl phenol (ICI 35868) during nitrous oxide anaesthesia in man. *Br. J. Anaesth.* 55, 105—111.

Prys-Roberts, C., Sear, J.W., Low, J.M., Phillips, K.C. and Dagnino, J. (1983b) Hemodynamic and hepatic effects of methohexital infusion during nitrous oxide anesthesia in humans. *Anesth. Analg.* 62, 317—323.

Raeder, J.C., Hole, A., Arnulf, V. and Hougens Grynne, B. (1987) Total intravenous anaesthesia with midazolam and flumazenil in outpatient clinics. A comparison with isoflurane or thiopentone. *Acta Anaesthesiol. Scand.* 31, 634—641.

Raeder, J.C., Nilsen, O.G. and Hole, A. (1988) Pharmacokinetics of midazolam and alfentanil in outpatient general anaesthesia. A study with concomitant thiopentone, flumazenil or placebo administration. *Acta Anaesthesiol. Scand.* 42, 467—472.

Rees, D.J. and Howell, M.L. (1986) Ketamine-atracurium by continuous infusion as the sole anesthetic for pulmonary surgery. *Anesth. Analg.* 65, 860—864.

Reiter, V., Fay, R., Pire, J.C., Lamiable, D. and Rendoing, J. (1989) Propofol à debit continu au cours des transplantations renales chez l'adulte. *Cahi. Anesthesiol.* 37, 23—31.

Richards, M.J., Skues, M.A., Jarvis, A.P. and Prys-Roberts, C. (1990) Total intravenous anaesthesia with propofol and alfentanil: dose requirements for propofol. *Br. J. Anaesth.* 65, 157—163.

Riddell, J.G., McAllister, C.B., Wilkinson, G.R., Wood, A.J.J. and Roden, D.M. (1984) A new method for constant plasma drug concentrations: application to lidocaine. *Ann. Int. Med.* 100, 25—28.

Rigg, J.R.A. and Wong, T.Y. (1981) A method for achieving rapidly steady-state blood concentrations of i.v. drugs. *Br. J. Anaesth.* 53, 1247—1257.

Roberts, F.L., Dixon, J., Lewis, G.T.R., Tackley, R.M. and Prys-Roberts, C. (1988) Induction and maintenance of propofol anaesthesia. A manual infusion scheme. *Anaesthesia* 43, Suppl., 14—17.

Robinson, F.P. and Patterson, C.C. (1985) Changes in liver function tests after propofol (Diprivan). *Postgrad. Med. J.* 61, Suppl. 3, 160—164.

Robson, D.J., Blow, C., Gaines, D., Flanagan, R.J. and Henry, J.A. (1984) Accumulation of chlormethiazole during intravenous infusion. *Intensive Care Med.* 10, 315—316.

de Ruiter, G., Popescu, D.T., de Boer, A.G., Smeekens, J.B. and Breimer, D.D. (1981) Pharmacokinetics of etomidate in surgical patients. *Arch. Int. Pharmacodyn. Ther.* 249, 180—188.

Runciman, W.B., Ilsley, A.H., Ryall, R.G., Parkin, K.S. and Heinrich, R. (1981) Intravenous chlormethiazole — haemolysis with concentrated solutions. *Anaesth. Intensive Care* 9, 34—39.

Russell, G.N., Wright, E.L., Fox, M.A., Douglas, E.J. and Cockshott, I.D. (1989) Propofol-fentanyl anaesthesia for coronary artery surgery and cardiopulmonary bypass. *Anaesthesia* 44, 205—208.

Saidman, L.J. and Eger, E.I., ii (1966) The effect of thiopental metabolism on the duration of anesthesia. *Anesthesiology* 27, 118—126.

Sanders, L.D., Isaac, P.A., Yeomans, W.A., Clyburn, P.A., Rosen, M. and Robinson, J.O. (1989) Propofol induced anaesthesia. Double-blind comparison of recovery after anaesthesia induced by propofol or thiopentone. *Anaesthesia* 44, 200—204.

Schüttler, J., Wilms, M., Lauven, P.M., Schwilden, H. and Stoeckel, H. (1980) Pharmakokinetische untersuchungen uber etomidat beim menschen. *Anaesthesist* 29, 658—661.

Schüttler, J., Schwilden, H. and Stoekel, H. (1983a) Pharmacokinetics as applied to total intravenous anaesthesia. Theoretical considerations. *Anaesthesia* 38, Suppl., 51—52.

Schüttler, J., Wilms, M., Stoeckel, H., Schwilden, H. and Lauven, P.M. (1983b) Pharmacokinetic interaction of etomidate and fentanyl. *Anesthesiology* 59, A 247.

Schüttler, J., Schwilden, H. and Stoeckel, H. (1985) Infusion strategies to investigate the pharmacokinetics and pharmacodynamics of hypnotic drugs: Etomidate as an example. *Eur. J. Anaesthesiol.* 2, 133—142.

Schüttler, J., Schwilden, H. and Stoeckel, H. (1986) Pharmacokinetic-dynamic modeling of Diprivan. *Anaesthesiology* 65, A 549.

Schüttler, J., Stanski, D.R. and White, P.F. et al. (1987) Pharmacodynamic modeling of the EEG effects of ketamine and its enantiomers in man. *J. Pharmacokinet. Biopharm.* 15, 241—253.

Schüttler, J., Kloos, K., Schwilden, H. and Stoeckel, H. (1988) Total intravenous anaesthesia with propofol and alfentanil by computer assisted infusions. *Anaesthesia* 43, Suppl., 2—7.

Schweitzer, S.A. (1978) Chlormethiazole (Heminevrin) infusion as supplemental sedation during epidural block. *Anaesth. Intensive Care* 6, 248—250.

Schwilden, H., Schüttler, J. and Stoekel, H. (1983) Pharmacokinetics as applied to total intravenous anaesthesia. Practical implications. *Anaesthesia* 38, Suppl., 53—56.

Schwilden, H., Stoeckel, H., Schüttler, J. and Lauven, P.M. (1986) Pharmacological models and their use in clinical anaesthesia. *Eur. J. Anaesthesiol.* 3, 175—208.

Schwilden, H., Schüttler, J. and Stoeckel, H. (1987) Closed-loop feedback control of methohexital anesthesia by quantitative EEG analysis in humans. *Anesthesiology* 67, 341—347.

Scott, J.C. and Stanski, D.R. (1987) Decreased fentanyl and alfentanil dose requirements with age. A simultaneous pharmacokinetic and pharmacodynamic evaluation. *J. Pharmacol. Exp. Ther.* 240, 159—166.

Scott, J.C., Cooke, J.E. and Stanski, D.R. (1991) Electroencephalographic quantitation of opioid effect: comparative pharmacodynamics of fentanyl and sufentanil. *Anesthesiology* 74, 34—42.

Seow, L.T., Mather, L.E. and Roberts, J.G. (1981) An integrated study of the pharmacokinetics and pharmacodynamics of chlormethiazole in healthy young volunteers. *Eur. J. Clin. Pharmacol.* 19, 263—269.

Sear, J.W. (1983) General kinetic and dynamic principles and their application to continuous infusion anaesthesia. *Anaesthesia* 38, Suppl, 10—25.

Sear, J.W. (1987a) Toxicity of i.v. anaesthetics. *Br. J. Anaesth.* 59, 24—45.

Sear, J.W. (1987b) Variability in drug disposition. In: Proceedings of VII European Congress of Anaesthesiology. *Beitr. Anasthesiol. Intensivmed.* 21, 165—174.

Sear, J.W. (1989) Drug infusions in intensive care. *Intensive Ther. Clin. Monit.* 10, 306—315.

Sear, J.W. and McGivan, J.D. (1979) The cytotoxicity of intravenous anaesthetic agents on the isolated rat hepatocyte. *Br. J. Anaesth.* 51, 733—739.

Sear, J.W. and Prys-Roberts, C. (1979) Dose-related haemodynamic effects of continuous infusions of Althesin. *Br. J. Anaesth.* 51, 867—873.

Sear, J.W., Prys-Roberts, C., Gray, A.J.G., Walsh, E.M., Curnow, J.S.H. and Dye, J. (1981) Infusions of minaxolone to supplement nitrous oxide-oxygen anaesthesia. A comparison with Althesin. *Br. J. Anaesth.* 53, 339—350.

Sear, J.W., Allen, M.C., Gales, M., McQuay, H.J., Kay, N.H., McKenzie, P.J. and Moore, R.A. (1983a) Suppression by etomidate of normal cortisol response to anaesthesia and surgery. *Lancet* ii, 1028.

Sear, J.W., Phillips, K.C., Andrews, C.J.H. and Prys-Roberts, C. (1983b) Dose-response relationships for infusions of Althesin or methohexitone. *Anaesthesia* 38, 931—936.

Sear, J.W., Prys-Roberts, C. and Dye, A. (1983c) Hepatic function after anaesthesia for major vascular reconstructive surgery — a comparison of four anaesthetic techniques. *Br. J. Anaesth.* 55, 603—609.

Sear, J.W., Prys-Roberts, C. and Phillips, K.C. (1984a) Age influences the minimum infusion rate ($ED_{50}$) for continuous infusions of Althesin and methohexitone. *Eur. J. Anaesthesiol.* 1, 319—325.

Sear, J.W., Walters, F.J.M., Wilkins, D.G. and Willatts, S.M. (1984b) Etomidate by infusion for neuroanaesthesia. Kinetic and dynamic interactions with nitrous oxide. *Anaesthesia* 39, 12—18.

Sear, J.W., Edwards, C.R.W. and Atherden, S. (1988a) Dual effect of etomidate on mineralocorticoid biosynthesis. *Acta Anaesthesiol. Belg.* 39, 87—94.

Sear, J.W., Shaw, I., Wolf, A. and Kay, N.H. (1988b) Infusion of propofol to supplement nitrous oxide-oxygen for maintenance of anaesthesia. A comparison with halothane. *Anaesthesia* 43, Suppl., 18—22.

Servin, F., Desmonts, J.M., Haberer, J.P., Cockshott, I.D., Plummer, G.F. and Farinotti, R. (1988) Pharmacokinetics and protein binding of propofol in patients with cirrhosis. *Anesthesiology* 69, 887—891.

Shafer, A., Doze, V.A., Shafer, S.L. and White, P.F. (1988) Pharmacokinetics and pharmacodynamics of propofol infusions during general anesthesia. *Anesthesiology* 69, 348—356.

Shapiro, H.M. (1985) Barbiturates in brain ischaemia. *Br. J. Anaesth.* 57, 82—95.

Sheiner, L.B., Stanski, D.R., Vozeh, S., Miller, R.D. and Ham, J. (1979) Simultaneous modeling of pharmacokinetics and pharmacodynamics: application to D-tubocurarine. *Clin. Pharmacol. Ther.* 25, 358—371.

Shen, D. and Gibaldi, M. (1974) Critical evaluation of the use of effective protein fractions in developing pharmacokinetic models for drug distribution. *J. Pharm. Sci.* 63, 1698—1703.

Simons, P.J., Cockshott, I.D., Douglas, E.J., Gordon, E.A., Hopkins, K. and Rowland, M. (1988) Disposition in male volunteers of a subanaesthetic intravenous dose of an oil in water emulsion of $^{14}$C-propofol. *Xenobiotica* 18, 429—440.

Spelina, K.R., Coates, D.P., Monk, C.R., Prys-Roberts, C., Norley, I. and Turtle, M.J. (1986) Dose requirements of propofol by infusion during nitrous oxide anaesthesia in man. I: Patients premedicated with morphine. *Br. J. Anaesth.* 58, 1080—1084.

Spence, A.A. (1987) Environmental pollution by inhalation anaesthetics. *Br. J. Anaesth.* 59, 96—103.

Stanski, D.R., Hudson, R.J., Homer, T.D., Saidman, L.J. and Meathe, E. (1984) Pharmacodynamic modeling of thiopental anesthesia. *J. Pharmacokinet. Biopharm.* 12, 223—240.

Tackley, R.M., Lewis, G.T.R., Prys-Roberts, C., Boaden, R.W., Dixon, J. and Harvey, J.T. (1989) Computer controlled infusion of propofol. *Br. J. Anaesth.* 62, 46—53.

Tatti, B., Neidhart, P. and Forster, A. (1989) Comparison of the sedative and hemodynamic effects of zolpidem and midazolam in intensive care patients. *Anesthesiology* 71, A 158 (abstract).

Thomson, I.A., Hughes, R.L., Fitch, W. and Campbell, D. (1982) Effects of nitrous oxide on liver haemodynamics and oxygen consumption in the greyhound. *Anaesthesia* 37, 548—553.

Thomson, I.A., Fitch, W., Hughes, R.L., Campbell, D. and Watson, R. (1984) Effects of certain iv. anaesthetics on liver blood flow and hepatic oxygen consumption in the greyhound. *Br. J. Anaesth.* 58, 69—80.

Todd, M.M., Drummond, J.C. and U, H.S. (1984) The hemodynamic consequences of high-dose methohexital anesthesia in humans. *Anesthesiology* 61, 495—501.

Todd, M.M., Drummond, J.C. and U, H.S. (1985) The hemodynamic consequences of high-dose thiopental anesthesia. *Anesth. Analg.* 64, 681—687.

Toner, W., Howard, P.J., McGowan, W.A.W. and Dundee, J.W. (1980) Another look at acute tolerance to thiopentone. *Br. J. Anaesth.* 52, 1005—1008.

Turtle, M.J., Cullen, P., Prys-Roberts, C., Coates, D., Monk, C.R. and Faroqui, M.H. (1987) Dose requirements of propofol by infusion during nitrous oxide anaesthesia in man. II: Patients premedicated with lorazepam. *Br. J. Anaesth.* 59, 283—287.

Vandermeersch, E., van Hemelrijck, J., Byttebier, G. and Van Aken, H. (1989) Pharmacokinetics of propofol during continuous infusion for pediatric anesthesia. *Acta Anaesthesiol. Belg.* 40, 161—165.

Vandesteene, A., Tremport, V., Deloof, T., Engelman, E., Wathieu, J.P. and de Rood, M. (1988) Influence of propofol on EEG. Abstract 163; *Proceedings of 5th International Congress of the Belgian Society of Anaesthesia and Reanimation,* Brussels, 1988.

Van Hamme, M.J., Ghoneim, M.M. and Ambre, J.J. (1978) Pharmacokinetics of etomidate, a new intravenous anesthetic. *Anesthesiology* 49, 274—247.

Van Hemelrijck, J., Van Aken, H., Plets, C., Goffin, J. and Vermaut, G. (1989) the effects of propofol on intracranial pressure and cerebral perfusion pressure in patients with brain tumours. *Acta Anaesthesiol. Belg.* 40, 95—100.

van Lambalgen, A.A., Bronsveld, W. and van den Bos, G.C. (1982) Cardiovascular and biochemical changes in dogs during etomidate-nitrous oxide anaesthesia. *Cardiovasc. Res.* 15, 599—606.

Vaughan, D.P. and Tucker, G.T. (1975) General theory for rapidly establishing steady-state drug concentrations using two consecutive constant rate intravenous infusions. *Eur. J. Clin. Pharmacol.* 9, 235—238.

Versichelen, L., Rolly, G. and Beerens, J. (1983) Alfentanil/etomidate anaesthesia for endolaryngeal microsurgery. *Anaesthesia* 38, Suppl., 57—60.

Vree, T.B., Baars, A.M. and de Grood, P.M.R.M. (1987) High-performance liquid chromatographic determination and preliminary pharmacokinetics of propofol and its metabolites in human plasma and urine. *J. Chromatogr. Biomed. Appl.* 417, 458—464.

Wagner, J.G. (1976) Linear pharmacokinetic equations allowing direct calculation of many needed pharmacokinetic parameters from the coefficients and exponents of polyexponential equations which have been fitted to the data. *J. Pharmacokinet. Biopharm.* 4, 443—467.

Wagner, R.L. and White, P.F. (1984) Etomidate inhibits adrenocortical function in surgical patients. *Anesthesiology* 61, 647—651.

Ward, S., Neill, E.A.M., Weatherley, B.C. and Corall, I.M. (1983) Pharmacokinetics of atracurium besylate in healthy patients (after a single bolus dose). *Br. J. Anaesth.* 55, 113—118.

Watt, I. and Ledingham, I.M.cA. (1984) Mortality amongst multiple trauma patients admitted to an intensive therapy unit. *Anaesthesia* 39, 973—981.

Welles, J.S., McMahon, R.E. and Doran, W.J. (1963) The metabolism and excretion of methohexital in the rat and dog. *J. Pharmacol. Exp. Ther.* 139, 163—171.

White, P.F. (1984) Continuous infusions of thiopental, methohexital or etomidate as adjuvants to nitrous oxide for outpatient anesthesia. *Anesth. Analg.* 63, 282.

White, P.F., Dworksy, W.A., Horai, Y. and Trevor, A.J. (1983) Comparison of continuous infusion of fentanyl or ketamine versus thiopental — determining the mean effective serum concentrations for outpatient anesthesia. *Anesthesiology* 59, 564—569.

White, P.F., Schuttler, J., Shafer, A., Stanski, D.R., Horai, Y. and Trevor, A.J. (1985) Comparative pharmacology of the ketamine isomers. Studies in volunteers. *Br. J. Anaesth.* 57, 197—203.

Wilson, E., Mackenzie, N. and Grant, I.S. (1988) A comparison of propofol and midazolam to provide sedation in patients who receive spinal anaesthesia. *Anaesthesia* 43, Suppl., 91—93.

Wilson, J., Stephen, W.G. and Scott, D.B. (1969) A study of the cardiovascular effects of chlormethiazole. *Br. J. Anaesth.* 41, 840—843.

Yamaoka, K., Nakagawa, T. and Uno, T. (1978) Statistical moments in pharmacokinetics. *J. Pharmacokinet. Biopharm.* 6, 547—558.

Zsigmond, E.K. and Domino, E.F. (1980) Ketamine — clinical pharmacology, pharmacokinetics and current clinical uses. *Anesthesiol. Rev.* 7, 13—33.

*B. Kay (ed.) Total Intravenous Anaesthesia*



# 3

# *Benzodiazepines and their reversal*

A. Nilsson

## MECHANISM OF ACTION

Benzodiazepines act by enhancing the inhibitory effects of gamma amino butyric acid (GABA) on neuronal transmission. GABA neurons are widely distributed throughout the central nervous system. When GABA is released into the synaptic cleft it interacts with receptors made by glycoproteins protruding from the postsynaptic cell membrane. Activation of this receptor, i.e. a reversible coupling of the released GABA molecule to the receptor, leads to conformational change of the receptor protein. Since the receptor is included in a protein molecule complex forming an ion-channel, permeable to $Cl^-$ ions, this change in confirmation leads to an increase in ion flux into the postsynaptic cell. The influx results in a hyperpolarisation of the cell and makes it less prone to react on excitatory stimulation. GABA is inactivated through active cellular transport (uptake) into GABA-ergic nerve endings and glial cells, where it can be metabolised. GABA is the most important inhibitory neurotransmitter, forming up to one third of all mammalian brain synapses and is of vital importance in the function of the CNS. Depression of GABA-ergic synaptic function will result in hyperexcitability with convulsions and death (Heafely, 1987).

The GABA receptor is found within a protein complex forming an ion channel. Within this complex receptors for other ligands such as benzodiazepines and barbiturates have been found. They interact with this system by modulating the response of the postsynaptic cell to GABA-ergic stimulation, i.e. increased channel opening leading to a greater $Cl^-$ ion influx. Barbiturates are also believed to have a direct action upon the ion-channel (Fig. 3.1). Studies of interactions between midazolam and thiopentone have indicated a supra-additive (synergistic) effect (Tverskoy et al., 1988). It has been postulated that this is an effect of allosteric modification of the benzodiazepine receptor, caused by the thiopentone binding to its receptor site, leading to increased affinity for the benzodiazepines.

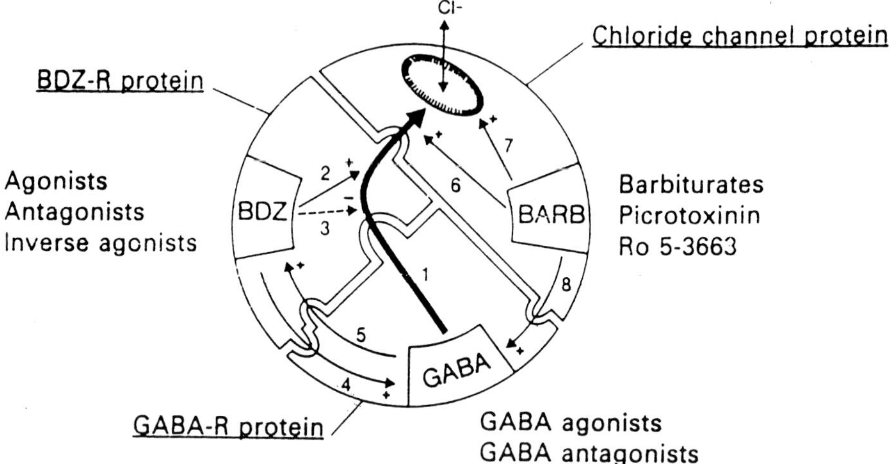


Fig. 3.1. Proposed model of subsynaptic GABA receptor (GABA-R) benzodiazepine receptor (BDZ-R)-chloride channel complex. The large, heavy arrow (1) indicates that activation of the GABA receptor leads to an opening of the chloride channel. The channel opening can be increased (2) or decreased (3) by binding of benzodiazepine agonists or inverse agonists. Binding to one receptor also enhances binding of ligands to another receptor through conformational changes (4,5,8). Barbiturates have a similar modulating effect (6) and also a proposed direct action on the chloride channel (7). (From Polc et al., 1982.)

By radioimmunoassay two types of benzodiazepine receptors have been found. One type mediates the well-known effects of benzodiazepines in the CNS while the second type is a high-affinity binding site on non-neuronal cells both within the CNS (glial cells) and in extra-cerebral tissues. No other function than binding has conclusively been found for these sites and they are not considered further (Haefely, 1987).

The benzodiazepine receptor in the CNS has been thoroughly investigated and it has been shown that it is an allosteric modulatory site of the GABA-receptor complex. The unique feature of the benzodiazepine receptor is the existence of three types of ligands with different qualitative effects on the GABA-receptor function.

The classical benzodiazepine action is enhancement of GABA-ergic transmission. The concentration-response curve for chloride conduction is shifted to the left. This shift depends on the concentration of the agonist. Recordings from a single GABA-receptor operated chloride channel using patch-clamp technique has revealed that the effect of a small dose of GABA in the presence of the benzodiazepine agonist is identical to the effect of a larger dose of GABA in the absence of a benzodiazepine agonist. The maximal shift of the GABA concentration-response curve that can be obtained by a benzodiazepine agonist is about 2- to 3-fold, hence rather modest (Mathers, 1987). Also, a ceiling effect can be seen where the effect of the agonist does not increase although the concentration is increased.

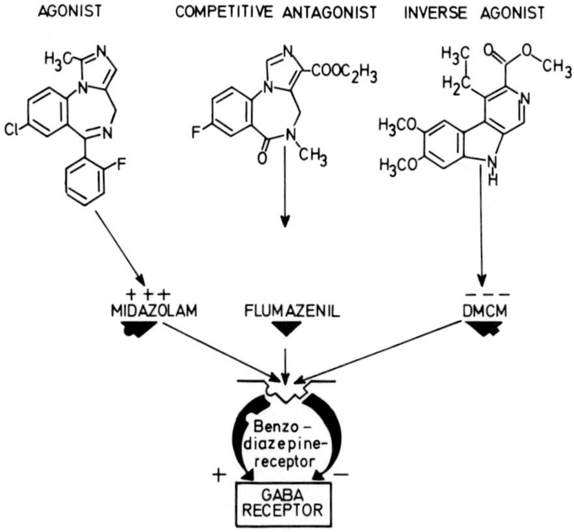


Fig. 3.2. Schematic representation of the different modes of interaction of the three basic types of benzodiazepine receptor ligands and their influence on the GABA receptor. (DMCM = dimethoxy-β-carbolin-methylester). (Modified from Amrein et al., 1987.)

This is believed to be an effect of saturation of the available receptor sites (Hall et al., 1988). This positive modulatory action of benzodiazepine agonists on GABA-receptor function is not difficult to transfer to the neuronal activities that can be seen clinically.

In the early eighties high affinity ligands for the benzodiazepine-receptor were found that produced opposite effects to the classical ligands (i.e. they were anxiogenic, convulsant and vigilance increasing). The first compounds of this kind were β-carbolines but similar properties were subsequently found in molecules of the benzodiazepine group. They act by reducing GABA binding and hence depress channel opening. Since no evidence exists that they act by different receptors and they fulfil the criteria of an agonist, i.e. binding to the receptor site and subsequent conformational changes, they are called 'inverse agonists' (Haefely, 1987)

The third group of ligands that bind to the benzodiazepine-receptor is clinically represented by flumazenil, a benzodiazepine molecule with a high binding affinity for the receptor. The binding of flumazenil to the receptor does not cause any conformational changes affecting the channel opening. By its high affinity for the receptor it acts as a competitive antagonist to both agonist and inverse agonists.

Several compounds with partial agonistic or inverse agonistic properties have been synthesized but their clinical importance is at present unclear. Figure 3.2 gives a schematic overview of the various classes of the ligands and their action on the GABA receptor.

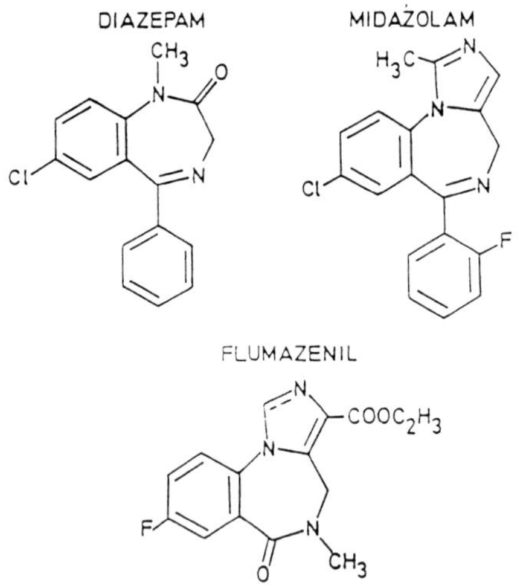

DIAZEPAM

MIDAZOLAM

FLUMAZENIL

Fig. 3.3. Structural formulae of benzodiazepine receptor ligands.

## NEUROLOGICAL EFFECTS

Although there is a variation in receptor affinity and intrinsic activity among the agonists, there is a similarity in action, especially when looking at drugs of interest to the anaesthesiologist. The effect is dose-related, increases in dosage lead to more pronounced CNS-depressive actions but there also seems to be a ceiling effect where increased dosage does not give more effect (Hall et al., 1988). This appears in a dose range above the usual clinical doses. The CNS depressant action of the benzodiazepines results in a dose-related depression of cerebral blood flow and cerebral oxygen consumption (Hoffman et al., 1986; Wolff, 1990).

At low doses the benzodiazepines are anxiolytic and anticonvulsant, increasing plasma concentration gives a sedative and amnesic effect. With high concentrations a state of hypnosis is achieved although the subjects often react to strong stimuli. As a consequence of the dose-related response there will be a variation in the duration of action of various effects. If a benzodiazepine is given in high dosage to induce and maintain a hypnotic effect it is not surprising that the period of postoperative sedation can be rather long (Fig. 3.4).

Another striking feature is the variability in response to a certain dosage, this is not only due to differences in pharmacokinetics but also related to pharmacodynamic variation. The latter effect may be caused by age-related changes in the receptor population but genetic differences also contribute to this variability (Short et al., 1987).

The CNS-depressant action of the benzodiazepines can be influenced by the co-administration of other drugs. Premedication or administration of an opioid immediately prior to induction of anaesthesia with a benzodiazepine allows a dosage

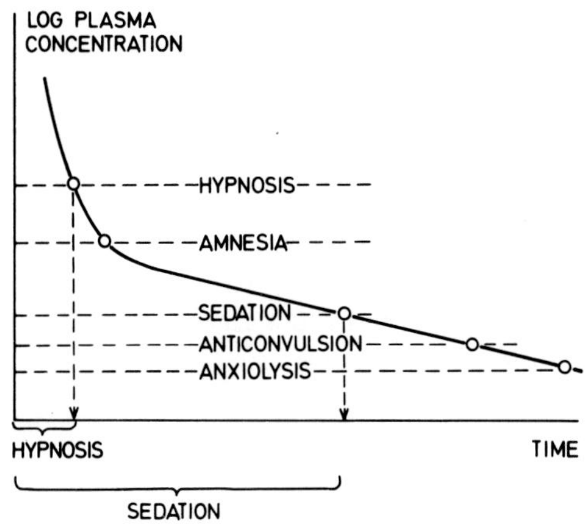


Fig. 3.4. Schematic representation of threshold concentrations of benzodiazepine agonist-mediated effects. (From Paalzow 1985.)

reduction of the latter (Kanto et al., 1982). This interaction can also be demonstrated in the postoperative period where an opioid, for example alfentanil, can interfere with the dose-response curve for sedation, whereas amnesia, another effect produced by midazolam, is unaffected (Persson et al., 1988).

Tolerance to the depressant effects of the benzodiazepines does occur after long-term use and might be of clinical importance. Cross-tolerance against alcohol is a well-known clinical phenomenon. Also, aminophylline has antagonistic properties which can lead to a need for an increased dosage of benzodiazepines (Stirt, 1981; Arvidsson et al., 1984).

The amnesic action of the benzodiazepines makes them especially useful to cover the unpleasant experiences that are frequent during endoscopy and in dental practice. In this respect midazolam seems to produce a more profound and reliable amnesic effect than equipotent doses of diazepam (Berggren et al., 1983). Also, lorazepam given orally produces long-lasting amnesia. The amnesic effects of benzodiazepines is described as an impaired long-term episodic memory. The benzodiazepines may block the consolidation process indirectly, by depressing the facilitating actions of reticular and limbic catecholamine arousal systems. In practice, this means that strong stimuli can break through the amnesic action of the drugs, an important fact when assessing the results of amnesia studies with artificial stimulation such as picture recall etc. (O'Boyle et al., 1987). Also, since short-term recall is relatively unaffected, a person can be seemingly awake and converse adequately and still be unable to recall this event later. This is a very important fact to remember when giving instructions to a patient that has been under sedation with these drugs. Relevant information should be given in writing and/or to an accompanying person.

Benzodiazepines have no analgesic action, midazolam has been shown to have a modulatory effect on pain threshold when coadministered with opioids intrathecally (Moreau and Pieri 1987; Serrao et al., 1988). The sedative and anxiolytic effects of benzodiazepines are often used to reduce discomfort in the postoperative period.

Diazepam is a well-established drug in the treatment of epilepsy of various origins and midazolam has proved equally potent in this aspect (Jawad et al., 1986). Experimental studies have shown that pretreatment with diazepam or midazolam will raise the threshold for local anaesthetic induced seizures. The effect of benzodiazepines on cardiovascular collapse following high i.v. concentrations of local anaesthetics is unclear (Bernards et al., 1988).

## CARDIOVASCULAR AND RESPIRATORY EFFECTS

The cardiovascular effects of benzodiazepines are generally considered to be mild. As a consequence, they have been widely used in elderly patients and in patients with heart conditions (Samuelson et al., 1981; Dundee et al., 1984; Reitan and Soliman, 1987). Both midazolam and diazepam cause a fall in systemic vascular resistance. This effect is most evident when the vascular resistance is increased due to hypertension and/or situations of mental stress (prior to an operation) (Samuelson et al., 1981; Muller et al., 1981). Another situation where this effect is of clinical importance is in hypovolemic shock and preshock, where the benzodiazepines should be given slowly in small doses. In combination with fentanyl or other opioids there can be an additive negative inotropic effect leading to more profound hypotension (Reves et al., 1984). Recently the combination of midazolam and sufentanil was evaluated in patients undergoing elective coronary bypass grafting (Raza et al., 1988). Although midazolam caused a reduction in systemic vascular resistance and blood pressure, the authors concluded that the combination resulted in no adverse haemodynamic effects.

Compensatory mechanisms following the fall in systemic vascular resistance are mobilisation of blood from the splanchnic area and tachycardia, the latter usually of little clinical importance (Reeves et al., 1985).

The general effect of benzodiazepines on coronary blood flow has been presented as a decrease related to the decrease in oxygen demand. Usually, a smaller vasodilator effect can be seen. It is important to control coronary perfusion pressure and prevent tachycardia when using these drugs in patients with severe coronary disease (Reiz, 1988). Studies with radionuclide ventriculography in patients with coronary artery disease did not show any effect on left ventricular ejection fraction and did not indicate regional myocardial dysfunction after i.v. bolus doses of diazepam, flunitrazepam or midazolam (Lepage et al., 1986).

The anxiolytic and amnesic properties as well as the cardiovascular stability has made the benzodiazepines popular as sedatives for cardioversion.

The effects on ventilation of benzodiazepines may be divided into two aspects, the effects on muscular tone and on the carbon dioxide response. Since the centrally depressant action of the benzodiazepines also include an effect on muscular tone there is an increased risk of airway obstruction, especially when benzodiazepines are given for i.v. sedation in the upright or semi-upright position (Dundee and Wyant, 1988). This effect is probably of greater clinical importance than the slight decrease in tidal volume that follows administration of benzodiazepines, although the effect on carbon dioxide response was noticeable at very low midazolam concentrations (Sunzel et al., 1988). The decrease in tidal volume is compensated by an increase in respiratory frequency, which in turn can be counteracted by the action of opioids (Berggren et al., 1987). Thus, respiratory depression is more likely to be present when benzodiazepines and opioids are combined (Dailland et al., 1988; Tverskoy et al., 1989). Another important factor that has been investigated is the response to hypoxia under hypercapnic conditions (Alexander et al., 1988). Midazolam in sedative doses given to hypercapnic volunteers resulted in a depressed reaction to hypoxia and these results emphasise the need for oxygen administration to and close supervision of patients given i.v. sedation.

## PHARMACOKINETIC CONSIDERATIONS

The pharmacokinetic parameters of the anaesthesiologically most important benzodiazepines are listed in Table 3.1.

Since diazepam and midazolam are the most commonly used i.v. benzodiazepine agonists, they will be discussed in most detail. They differ mainly in their clearance values, diazepam having a rather low value and midazolam being characterised as a drug with intermediate clearance. A drug with a higher clearance value is more dependent on changes in liver blood flow, while the intrinsic capacity of the liver is more significant for a drug with low clearance values (Rowland and Tozer, 1980). In cirrhotic patients plasma clearance of midazolam was reduced with an overall result of prolonged half-life (from 135 min in control patients to 168 min in cirrhotic patients) (Trouvin et al., 1988). The intrinsic activity of the liver can be influenced by administration of other drugs or substances (smoking, alcohol etc.)

TABLE 3.1

Pharmacokinetics of the most commonly used injectible benzodiazepines

| | $Vd$ (l/kg) | $Cl_p$ (ml/min) | $t_{1/2}\,\beta$ (h) | Protein binding (%) |
|---|---|---|---|---|
| Diazepam | 1.2 | 20—47 | 21.0—37.0 | 98 |
| Flunitrazepam | 4.0 | 140—350 | 13.0—19.0 | 80 |
| Midazolam | 1.1—1.7 | 266—633 | 1.5—4.0 | 95 |
| Flumazenil | 0.6—1.6 | 516—1300 | 0.7—1.3 | 36—46 |

leading to increased or decreased capacity of drug metabolism. The difference in clearance values between midazolam and diazepam is also the main reason for the difference in elimination half-life ($t_{1/2}$ = 0.693 *Vd/Cl*). This derived parameter is interesting since it provides information about the time it will take until a drug given at a constant rate reaches a steady state concentration (95% of $C_{ss}$ within 3—4 half-lives). Also, it gives information about recovery characteristics, since after prolonged administration it is mainly the elimination process that governs the reduction of plasma concentration of the drug. After a single i.v. injection or a short infusion period it is mainly the effect of distribution of the drug that determines the duration of effect. Consequently, there is less difference in the duration of effect of a single dose of midazolam compared to diazepam than of repeated administrations or infusion of these drugs (Stanski and Hudson, 1985).

Another important effect is the influence of metabolites, diazepam having pharmacologically active metabolites, desmethyldiazepam and oxazepam; the former with a long elimination half-life may contribute to prolonged effect (Dundee and Wyant, 1988). Midazolam has one pharmacologically active break-down product α-hydroxymidazolam, but this is rapidly conjugated ($t_{1/2}$ < 1 h) and of less clinical importance (Crevoisier et al., 1983). The influence of age on pharmacokinetics must also be considered, the elimination half-life of midazolam showed little variation with age, thus comparing favourably with diazepam (Avram et al., 1983).

Flumazenil, the competitive antagonist, has a smaller volume of distribution than the agonists and a high clearance value leading to a short elimination half-life (Klotz et al., 1984). The consequences of this will be discussed later in this chapter.

Midazolam has been suggested as an alternative to thiopentone as an induction agent for elective caesarean section anaesthesia (Crawford et al., 1989). This study was also followed up with investigations of neonatal behaviour (Ravlo et al., 1989) with only minor differences in behaviour between children where anaesthesia had been induced by either thiopentone or midazolam. In a study of placental transfer and elimination of midazolam and thiopentone in neonates (Bach et al., 1989) there was an elimination half-life of 6.3 h for midazolam (compared to 14.7 h for thiopentone). The placental transfer, expressed as the umbilical/maternal concentration ratio, was less for midazolam (0.66) than for thiopentone (0.96). Despite these findings the use of midazolam in this clinical situation is limited and the amnesic effect, perhaps being advantageous peroperatively, might be a considerable drawback during recovery, although this was not considered in the extensive study cited above.

## INDUCTION OF ANAESTHESIA

When used for induction of anaesthesia the most striking feature of the benzodiazepines is their variability in response. This is specially marked in young individuals, when unpremedicated and when the drug is given as sole induction agent. One reason for this variation may be that these drugs are highly protein-bound leaving only a minor, pharmacologically active free fraction. A correlation between plasma albumin concentration and induction time of midazolam has been demonstrated, and this is partly the reason why midazolam is a more effective induction agent in the elderly, undernourished or chronically ill patient. Manipulation of plasma protein binding by pretreatment with probenicid or aspirin will reduce onset time (Dundee and Wyant, 1988) but is not used in routine practice.

Since in clinical practice recovery from equivalent doses of midazolam is more rapid than when diazepam or flunitrazepam has been administered, this is the drug of choice in most circumstances (Galletly et al., 1988; Dundee and Wyant, 1988). This is especially important when large or repeated doses are given (see pharmacokinetics).

The induction of anaesthesia with benzodiazepines results in a gradual increase in sedation leading to hypnosis without very much excitation or respiratory upset. Provided that the airway is protected, midazolam induction, although somewhat slower in onset, results in a smooth transition to inhalational anaesthesia with significantly less apnoea than a traditional dose of thiopentone (Nilsson et al., 1984).

The induction properties of midazolam are greatly influenced by premedication or simultaneous administration of an opioid (Kanto et al., 1982; Reeves et al., 1985; Dundee and Wyant, 1988; Vinik et al., 1989). It has been demonstrated that such coadministration reduces both induction time and dosage. This is particularly important in younger subjects since the alternative, larger doses of benzodiazepines, will result in prolonged recovery.

It is rather difficult to establish the ratio between equipotent doses of midazolam and diazepam, this depends on the effect studied and is also related to the preparation of diazepam used. It has been stated that midazolam is approximately two to three times as potent as the lipid emulsion of diazepam with regard to sedative effects (Galletly et al., 1988). The diazepam preparations containing organic solvents such as propylene glycol have been claimed to be more potent but cause a higher incidence of venous irritation (Fee et al., 1984) and are thus inferior for intravenous administration.

The large interindividual range of dosages needed for induction, especially in relation to age and coadministered drugs, makes a general dosage recommendation useless. Many studies have been performed comparing the induction properties of midazolam and thiopentone (Nilsson et al., 1984; Reeves et al., 1985; Dundee and Wyant, 1988). The usual finding is that the onset time of midazolam in doses of 0.2—0.3 mg/kg is generally slower than with thiopentone 4—5 mg/kg. A somewhat better cardiovascular stability following benzodiazepine induction has been claimed (see above) but the most important feature of thiopentone is the speed of recovery after a single i.v. bolus dose (Reitan et al., 1986; Raeder et al., 1988). Although many patients may prefer the gradual recovery experienced after midazolam this is a relative drawback of the drug in comparison with thiopentone and propofol, especially in a busy outpatient setting.

A premedication including an opioid and/or beginning the induction sequence with an opioid is advisable and then small incremental doses are given slowly i.v. until the desired endpoint is reached. Depending on the following procedure this endpoint varies, but prior to inhalational anaesthesia absence of response to verbal commands is usually satisfactory. To obtain loss of eyelid or eyelash reflexes often demands greater dosage but may be necessary if tracheal intubation is to follow. To give more midazolam than 0.5 mg/kg as a bolus dose is generally not recommended, for an old, poor-risk patient a total dose as little as 2—3 mg can be sufficient. Midazolam has been claimed to reduce the cardiovascular response to intubation (Boralessa et al., 1983) and when midazolam was combined with fentanyl the pressure response was of little clinical significance although the patients reacted in both EEG and frontal EMG to laryngoscopy and intubation (Nilsson et al., 1986).

One important difference between benzodiazepines and other induction agents such as thiopentone or propofol is that the benzodiazepines are selectively hypnotic and do not cause the profound unconsciousness that make these other agents usable as sole agents for minor procedures (for instance dilatation and curettage). The benzodiazepines must be combined with opioids and/or nitrous oxide or another inhalational agent if any noxious procedures are intended.

## BENZODIAZEPINES FOR MAINTENANCE OF ANAESTHESIA

Apart from being used to temporarily increase hypnosis during anaesthesia by giving bolus doses, attempts have been made to use benzodiazepines for maintenance of the hypnotic effect during anaesthesia.

When nitrous oxide is omitted the plasma concentration of the hypnotic must be relatively high (see below). A technique with repeated bolus doses will result in fluctuations of the plasma concentration and hence the effect (Crevat-Pisano et al., 1986). This can only be accepted for brief periods, and for anaesthesia of some length, the use of an infusion technique is necessary. As a consequence of the pharmacokinetic differences between the drugs discussed earlier in this chapter, only midazolam is considered for this technique, since rapid recovery is usually of importance.

For the successful administration of an infusion there are two pre-requisites that have to be fulfilled. One must know the concentration at which the desired effect is achieved and also the pharmacokinetics of the drug to be used (Sear, 1983). It was earlier demonstrated that a steady state concentration of midazolam of 500—600 ng/ml produced an intense hypnotic effect (Lauven et al., 1985). The CNS effects of benzodiazepines can be augmented by the concomitant use of opioids and studies of midazolam given as an infusion for abdominal hysterectomy showed that a concentration above 250—300 ng/ml kept the patient unconscious when midazolam was coadministered with fentanyl or alfentanil (Nilsson et al., 1986, 1988). The patients were given muscle relaxants and ventilated with oxygen in air, the method consequently described as a total intravenous technique (TIVA). Other studies (Möller et al., 1986; Klausen et al., 1988) have produced similar results and attempts to reduce the midazolam concentration below 200 ng/ml have resulted in reports of awareness (Klausen et al., 1988; also personal observation). Blocking the noxious stimuli from lower abdominal surgery by the use of an epidural blockade (Persson et al., 1988) provided the information that arousal from midazolam anaesthesia could be seen at a plasma concentration around 175—200 ng/ml (Fig. 3.8).

Using a system with computer-assisted continuous infusion (CACI) maintenance of anaesthesia has been reported with lower plasma levels of midazolam (50—85 ng/ml) (Reeves et al., 1989). In these trials midazolam was co-administered with fentanyl or sufentanil. The computer controlled infusion pump varied the infusion rate repeatedly in order to achieve and maintain the desired plasma concentration using a given set of pharmacokinetic data. Apart from displaying dosage rate and estimated plasma concentration this instrument is also capable of predicting recovery time etc. and may be a prototype for future infusion devices.

The pharmacokinetics of midazolam and alfentanil were not changed in patients undergoing lower abdominal surgery with a combination of these drugs (Persson et al., 1987, 1988) when compared to studies in volunteers and other patients undergoing surgery, but other workers (Harper et al., 1985) have reported changes in pharmacokinetics during surgery and intensive care with a prolonged elimination half-life (Bodenham et al., 1988). Changes in liver blood flow and protein concentration during surgery may contribute to these changes.

The principles for infusion of hypnotics are considered in Chapter 2. With the knowledge of the target value of midazolam (approx 300 ng/ml) and the pharmacokinetics a dosage regimen using a bolus injection of 0.25 mg/kg gives a rapid induction, provided that the patient has been given an opioid premedication. This is followed by a rapid constant rate infusion of 0.65 mg/kg per h given for 15 min to avoid any temporary fall in the plasma concentration versus time profile. A maintenance with an infusion rate of 0.125 mg/kg per h follows the loading infusion, this will result in a steady state concentration of midazolam of approx. 300 ng/ml from 45 min after commencement of the induction and onwards (Persson et al., 1987) (Fig. 3.5). The dosage recommendation above must naturally be weighed against the general condition of the patient, type of surgery employed etc. Once surgery starts it must be the individual need of the patient that governs the administration of the drug. Incremental doses of midazolam, 2.5—5 mg, can be given to temporarily increase the hypnotic depth. During upper abdominal surgery or other stressful surgical procedures the proposed infusion rate may be unsatisfactory (personal observations) and can be temporarily doubled. The use of higher infusion rates (0.66 mg/kg per h during the initial 30 min followed by 0.48 mg/kg per h for 30 min and 0.36 mg/kg per h for maintenance until 15 min before end of surgery) for hypnosis during superficial body surgery has been described by others (Breimer et al., 1988) aiming at a plasma concentration of 400—600 ng/ml. Upward changes in infusion rate are best preceded by a bolus dose to rapidly increase the concentration of the drug. Cardiovascular responses to intense surgical stimuli are best treated by additional analgesic. If the patient is unresponsive during periods of intense stimulation, overdosage must be considered and the infusion must be reduced or temporarily stopped.

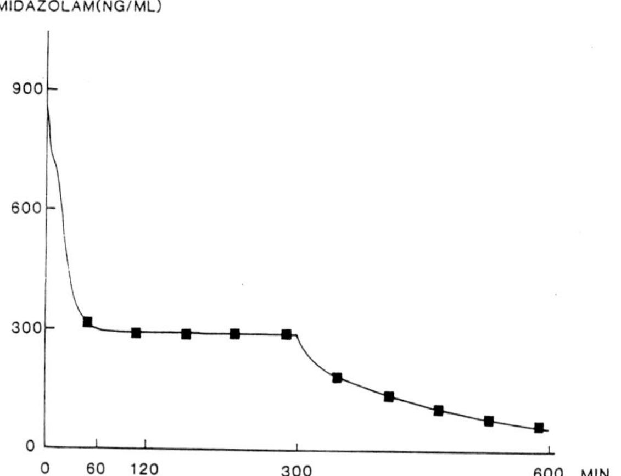


Fig. 3.5. Simulated concentration-time profile for midazolam after two consecutive infusion rates combined with a bolus injection. The bolus injection was 0.3 mg/kg while the infusion rates were 0.68 mg/kg per h for 15 min followed by 0.125 mg/kg per h over the next 285 min. (From Persson et al., 1987.)

It must be emphasised that dosage recommendations are based on mean values of the pharmacokinetics. Apart from the often large interindividual differences, drug distribution and elimination can be altered by the cardiovascular response to anaesthesia and surgical manipulation, changes in protein binding, etc.

If a slower induction is preferred or acceptable, a double infusion regimen can be used. Anaesthesia is induced by midazolam 0.42 mg/kg over 5 min. Once the patient stops reacting to verbal commands, opioids and muscle relaxants are given. The maintenance infusion starts at the same rate as above (Persson et al., 1987; Nilsson et al., 1988) (Fig. 3.6). One advantage with the loading infusion as compared to a bolus injection is that it gives some impression about the patient's response to the drug. Also, as has been demonstrated for propofol (Roberts et al., 1988) this may lead to less cardiovascular effects although this has not been proved in clinical trials.

Midazolam must be combined with an analgesic (opioid, ketamine) or local/regional anaesthesia since it has no analgesic properties. When using opioids this usually requires intubation and controlled ventilation. The analgesic requirement in combination with midazolam-induced hypnosis seems to be in the same range as when supplementing nitrous oxide anaesthesia (De Castro, 1987).

Midazolam does not have any effect on the adrenocortical response to trauma when used as an induction agent (Dawson and Sear, 1986). When used for maintenance of anaesthesia in combination with alfentanil there was no difference in the cortisol levels during and after surgery when compared to thiopentone, alfentanil, nitrous oxide anaesthesia (Nilsson et al., 1988). In both groups cortisol values were within normal fasting levels during surgery and they were elevated in the immediate postoperative period when influence of anaesthesia was reduced (Fig. 3.7).

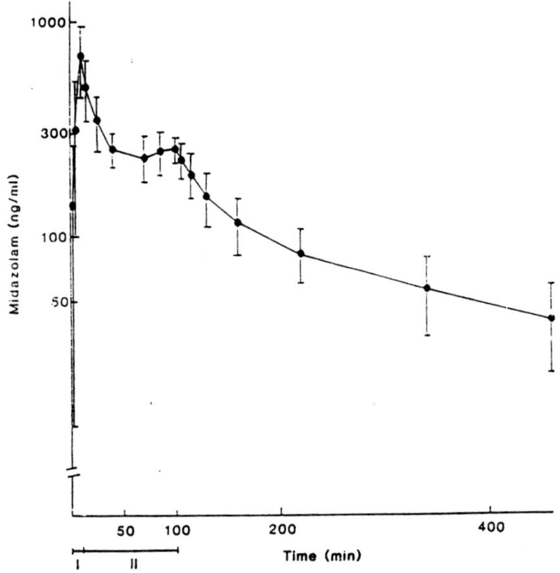


Fig. 3.6. Observed plasma concentrations in a group of patients ($n$ = 10) given a midazolam loading infusion of 0.42 mg/kg per h over 10 min (I), followed by a maintenance infusion of 0.125 mg/kg per h for the next 110 min (II) Mean values ± S.D. (Persson, M.P. and Nilsson, A., unpublished data).

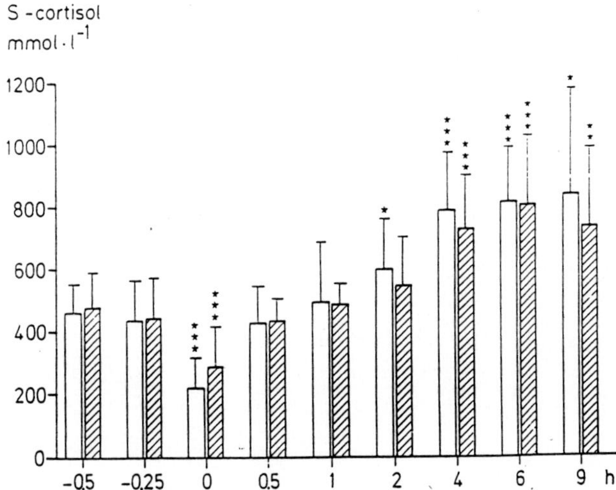


Fig. 3.7. Serum cortisol concentrations before induction (−0.05, −0.25 h), before (=) and after incision in patients undergoing abdominal hysterectomy (duration of anaesthesia approx. 2 h). Striped bar, anaesthesia with midazolam/alfentanil infusions. $O_2$ and air, atracurium. Open bar, thiopentone induction, alfentanil infusion, $O_2$ and $N_2O$ atracurium. *Indicates statistically significant differences from base-line measurements. *$P < 0.05$, **$P < 0.01$, ***$P < 0.001$. No significant differences between groups. (From Nilsson et al., 1988.)

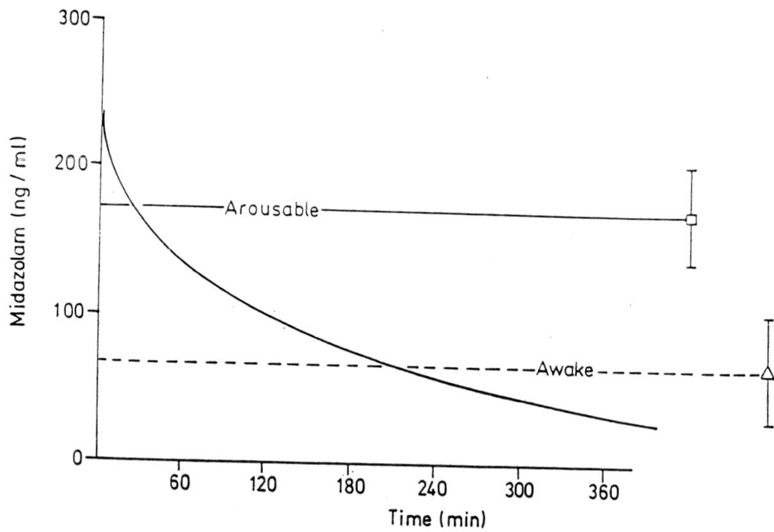


Fig. 3.8. Concentration-time profile of midazolam after an infusion at a concentration of approx. 250 ng/ml for 2 h. Threshold values (mean ± S.D.) for being arousable and awake are indicated. (Modified from Persson et al., 1988.)

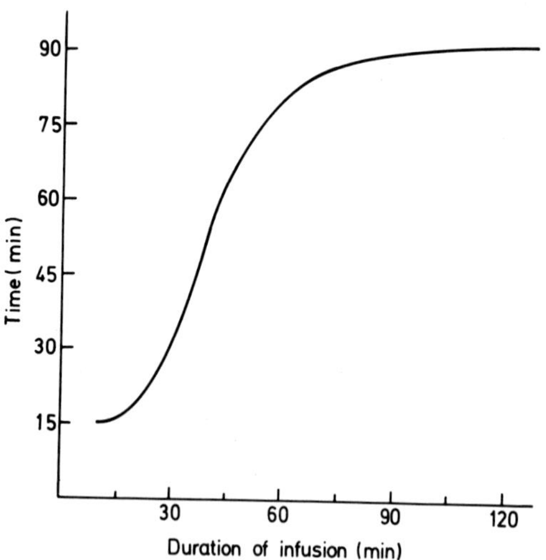


Fig. 3.9. Time for the plasma concentration of midazolam to decline by 50% as a function of the duration of the infusion regimen. (From Persson, 1987.)

Recovery from midazolam anaesthesia is partly dependent on the dosage and partly the duration of administration. The studies on postoperative concentration-effect relationships of midazolam (Persson et al., 1988) indicated that the subjects were arousable at a plasma concentration of around 200 ng/ml. The plasma concentration must fall to 75 ng/ml before the subjects are awake enough to leave the postoperative unit (Fig. 3.8). The co-administration of alfentanil peroperatively and ketobemidon during the postoperative phase resulted in a shift to the left of the concentration-response curve with regard to sedation. Amnesia was not affected. The differences in drug demand during surgery compared with recovery results in prolonged sedation extending over several hours after a 2 h infusion (Nilsson et al., 1988). The relation between the duration of infusion and decay of the plasma concentration (Persson, 1987) is presented in Fig. 3.9. Although midazolam is the most rapidly eliminated benzodiazepine presently available, prolonged recovery is the main disadvantage of its use as a maintenance agent in TIVA for routine surgery. There is probably not very much to gain by reducing the rate of administration of midazolam towards the end of surgery. Another solution to this problem may be the use of the new benzodiazepine antagonist flumazenil and this will be described later.

Midazolam infusions have also been employed as hypnotics in combination with opioids and nitrous oxide (Shapiro et al., 1988). When nitrous oxide is administered the dosage can be reduced and less postoperative drowsiness is seen. Midazolam 0.1 mg/kg per h was successfully given together with sufentanil and nitrous oxide during major surgery on patients susceptible to malignant hyperthermia (Tuman et al., 1988).

Benzodiazepines are also frequently used for sedation as a complement to local anaesthesia. The desired level of sedation is often variable and repeated injections of small doses usually offer the best solution. As previously stated, there is little difference in recovery time after a bolus dose of midazolam compared to diazepam but higher and repeated dosages favours the use of midazolam. The higher potency and steeper dose-effect relationship for midazolam emphasises the importance of a careful titration to avoid oversedation (White et al., 1988). This is especially important in the elderly population. The availability of a more diluted (1 mg/ml) solution of midazolam in some markets is helpful in this respect.

Sometimes a more profound sedation in combination with spinal or epidural anaesthesia for major procedures can be beneficial and an infusion can be a good alternative in these situations. After bolus titration to desired effect an infusion rate of midazolam of 0.05—0.2 mg/kg per h is usually satisfying. Since benzodiazepines may cause some respiratory depression or loss of airway control, careful monitoring and oxygen administration is necessary, especially if the drugs are co-administered with opioids.

Prolonged infusions of midazolam at a level that gives deep sedation will also result in delayed recovery (Wilson et al., 1988).

The cardiovascular and psychotomimetic side-effects of ketamine can be reduced by simultaneous administration of diazepam or midazolam. The use of ketamine is described in Chapter 6.

## ANTAGONISM OF BENZODIAZEPINE ACTION

Both physostigmine (Nilsson and Himberg, 1982; Caldwell and Gross, 1982) and aminophylline (Stirt, 1981; Arvidsson et al., 1984) have been described as benzodiazepine antagonists. Neither drug is specific in action and this is probably the reason for variable reports regarding their effectiveness (Sleigh, 1986; Breimer et al., 1988). With the discovery of flumazenil, a benzodiazepine compound with high receptor affinity and very little intrinsic activity, a selective antagonist became a reality (Amrein et al., 1987). Initially, flumazenil was regarded as a competitive antagonist capable of blocking all CNS-effects produced by benzodiazepine agonists (and inverse agonists). In clinical practice this seems to be true, but in various experiments weak inverse agonist and agonist effects have been reported (Brogden and Goa, 1988) including a weak anticonvulsant effect. This latter effect has focused interest on the drug as an antiepileptic, given in large doses orally (Scollo-Lavizzari, 1988).

In early studies, as much as 5—10 mg of flumazenil was given i.v. (Brogden and Goa, 1988) but it was soon found that the drug is effective in doses as little as 0.4—1.0 mg i.v. in most clinical settings. In volunteers, up to 100 mg has been given without symptoms of anxiety, convulsions or other side-effects (Darragh et al., 1983).

The effectiveness of flumazenil in reversing the effects of benzodiazepine agonists and inverse agonists is well established (Amrein et al., 1987, Brogden and Goa, 1988). The drug is also a useful tool in mixed intoxications where benzodiazepines are included (Geller et al., 1984; O'Sullivan and Wade, 1987; Baehrendtz and Höjer, 1988).

For comprehensive reviews of pharmacology and early clinical trials the reader is referred to Amrein et al., (1987) and Brogden and Goa (1988).

## FLUMAZENIL IN ANAESTHESIA

Recovery from the hypnotic-sedative action of benzodiazepines is usually a rather slow process, especially after large and/or repeated dosages. Flumazenil is a competitive antagonist and administration i.v. leads to an immediate recovery with effect on sedation, amnesia, co-operation and orientation. Although flumazenil is a weak anticonvulsive, the dosage recommendations for flumazenil favour a slow titration in divided doses to avoid an abrupt termination of agonistic effects with the possible risk of withdrawal convulsions and anxiety (Amrein, 1987). Withdrawal phenomena are more likely to be seen in patients on long-term treatment with benzodiazepines. Anxiety and other unspecific reactions have incidently been reported and are at least partly related to prompt awakening in a strange surrounding such as an operating theatre or a casualty ward (Amrein et al., 1987). Postoperative anxiety could also be related to pain but in a comparative study (Nilsson et al., 1988) there were no significant differences in time or amount of analgesic demands when flumazenil was used to reduce postoperative sedation after total i.v. anaesthesia with midazolam and alfentanil.

Since the action of flumazenil is rapid (maximum effect within minutes) neuromuscular blockade must be reversed before attempting to reverse benzodiazepine effects. If a technique with relatively large doses of midazolam and an opioid such as fentanyl, sufentanil or alfentanil has been used for induction and maintenance of anaesthesia (Nilsson et al., 1986, 1988; Radakovic et al., 1988), respiratory depression is a common side effect at the end of the procedure. In this situation careful titration of flumazenil may restore adequate respiration without the use of opioid antagonism. By using the reversal agents in this order, unnecessary pain and discomfort may be avoided.

Initially a bolus dose of 0.2 mg of flumazenil is given; if no response to this injection is seen after 1 min, 0.1—0.2 mg is given every minute until effective. Administration of more than 1.0 mg (in rare cases 2.0 mg) is not necessary and in case of no improvement, other causes of sedation, e.g. overdosage of opioids, must be considered.

The lack of effect on stress mediators such as catecholamines, vasopressin and $\beta$-endorphins after reversal of midaxolam induced sedation (White et al., 1988) favours the use of antagonism. Also, the hyperglycaemic and cortisol response after reversal of total i.v. anaesthesia with midazolam/alfentanil was comparable to nitrous oxide/alfentanil anaesthesia (Nilsson et al., 1988).

The influence of flumazenil on cerebral blood flow (CBF) was studied in volunteers (Forster et al., 1987). It was found that flumazenil was able to antagonize the cerebrovascular effects of midazolam induced hypnosis, whereas flumazenil had no effect on CBF on its own (Wolff, 1990). Flumazenil has also been used to facilitate postoperative observation after neurosurgery in patients receiving midazolam infusion combined with nitrous oxide and fentanyl during surgery. A total dose of 1.0 mg flumazenil lead to a prompt improvement in Glasgow Coma Scale but this was later followed by a decline, calling for further injections of the antagonist (Chiolero et al., 1986). However, an experimental study of dogs given high-dose infusions of midazolam showed significant increases in CBF and intracranial pressure (ICP) on reversal (Fleisher et al., 1988). Similar observations were made in an experimental study in goats during the reperfusion phase following incomplete global ischaemia (Kochs et al., 1988). In patients with increased and unstable ICP, who were being sedated with midazolam during mechanical ventilation, reversal with flumazenil caused severe increases in ICP and a concomitant decrease of cerebral perfusion pressure (CPP). In patients with good control of ICP before reversal there was no change in ICP or CPP (Chiolero et al., 1988). Until further experience has been gained concerning the effects on cerebral perfusion and duration of reversal, flumazenil must be used with caution in patients with increased ICP.

With the availability of flumazenil, being a potent, selective antagonist devoid of serious side effects, interest has focused on extended and new usages of the agonists. This must not lead to oversedation and careless administration of benzodiazepines (unsigned, Lancet, July 16, 1988, 140—142). However, there are situations where the possibility of deep sedation rapidly reversed with flumazenil is beneficial, for instance when using benzodiazepines for total i.v. anaesthesia (Hennis et al., 1988) and during unpleasant examinations of short duration (Geller et al., 1988).

The major problems with flumazenil when reversing intense sedation is the duration of the effect (Sage et al., 1987; Rodrigo and Rosenquist, 1987; Claeys et al., 1988; Nilsson et al., 1988). Flumazenil has a high clearance and a small volume of distribution which leads to an elimination half-life of less than 1 h ( Klotz et al., 1984). Since all benzodiazepine agonists have longer elimination half-lives, there is a risk of reappearance of sedation, amnesia etc. There is a complex relation between dosage, duration of administration, receptor affinity for the agonist used, time interval before attempted reversal and dose of antagonist. When interpreting results from different studies various assessments of sedation, amnesia etc., employed over different time scales, contributes to confusion.

The complexity of flumazenil duration can be illustrated by two clinical studies where approximately the same mean total dose (36—39 mg) of midazolam was given intermittently for short (5—36 min) procedures (Wolff et al., 1986) or as an infusion over approximately 2 h (Nilsson et al., 1988). Although the median dose of flumazenil was lower (0.4 mg) in the study by Wolff and co-workers they did not record any signs of resedation during the observation period (Fig. 3.10) whereas

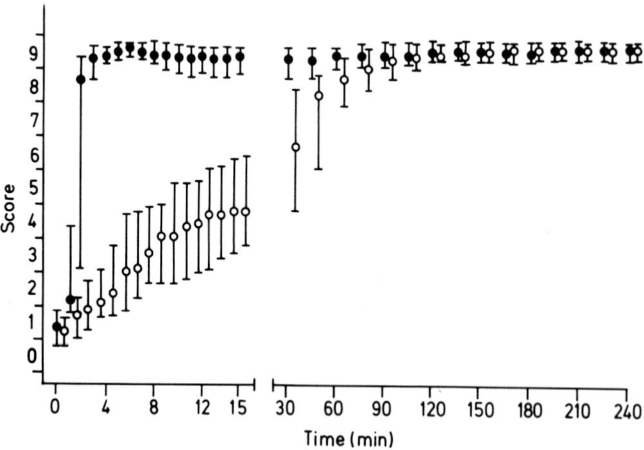


Fig. 3.10. Recovery scores on a modified Steward scale 0—9 (9 = fully awake, eyes open, conversing, with full airway control and cooperation; 0 = unresponsive, needing airway support). Patients ($n$ = 100) were anaesthetised with midazolam bolus injections for minor gynaecological surgery. Flumazenil (median dose 0.4 mg) (closed circles) or placebo (open circles) given for reversal. Median (interquartile range). (From Wolff et al., 1986.)

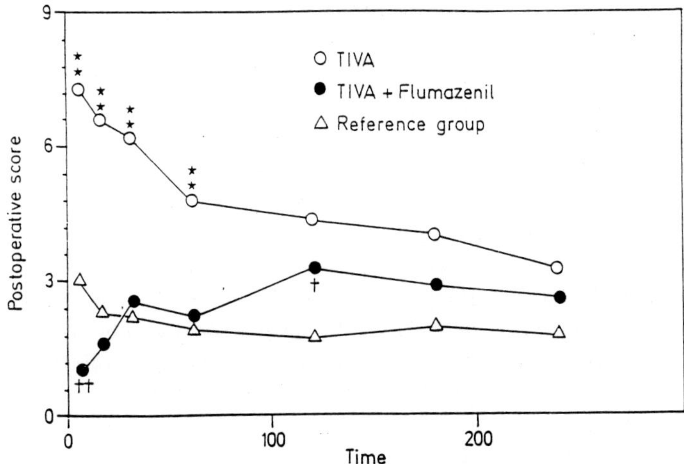


Fig. 3.11. Post-operative performance scores after total intravenous anaesthesia with infusions of midazolam/alfentanil with and without reversal with flumazenil 1.0 mg i.v. Reference group anaesthetised with thiopentone induction, alfentanil, nitrous oxide in oxygen. (0 = fully alert, no amnesia, orientated and cooperative; 9 = unresponsive). *Indicates statistically significant differences between the TIVA groups (**$P < 0.01$). †Indicates statistically significant differences between TIVA + flumazenil group and reference group (†$P < 0.05$, ‡$P < 0.01$). (From Nilsson et al., 1988.)

in the group given midazolam infusion, resedation was a frequent phenomenon (Fig. 3.11). One explanation of this difference may be that after cessation of an infusion, more drug has been distributed and the speed of recovery is more dependent on the elimination process (Persson, 1987). Also, concomitant opioid administration potentiates the sedative effect of midazolam (Persson et al., 1988).

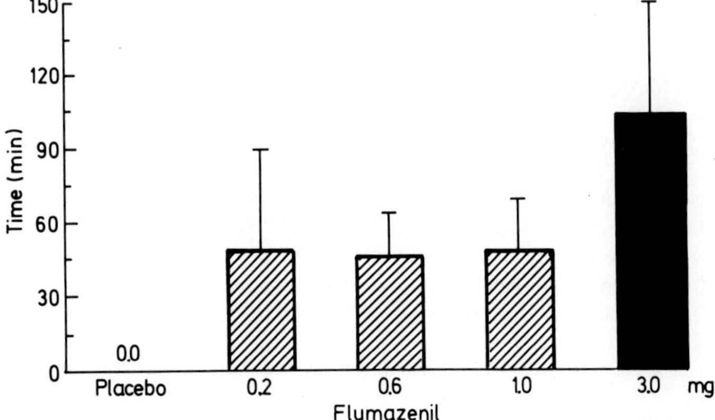


Fig 3.12. Mean time (±SD) of reversal following different i.v. doses of flumazenil in volunteers given a steady-state infusion of midazolam. (From Dunton et al., 1988.)

In an interesting report (Dunton et al., 1988) low doses of flumazenil (0.007—0.014 mg/kg) were found to consistently reverse diazepam and lorazepam induced sedation but the duration was short, approximately 45 min. The same report also includes a study where 0, 0.2, 0.6, 1.0 or 3.0 mg of flumazenil was given to volunteers having a constant degree of conscious sedation produced by an infusion of midazolam. The highest dose of flumazenil resulted in a reversal of sedation with a duration approximately twice as long as the other doses (Fig. 3.12).

Consequently, there is a possible conflict between the recommended dosage procedure with titration to least effective dose and the need to prolong the action of the antagonist. This is most likely to appear after administration of high and/or repeated doses of benzodiazepine agonists. Also, one must remember that the antagonism is competitive and it is possible to achieve a patient that is responsive and alert but with total amnesia. The effect of flumazenil on midazolam-induced ventilatory depression also seems to be of limited duration as presented in two recent reports (Dailland et al., 1988; Barakat et al., 1988).

Before more information about this complex problem has been gained it must be realised that use of flumazenil in both in- and outpatients does not reduce the duration of postoperative surveillance but nursing can be facilitated by making the patient responsive and mobile and by reducing the risk of loss of airway control, aspiration etc. The recovery staff involved must be informed that an antagonist has been used and that a second injection may be necessary. In the treatment of drug overdose, when the duration of a single bolus dose of flumazenil is usually insufficient to prevent resedation, the use of an infusion of 0.1—0.4 mg/h is recommended. Of course, infusions may be used postoperatively to maintain the reversal but for practical reasons this method is not applicable to routine anaesthesia.

## REFERENCES


Alexander, C.M. and Gross, J.B. (1988) Sedative doses of midazolam depress hypoxic ventilatory responses in humans. *Anesth. Analg.* 67, 377—382.

Amrein, R., Leishman, B., Bentzinger, C. and Roncari, G. (1987) Flumazenil in benzodiazepine antagonism. Actions and clinical use in intoxications and anaesthesiology. *Med. Toxicol.* 2, 411—429.

Arvidsson, S., Niemand, D., Martinell, S. and Ekström-Jodal, B. (1984) Aminophylline reversal of diazepam sedation. *Anaesthesia* 39, 806—809.

Avram, M.J., Fragan, R.J. and Caldwell, N.J. (1983) Midazolam kinetics in women of two age groups. *Clin. Pharmacol. Ther.* 34, 505—508.

Ausems, M.E., Hug, C.C. and de Lange, S. (1983) Variable rate infusion of alfentanil as a supplement to nitrous oxide anaesthesia for general surgery. *Anesth. Analg.* 62, 982—986.

Bach, V., Carl, P., Ravlo, O., Crawford, M.E., Jensen, A.G., Ohrt Michelsen, B., Crevoisier, C., Heizmann, P. and Fattinger, K. (1989) A randomized comparison between midazolam and thiopental for elective Cesarean section anaesthesia : 111. Placental transfer and elimination in neonates. *Anesth. Analg.* 68, 238—242.

Baehrendtz, S. and Höjer, J. (1988) Flumazenil in self-induced benzodiazepine poisoning. *Eur. J. Anaesthesiol.* Suppl. 2, 287—293.

Barakat, T., Lechat, J.P., Laurent, P., Fletcher, D., Clerque, F. and Viars, P. (1988) Ventilatory effects of flumazenil on midazolam-induced sedation. *Anesthesiology* 69, A817.

Berggren, L., Eriksson, I., Mollenholt, P. and Wickbom, G. (1983) Sedation for fiberoptic gastroscopy; a comparative study of midazolam and diazepam. *Br. J. Anaesth.* 55, 289—296.

Berggren, L., Eriksson, I. and Mollenholt, P. (1987) Cuanges in breathing pattern and chest wall mechanics after benzodiazepines in combination with meperidine. *Acta. Anaesthesiol. Scand.* 31, 381—386.

Bernards, C.M., Carpenter, R.L., Rup. S.M., Brown, D.L., Morse, B.V., Morell, R.C. and Thompson, G.E. (1988) The effect of benzodiazepine premedication on the toxicity of bupivacaine. *Anesthesiology* 69, No 3A A871.

Bodenham, A., Shelly, M.P. and Park, G.R. (1988) The altered pharmacokinetics and pharmacodynamics of drugs commonly used in critically ill patients. *Clin. Pharmacokinet.* 14, 347—373.

Boralessa, H., Senior, D.F. and Whitwam, J.G. (1983) Cardiovascular response to intubation. *Anaesthesia* 38, 623—627.

Breimer, L.T., Hennis, P.J., Bovill, J.G. and Spierdijk, J. (1988) The efficacy of flumazenil versus physostigmine after midazolam-alfentanil anaesthesia in man. *Eur. J. Anaesthesiol.*, Suppl. 2. 109—116.

Brogden, R.N. and Goa, K.L. (1988) Flumazenil. A preliminary review of its benzodiazepine antagonist properties, intrinsic activity and therapeutic use. *Drugs* 35, 448—467.

Caldwell, C.B. and Gross, J.B. (1982) Physostigmine reversal of midazolam induced sedation. *Anesthesiology* 57, 125—127.

Chiolero, R., Ravussin, P., Chassot, P.G., Neff, R. and Freeman, J. (1986) Ro 15—1788 for rapid recovery after craniotomy. *Anesthesiology* 65, A466.

Chiolero, R.L., Ravussin, P., Anderes, J.P. Lederman, P. and de Tribolet, N. (1988) The effects of midazolam reversal by Ro 15—1788 on cerebral perfusion pressure in patients with severe head injury. *Intensive Care Med.* 14, 196—200.

Claeys, M.A., Camu, F., Schneider, L. and Gepts, E. (1988) Reversal of flunitrazepam with flumazenil: duration of antagonist activity. *Eur. J. Anaesthesiol.* Suppl. 2, 209—217.

Crawford, M.E., Carl, P., Bach, V., Ravlo, O., Ohrt Michelsen, B. and Werner, M. (1988) A randomized comparison between midazolam and thiopental for elective cesarean section anesthesia: I. Mothers. *Anesth. Analg.* 68, 229—233.

Crevat-Pisano, P., Dragna, S., Granthil, C., Coassolo, P., Cano, J. P. and Francois, G. (1986) Plasma concentrations and pharmacokinetics of midazolam during anaesthesia. *J. Pharm. Pharmacol.* 38, 578—582.

Crevoisier, C., Ziegler, W.H., Eckert, M. and Heizmann, P. (1983) Relationship between plasma concentration and effect of midazolam after oral and intravenous administration. *Br. J. Clin. Pharmacol.* 16, 51S—61S.

Dailland, Ph., Lirzin, J.D., Jugan, E., Jacquinot, P., Jarrot, J.C. and Conseiller, Ch. (1988) Effect of Ro 15—1788 (flumazenil) on the $CO_2$ responsiveness after midazolam-fentanyl anesthesia. *Anesthesiology* 69, A815.

Darragh, A., Lambe, R., Kenny, M. and Brick, I. (1983) Tolerance of healthy volunteers to intravenous administration of the benzodiazepine antagonist Ro 15—1788. *Eur. J. Clin. Pharmacol.* 24, 569—570.

Dawson, D. and Sear, J.W. (1986) Influence of induction of anaesthesia with midazolam on the neuroendocrine response to surgery. *Anaesthesia* 41, 268—271.

De Castro, J. (1987) The use of midazolam and opioid associations in anesthesia (ataranalgesia). *Acta Anaesthesiol. Belg.* 38, Suppl. 1. 33—44.

Dundee, J.W., Halliday, N.J., Harper, K.W. and Brogden R.N. (1984) Midazolam. A review of its pharmacological properties and therapeutic use. *Drugs* 28, 519—543.

Dundee, J.W. and Wyant, G.M. (1988) *The Benzodiazepines, Intravenous Anaesthesia*, 2nd Edn. Churchill Livingstone, Edinburgh, London, Melbourne and New York, pp. 184—205.

Dunton, A.W., Schwam, E., Pitman, V., McGrath, J., Hendler, J. and Siegel, J., (1988) Flumazenil; US clinical pharmacology studies. *Eur. J. Anaesthesiol.*, Suppl. 2, 81—102.

Fee, J.P.H., Dundee, J.W., Collier, P.S. and Mclean, E. (1984) Bioavailability of intravenous diazepam. *Lancet* 2, 813.

Fleisher, J.E., Milde, J.H., Moyer, T.P. and Michenfelder, J.D. (1988) Cerebral effects of high-dose midazolam and subsequent reversal with Ro 15—1788 in dogs. *Anesthesiology* 68, 234—242.

Forster, A., Juge, O., Louis, M. and Nahory, A. (1987) Effects of a specific benzodiazepine antagonist Ro 15—1788 on cerebral blood flow. *Anesth. Analg.* 66, 309—313.

Galletly, D., Forrest, P. and Purdie, G. (1988) Comparison of the recovery characteristics of diazepam and midazolam. *Br. J. Anaesth.* 60, 520—524.

Geller, E., Niv, D., Rudick, V. and Vidne, B. (1984) The use of Ro 15—1788: a benzodiazepine antagonist in the diagnosis and treatment of benzodiazepine overdose. *Anesthesiology* 61, Suppl., A135.

Geller, E., Niv, D., Nevo, Y., Leykin, Y., Sorkin, P. and Rudick, V. (1988) Early clinical experience in reversing benzodiazepine sedation with flumazenil after short procedures. *Resuscitation* 16. Suppl. 549—556.

Haefely, W.E., (1987) Structure and function of the benzodiazepine receptor. *Chimia* 41., Suppl., 389—396.

Hall, R.I., Schwieger, I.M. and Hug, C.C. (1988) The anesthetic efficacy of midazolam in the enflurane-anesthetized dog. *Anesthesiology* 68, 862—866.

Harper, K.W., Collier, P.S., Dundee, J.W., Elliot, P., Halliday, N.J. and Lowry, K.G. (1985) Age and nature of operation influence the pharmacokinetics of midazolam. *Br. J. Anaesth.* 57, 866—871.

Hennis, P.J., van Haastert, F.A., Mulder, A.J. and Spierdijk, J. (1988) Antagonism of midazolam sedation by flumazenil: a placebo-controlled study in patients recovering from intravenous anaesthesia with high doses of midazolam *Eur. J. Anaesthesiol.* 5, 369—376.

Hoffman, W.E., Miletich, D.J. and Albrecht, R.F. (1986) The cerebrovascular and cerebral metabolic effects of midazolam and its interaction with $N_2O$. *Anesthesiology* 65, A355.

Jawad, S., Oxley, J., Wilson, J. and Richens, A. (1986) A pharmacodynamic evaluation of midazolam as an antiepileptic compound. *J. Neurol. Neurosurg. Psychiatry* 49, 1050—1054.

Kanto, J., Sjövall, S. and Vuori, A. (1982) Effect of different kinds of premedication on the induction properties of midazolam. *Br. J. Anaesth.* 54, 507—511.

Klausen, N.O., Juhl, O., Sörensen, J., Ferguson, A.H. and Neumann, P.B. (1988) Flumazenil in total intravenous anaesthesia using midazolam and fentanyl. *Acta Anaesthesiol. Scand.* 32, 409—412.

Klotz, U., Ziegler, G. and Reimann, I.W. (1984) Pharmacokinetics of the selective benzodiazepine antagonist Ro 15—1788 in man. *Eur. J. Clin. Pharmacol.* 27, 115—117.

Kochs, E., Roewer, N., Peter. A. and Schulte-am-Esch, J. (1988) Wirkungen von Flumazenil auf den globalen zerebralen blutfluss und den intrakraniellen druck in der reperfusionsphase nach globaler inkompletter zerebraler ischaemie. *Anesth. Intensivther. Notfallsmed.* 23, 159—162.

Lauven, P.M. Schwilden, H., Stoeckel, H. and Greenblatt, D.J. (1985) The effects of a benzodiazepine antagonist Ro 15—1788 in the presence of stable concentrations of midazolam. *Anesthesiology* 63, 61—64.

Lepage, J-Y., Blanloeil, Y., Pinaud, M., Helias, J., Auneau, C., Cozian, A. and Souron, R. (1986) Hemodynamic effects of diazepam, flunitrazepam and midazolam in patients with ischemic heart disease; assessment with a radionuclide approach. *Anesthesiology* 65, 678—683.

Mathers, D.A. (1987) The GABA receptor; new insights from single-channel recording. *Synapse* 1, 96—101.

Moreau, J.L. and Pieri, L. (1987) Modification of morphine antinociception by intrathecally (i.t.) administered benzodiazepine receptor ligands. *Br. J. Clin. Pharmacol.* 92, Suppl., 652P.

Möller, J.T. and Lybecker H. (1986) Total intravenous anaesthesia with midazolam and alfentanil. Beitrage zur Anaestheiologie und Intensivmedizin: V11 European Congress of Anaesthesiology, A780. Verlag Wilhelm Maudrich, Wien-München-Bern.

Muller von, H., Schleussner, E., Stoganov, M., Kling, D. and Hempelmann, G., (1981) Hämodynamische Wirkungen und charkteristika der Narkoseeinleitung mit Midazolam. *Arzneimittel-Forschung/Drug Research* 31, 2227—2232.

Nilsson, A., Lee., P.F.S. and Revenäs, B. (1984) Midazolam as induction agent prior to inhalational anaesthesia: a comparison with thiopentone. *Acta Anesthesiol. Scand.* 28, 249—251.

Nilsson, A., Tamsen, A., and Persson, P. (1986) Midazolam-fentanyl anesthesia for major surgery. Plasma levels of midazolam during prolonged total intravenous anesthesia. *Acta. Anaesthesiol. Scand.* 30, 66—69.

Nilsson, A., Persson, M.P. and Hartvig, P (1988) Effects of flumazenil on postoperative recovery after total intravenous anaesthesia with midazolam and alfentanil. *Eur. J. Anaesthesiol.*, Suppl. 2, 251—256.

Nilsson, A., Persson, M.P., Hartvig, P. and Wide, L. (1988) Effect of total intravenous anaesthesia with midazolam/alfentanil on the adrenocortical and hyperglycaemic response to abdominal surgery. *Acta. Anaesthesiol. Scand.* 32, 379—382.

Nilsson, E. and Himberg, J.J. (1982) Physostigmine for postoperative somnolence after diazepam nitrous oxide anaesthesia. *Acta Anaesthesiol. Scand.* 26, 9—14.

O'Boyle, C.A., Barry, H., Fox. E., Harris, D and McCreary, C. (1987) Benzodiazepine-induced event amnesia following a stressful surgical procedure. *Psychopharmacology* 91, 244—247.

O'Sullivan, G.F. and Wade, D.N. (1987) Flumazenil in the management of acute drug overdose with benzodiazepines and other agents. *Clin. Pharmacol. Ther.* 42, 254—259.

Paalzow, L. (1985) Proceedings from a symposium of the Swedish Association of Anaesthetists, Uppsala.

Persson, M.P. (1987) Rate-controlled intravenous infusion of midazolam and opioid analgesics in surgical patients. Ph.D. thesis, University of Uppsala, Sweden.

Persson, M.P., Nilsson, A., Hartvig, P. and Tamsen, A. (1987) Pharmacokinetics of midazolam in total i.v. anaesthesia. *Br. J. Anaesth.* 59, 548—556.

Persson, M.P., Nilsson, A., Hartvig, P. (1988) Relation of sedation and amnesia to plasma concentrations of midazolam in surgical patients. *Clin. Pharmacol. Ther.* 43, 324—331.

Polc, P., Bonetti, E.P., Schaffner, R. and Haefley, W. (1982) A three-state model of the benzodiazepine receptor explains the interaction between the benzodiazepine antagonist Ro 15-1788, benzodiazepine tranquillizers, $\beta$-carbolines, and phenobarbitone. *Naunyn-Schmiedeberg's Arch. Pharmacol.* 321, 260.

Radakovic, D., Toia, D. and Bentzinger, C., (1988) Double-blind, placebo-controlled study of the effects of R0 15—1788 (Flumazenil, Anexate) on recovery of ventilatory function after total i.v. anaesthesia with midazolam-alfentanyl. *Eur. J. Anaesthesiol.* Suppl. 2, 279—282.

Raeder, J.C., Hole, A., Arnulf, V. and Hougens Grynne, B. (1988) Total intravenous anaesthesia with midazolam and flumazenil in outpatient clinics. A comparison with isoflurane or thiopentone. *Acta Anaesthesiol. Scand.* 31, 634—641.

Ravlo, O., Carl, P., Crawford, M.E., Bach, V., Ohrt Michelsen, B. and Kierkegaard Nielsen, H. (1989) A randomised comparison between midazolam and thiopental for elective cesarean section anesthesia; II. Neonates. *Anesth. Analg.* 68, 234—237.

Raza, S.M.A., Masters, R.W., Vasireddy, A.R. and Zsigmond, E.K. (1988) Haemodynamic stability with midazolam -sufentanil analgesia in cardiac surgical patients. *Can. J. Anaesthesiol.* 35, 518—525.

Reeves, J.G., Glass, P. and Jacobs, J.R. (1989) Alfentanil and midazolam: New anesthetic drugs for continuous infusion and an automated method of administration. *Mt. Sinai. J. Med.* 56, 99—107.

Reitan, J.A. Porter, W. and Braunstein M. (1986) Comparison of psychomotor skills and amnesia after induction of anesthesia with midazolam or thiopental. *Anaesth. Analg.* 65, 933—937.

Reitan, J.A., and Soliman, I.E. (1987) A comparison of midazolam and diazepam for induction of anaesthesia in high-risk patients. *Anaesth. Intensive Care* 15, 175—178.

Reiz. S. (1988) Myocardial ischemia associated with general anaesthesia. *Br. J. Anaesth.* 61, 68—84.

Reves, J.G., Kissin, I., Fournier, S.E. and Smith, L.R. (1984) Additive negative in-tropic effect of a combination of diazepam and fentanyl. *Anesth. Analg.* 63, 97.

Reves, J.G., Fragen, R.J., Vinik, H.R. and Greenblatt, D.J. (1985) Midazolam: pharmacology and uses. *Anesthesiology* 62, 310—324.

Roberts, F.L., Dixon, J., Lewis, G.T.R., Tackley, R.M. and Prys-Roberts, C. (1988) Induction and maintenance of propofol anaesthesia. A manual infusion scheme. *Anaesthesia* 43, Suppl., 14—17.

Rodrigo, M.R.C. and Rosenquist, J.B. (1987) The effect of Ro 15—1788 (Anexate) on conscious sedation produced with midazolam. *Anaesth. Intensive Care* 15, 185—192.

Rowland, M. and Tozer, T.N. (1980) *Clinical Pharmacokinetics: Concepts and Applications.* Lea & Febiger, Philadelphia.

Sage, D.J., Close, A., Boas, R.A. (1987) Reversal of midazolam sedation with Anexate. *Br. J. Anaesth.* 59, 459—464.

Samuelson, P.N., Reves, J.G., Kouchoukos, N.T., Smith, L.R. and Dole, K.M. (1981) Hemodynamic responses to anesthetic induction with midazolam or diazepam in patients with ischemic heart disease. *Anesth. Analg.* 60, 802—809.

Scollo-Lavizzari, G (1988) The clinical anti-convulsant effects of flumazenil, a benzodiazepine antagonist. *Eur. J. Anaesthesiol.* Suppl. 2, 129—138.

Sear, J.W. (1983) General kinetic and dynamic principles and their application to continuous infusion anaesthesia. *Anaesthesia* 38, Suppl. 10—25.

Serrao, J.M., Goodchild, C.S. and Gent, J.P. (1988) Naloxone reverses the analgesic effect of intrathecal midazolam: a comparison with mu and kappa opioid agonists, In: 9th World Congress of Anaesthesiologists, May 22—28, 1988, Washington D.C., *Abstracts,* Vol. 2, A 732.

Shapiro, J.D., el-Ganzouri. A., White, P.F. and Ivankovich, A.D. (1988) Midazolam-alfentanil anesthesia for phaechromocytoma resection. *Can. J. Anaesthesiol.* 35, 190—194.

Short, T.G., Forrest, P. and Galletly, D.C. (1987) Paradoxical reactions to benzodiazepines — a genetically determined phenomenon? *Anesth. Intensive Care* 15, 330—331.

Sleigh, J.W. (1986) Failure of aminophylline to antagonize midazolam sedation. *Anesth. Analg.* 65, 540.

Stanski, D.R. and Hudson, R.J., (1985) Midazolam pharmacology and pharmacokinetics. *Anesthesiol. Rev.* 12, Suppl., 21—23.

Stirt, J.A. (1981) Aminophylline is a diazepam antagonist. *Anesth. Analg.* 60, 767—768.

Sunzel, M., Paalzow, L., Berggren, L. and Eriksson, I. (1988) Respiratory and cardiovascular effects in relation to plasma levels of midazolam and diazepam. *Br. J. Clin. Pharmacol.* 25, 561—569.

Trouvin, J.H., Farinotti, R., Harberer, J.P., Servin, F., Chauvin M., and Duvaldestin, P., (1988) Pharmacokinetics of midazolam in anaesthetized cirrhotic patients. *Br. J. Anaesth.* 60, 762—767.

Tuman, K.J., Spiess, B.D., Wong, C.A. and Ivankovich, A.D. (1988) Sufentanil-midazolam anesthesia in malignant hyperthermia. *Anesth. Analg.* 67, 405—408.

Tverskoy, M., Fleyshman, G., Bradley, E.L. and Kissin, I. (1988) Midazolam-thiopental anesthetic interactions in patients. *Anesth. Analg.* 67, 342—345.

Tverskoy, M., Fleyshman, G., Ezry, J., Bradley, E.L. and Kissin, I. (1989) Midazolam-morphine sedative interaction in patients. *Anesth. Analg.* 68, 282—285.

Vinik, H.R., Bradley, Jr., E.L. and Kissin, I. (1989) Midazolam-alfentanil synergism for anesthetic induction in patients. *Anesth. Analg.* 69, 213—217.

White, P.F., Shafer, A., Boyle, W.A. and Doze, V.A. (1988) Stress response following reversal of benzodiazepine-induced sedation. *Eur. J. Anaesthesiol.* Suppl. 2, 173—176.

White, P.F., Vasconez, L.O., Mathes, S.A., Way, W.L. and Wender, L.A. (1988), Comparison of midazolam and diazepam for sedation during plastic surgery. *Plast. Reconstr. Surg.* 81, 703—710.

Wilson, E., Mackenzie, N. and Grant, I.S. (1988) A comparison of propofol and midazolam by infusion to provide sedation in patients who receive spinal anaesthesia. *Anesthesia* 43, Suppl. 91—94.

Wolff, J., Claussen, T.G. and Mikkelsen, B.O. (1986) Ro 15—1788 for postoperative recovery. *Anaesthesia* 41, 1001—1006.

Wolff, J. (1990) Cerebrovascular and metabolic effects of midazolam and flumazenil. *Acta Anaesthesiol. Scand.* 34, Suppl. 92. 75—77.

*B. Kay (ed.) Total Intravenous Anaesthesia*



# 4

# *Opioid anaesthesia*

J.G. Bovill

## INTRODUCTION

Opioids, in low to moderate doses, are widely used as supplements to the induction and maintenance of general anaesthesia. In this setting they contribute to the analgesic component of anaesthesia, and by reducing the minimum alveolar concentration (MAC) of inhalational anaesthetics permit lower concentrations of these agents to be used. In recent years intravenously administered opioids, alone or combined with a hypnotic, have increasingly been used also for the maintenance of anaesthesia. The term 'total intravenous anaesthesia' is often used to describe this technique. However, with the possible exception of cardiac anaesthesia, intravenous opioids are frequently combined with nitrous oxide or low concentrations of an inhalational agent, e.g. enflurane. For the purposes of this chapter, I will use the term 'opioid anaesthesia' to refer to any anaesthetic technique in which an opioid, in moderate to high doses, makes a major contribution to the anaesthetic state, whether or not this is supplemented by other agents.

## ADVANTAGES AND DISADVANTAGES

The advantages claimed for opioid anaesthesia are improved haemodynamic stability, suppression of the stress response to surgery, absence of organ toxicity and lack of operating theatre pollution. Opioid anaesthesia is, however, associated with disadvantages, which for an individual patient must be balanced against the possible advantages. All opioids cause a dose-dependent depression of respiration which makes it difficult to use this technique in spontaneously breathing patients. Furthermore, since the drug is only slowly eliminated from the body after stopping an intravenous infusion, the risk of respiratory depression can extend for some hours into the postoperative period. The use of high doses of opioids intra-operatively will also contribute to an increased incidence of nausea and vomiting postoperatively. Finally, muscle rigidity induced by opioids may give rise to problems, not only during induction of anaesthesia but also occasionally for up to several hours after surgery.

## HISTORY AND DEVELOPMENT

The widespread acceptance of high-dose opioid anaesthesia among cardiac anaesthetists was a major stimulus to the introduction of opioid anaesthesia for non-cardiac surgery. The use of this technique for cardiac surgery developed in the 1960s from the observation by Lowenstein and his colleagues in Boston, MA, that patients requiring artificial ventilation after surgery for end-stage valvular disease tolerated intravenous doses of morphine for sedation, exceeding any previously reported in the literature, without detectable circulatory deterioration. This observation led them to administer morphine, in doses up to 3.0 mg/kg, as the sole anaesthetic for these patients (Lowenstein et al., 1969). It soon became apparent, however, that whereas this dose of morphine was adequate for these critically ill patients, in other less critically ill patients it did have serious disadvantages. Major problems included inadequate anaesthesia, even with extremely high doses of 8 to 11 mg/kg, episodes of hypotension due to histamine release and increased intra- and postoperative blood and fluid requirements (Lowenstein et al., 1971; Stanley et al., 1973). Attempts to overcome these problems by combining lower doses of morphine with a variety of supplements, e.g., nitrous oxide, halothane or diazepam proved unsatisfactory, resulting in significant myocardial depression, with decreases in cardiac output and falls in arterial blood pressure (Stoelting and Gibbs, 1973; Stoelting et al., 1974; Stanley et al., 1976).

Because of the above problems associated with the use of morphine, several other opioids were investigated in an attempt to find a suitable alternative. Pethidine, when given in doses that produced anaesthesia, caused significant hypotension, tachycardia and marked myocardial depression (Stanley and Liu, 1977). Hydromorphone, a hydrogenated-ketone derivative of morphine, that is 7 to 10 times as potent and 8 to 10 times as lipid soluble as morphine, was also investigated. Like morphine, hydromorphone did not reliably produce anaesthesia and supplementation with nitrous oxide and halothane was necessary for unconsciousness and complete suppression of sympathetic responses during surgery (Welti et al., 1984). The use of fentanyl as a total anaesthetic was reported by Stanley and Webster in 1978. Since then there have been extensive investigations of fentanyl, and more recently of its two newer congeners, sufentanil and alfentanil, in cardiac surgery (Bovill et al., 1984a; Sebel and Bovill, 1987). The fentanyl group of drugs has proved to be the most reliable and effective opioids for producing anaesthesia both for patients with valvular disorders and those undergoing coronary artery surgery.

## CHOICE OF OPIOID

A major advantage of fentanyl and its analogues for patients undergoing cardiac surgery is their lack of cardiovascular depression. This is of particular importance during the induction of anaesthesia, when episodes of hypotension can be crucial. Also the ability of opioids to obtund haemodynamic responses to laryngoscopy and intubation of the trachea is an important advantage. However, cardiovascular stability may be less evident during surgery, and in particular the period of sternotomy and aortic root dissection may be associated with significant hypertension and tachycardia, which is not always amenable to increasing doses of opioid.

There may be differences between the opioids in regard to haemodynamic stability during surgery. One study (Miller et al., 1988) concluded that both fentanyl and sufentanil provide similar haemodynamic stability during induction, whereas alfentanil caused haemodynamic instability and myocardial ischaemia. Alfentanil may also be less effective in suppressing reflex sympathetic and haemodynamic responses to stimuli than fentanyl or sufentanil (Swenzen et al., 1988). Howie et al. (1985) also found little difference between fentanyl and sufentanil anaesthesia in patients undergoing elective coronary artery surgery, although systemic vascular resistance was significantly lower in the sufentanil group. In patients undergoing valvular heart surgery all three opioids provided satisfactory anaesthesia (Bovill et al., 1984b).

However, controversy still surrounds the best choice of anaesthetic, at least for coronary artery surgery. Two recent studies, together involving over 2000 patients anaesthetized with either inhalational agents, or fentanyl or sufentanil, came to the conclusion that the choice of anaesthetic technique did not significantly influence the outcome after coronary artery surgery (Slogoff and Keats, 1989; Tuman et al., 1989).

### Use in children

High dose opioid anaesthesia has proved to be effective for cardiac surgery in infants (Hickey and Hansen, 1984; Robinson and Gregory, 1981). The ability of high-dose fentanyl and sufentanil to modify the pathological stress responses to surgery was considered a significant advantage of this technique, especially for neonates (Anand et al., 1987a,b). In older children between 4 and 12 years, sufentanil in bolus form in doses up to 20 μg/kg did not provide suitable anaesthesia (Moore et al., 1985). My personal experience, however, is that sufentanil given by continuous infusion, at a dose of 0.05—0.1 μg/kg per min, produces satisfactory anaesthesia in this population.

## OPIOID 'ANAESTHESIA'?

While opioids have been used as the primary drug for anaesthesia, e.g. for cardiac surgery, controversy still surrounds the question as to whether they are indeed capable of adequately producing a true state of anaesthesia. Some are firmly convinced that opioids do not produce unconsciousness or amnesia (Wong, 1983), and thus, according to the definition of anaesthesia proposed by Prys-Roberts (1987), are not anaesthetics.

This scepticism has been enhanced by isolated reports of awareness in patients given high doses of fentanyl for cardiac surgery (Mummaneni et al., 1980; Mark and Greenberg, 1983). It should be pointed out, however, that incidents of awareness are not confined to patients given opioids for anaesthesia. Numerous cases have been reported of patient awareness during apparently adequate general anaesthesia (Mainzer, 1979; Jones and Konieczko, 1986). Based on over ten years experience with the use of various opioids for cardiac anaesthesia, this author is convinced that opioids, in appropriate doses, are anaesthetics. Never have I failed to produce unconsciousness in a patient, and patients seldom respond, either haemodynamically or somatically to laryngoscopy or intubation of the trachea. Thus, according to Prys-Roberts' (1987) definition of the anaesthetic state, opioids are anaesthetics.

With the exception of morphine, which is by far the least effective of the opioids as an anaesthetic, opioids produced a marked change in the EEG characterized by slow, synchronized delta waves and the virtual absence of frequencies higher than 8—10 Hz (Sebel et al., 1981; Bovill et al., 1982; Smith et al., 1984; Smith et al., 1985). These changes, reflecting generalized cortical depression, i.e. anaesthesia (Rampil et al., 1980), are similar to those seen during surgical anaesthesia with conventional anaesthetic agents.

Increases in the EEG frequency power distribution during alfentanil anaesthesia may indicate pending or existing inadequate depth of anaesthesia (Stanski et al., 1987). EEG descriptors derived from aperiodic analysis rather than spectral analysis, such as the cumulative power to 3 Hz (CP3) may be the most sensitive indicators of a light level of opioid anaesthesia (Smith et al., 1985). The inhalational agents and the intravenous barbiturates, thiopentone and methohexitone, alter both the brain stem as well as the cortical part of the auditory evoked response, reflecting widespread CNS depression (Jones and Konieczko, 1986). In contrast fentanyl, in common with etomidate, althesin and nitrous oxide, has no effect on the brain stem but attenuates the amplitude of the cortical waves in the auditory response, evidence that fentanyl causes cortical depression.

The exact mechanism by which opioids cause cortical depression resulting in unconsciousness is not known. It is reasonable to assume that it in some way involves opioid receptors since it can be reversed by appropriate doses of naloxone (Murphy and Hug, 1983). It has also been speculated by Stone and DiFazio (1988) that the anaesthetic effect of very high concentrations of opioid may involve a membrane effect in addition to receptor interaction. Their conclusion was based on the similarity between the calculated brain lipid content of a variety of opioids associated with a 50% reduction in maximum spectra edge frequency of the EEG in man and 50% MAC reduction in animals. A non-receptor mechanism for the loss of the righting reflex induced by leucine enkephalin in amphibians has been proposed (Dodson and Miller, 1985). In rats, anaesthesia (no response to bone-crush injury) occurred at doses of lofentanil, a highly potent fentanyl analogue, that produced only about 25% of receptor occupancy (Stanley et al., 1983).

While high doses of opioids produce intense analgesia and unconsciousness, there is good experimental and clinical evidence that the anaesthesia produced is different to that produced by the classical anaesthetic agents. The dose-response curve for anaesthesia with opioids is not linear but reaches a plateau beyond a certain plasma concentration. One measure of a drugs ability to act as an anaesthetic is the degree by which it can reduce the MAC of a volatile anaesthetic. In a series of experiments the group lead by Hug from Atlanta, GA, has demonstrated that, for morphine, fentanyl, sufentanil and alfentanil, there is a ceiling effect in terms of their ability to reduce the MAC of enflurane in dogs (Murphy and Hug, 1982a,b; Hall et al., 1987a,b). This ceiling effect was around 65—70% reduction for each of these drugs. Morphine reduces halothane MAC by 84% in rats (Lake et al., 1985). By contrast, the mixed agonist-antagonists nalbuphine and butorphanol were only capable of reducing enflurane MAC by 8% and 11%, respectively (Murphy and Hug, 1982a). In a rat model, the maximum decrease in the MAC of halothane by nalbuphine was 20% (DiFazio et al., 1981).

The mixed agonist-antagonists are only minimally effective as anaesthetics in humans. Butorphanol 0.3 mg/kg (equivalent to 1.5—2.0 mg/kg morphine) does not render patients unconscious (Moldenhauer et al., 1981). In patients with coronary or valvular heart disease, nalbuphine 2 mg/kg did not produce anaesthesia (Lake et al., 1982). The difference between the mu-agonists and the mixed agonist-antagonists appears to be the result of the antagonist potential of the latter group. Drugs such as nalbuphine and butorphanol are primarily kappa-receptor agonists and antagonists at the mu-receptor. Selective kappa-receptor agonists reduce the MAC of halothane by about 70% (Althaus et al., 1987, 1988).

Hecker et al. (1983) reported that sufentanil reduced halothane MAC by about 90% in rats, with a plateau in the response curve occurring at a dose of 0.11 $\mu$g/kg per min. This is markedly different from the findings of Hall et al. (1987a) of a maximum reduction (70%) of enflurane MAC in dogs despite a dose of sufentanil ten times that used by Hecker et al. It is unlikely that these differences can be attributed to the differences in the inhalational anaesthetic used in the two studies. A possible explanation could be differences in responses to sufentanil between dogs and rats.

There is a remarkable similarity between the plasma concentrations of opioids associated with maximum MAC reduction in dogs and those that have maximum anaesthetic efficacy in dogs and humans. The plateau in the reduction of enflurane MAC in dogs occurred at fentanyl concentration about 30 ng/ml (Murphy and Hug, 1982b). Similar fentanyl concentrations result in maximum suppression of haemodynamic and somatic responses to application of a tail-clamp in dogs (Arndt et al., 1984). In patients undergoing cardiac surgery, concentrations of fentanyl greater than 20 ng/ml cause little further reduction in haemodynamic responses to sternotomy and aortic dissection (Sprigge et al., 1982; Wyands et al., 1984). There are comparable similarities between the studies reported above in dogs with sufentanil and findings in humans (Philbin et al., 1986). The plasma alfentanil concentrations required to produce equivalent anaesthetic effect in humans (Ausems et al., 1986) and dogs (Hall et al., 1987b) are also similar.

## ADJUVANT DRUG THERAPY

From the above discussion, it is evident that attempts to provide anaesthesia with high doses of opioids alone may be inappropriate. In routine clinical practice, however, opioids are seldom used in this way. The majority of patients receive premedication before surgery. Premedicant drugs reduce the MAC of inhalational agents and contribute significantly to the anaesthetic and haemodynamic effects of opioids (Hug et al., 1988; Thompson et al., 1988).

Younger patients with coronary artery disease undergoing cardiac surgery often exhibit a hyperdynamic circulation during sternotomy and aortic root dissection. Attempts to control this by increasing doses of opioids is often unsuccessful, for the reasons explained above. In this situation the judicious use of a volatile agent has a place. The use of low doses of enflurane or isoflurane in combination with fentanyl or sufentanil provides good anaesthesia with stable haemodynamics (Heikkila et al., 1987; Vermeyen et al., 1989). By allowing the total dose of the opioid to be reduced this technique may also reduce the period during which artificial ventilation is required postoperatively.

The combination of fentanyl and propofol has also been investigated for cardiac anaesthesia (Vermeyen et al., 1987; Russell et al., 1989). Because of the hypotensive effects of propofol, caution needs to be exercised with this technique and further experience is needed before it can be recommended for widespread use. There is evidence that the combination may have deleterious cardiovascular effects (Lepage et al., 1988). See also Chapter 12.

Benzodiazepines are often used as supplements to opioid anaesthesia. Diazepam causes a decrease in cardiac output and systemic vascular resistance when combined with fentanyl (Stanley and Webster, 1978). Anaesthesia with a combination of sufentanil, midazolam and nitrous oxide for cardiac surgery obtunded haemodynamic responses to surgical stimuli but resulted in marked hypotension in some patients during unstimulated periods (Windsor et al., 1988). Neither fentanyl nor diazepam, when given alone, produce important haemodynamic depression in patients. In the isolated rat heart preparation both fentanyl and diazepam, in doses about 400 times in excess of those encountered in patients, have a negative inotropic effect, but the combination of the two drugs produced an additive and not a supra-additive negative inotropy (Reeves et al., 1984). The changes observed in patients may be due to a reduction in plasma catecholamine levels (Tomicheck et al., 1983). The combination of sufentanil with midazolam and ketamine produced haemodynamic stability in cardiac surgical patients (Raza et al., 1989).

Presumably ketamine counteracts the peripheral vascular effects of the other two drugs.

The combination of nitrous oxide and high doses of opioids may have adverse haemodynamic and myocardial consequences. In patients with poor left ventricular function undergoing coronary artery surgery in whom anaesthesia was induced with fentanyl 50 μg/kg, addition of 50% nitrous oxide resulted in a significant decrease in cardiac index, an increase in systemic vascular resistance but no change in arterial blood pressure. These changes were not seen in patients with good ventricular function (Moffitt et al., 1984).

A study with an isolated papillary muscle preparation suggested that the negative inotropic effects of nitrous oxide and fentanyl were only additive (Motomura et al., 1984). However, there is evidence that the addition of nitrous oxide during fentanyl or sufentanil anaesthesia can produce regional myocardial dysfunction in dogs with stenotic coronary arteries (Philbin et al., 1985). In the absence of a critical coronary artery stenosis, no evidence of regional myocardial dysfunction was seen either with or without nitrous oxide. However, once a critical stenosis was produced in the left anterior descending (LAD) artery, the introduction of nitrous oxide caused rapid and significant dysfunction, measured by postsystolic shortening, in only the area of the LAD distribution. This evidence raises doubts about the wisdom of combining opioids and nitrous oxide in patients with coronary disease. Nonetheless, some investigators found no evidence of regional dysfunction or myocardial ischaemia when 66% nitrous oxide was added to the inspired gas mixture of patients anaesthetized with fentanyl (Cahalan et al., 1987).

## USE FOR NON-CARDIAC SURGERY

Intravenous opioids, alone or in combination with other drugs, are increasingly being used for non-cardiac surgery. Opioids are popular in neurosurgical anaesthesia because they do not affect the $CO_2$ reactivity of the cerebral blood vessels. They also have little effect on cerebral blood flow or intracranial pressure in ventilated patients. Sufentanil has become popular (McKay et al., 1984; Shupak et al., 1985), partly because of its favourable haemodynamic profile, and the possibility that postoperative respiratory depression may be less than with fentanyl (Clark et al., 1987). Alfentanil, in combination with droperidol, has also been used for neuroleptanalgesia for patients undergoing awake craniotomies, in which the patients cooperation intra-operatively was essential (Welling and Donegan, 1989). Alfentanil was chosen because of its more rapid onset and shorter duration of action. Alfentanil was given as an infusion of about 1.0—1.5 μg/kg per min, supplemented by additional boluses of alfentanil and droperidol.

### Infusion regimens

Not all of the many available opioids are suitable for use in total intravenous anaesthesia. The ideal drug for this application should have a rapid onset of action, a short elimination half-life and a broad therapeutic index. A rapid onset, i.e. minimal hysteresis between changes in plasma concentrations and desired effect, is essential to allow effective control during periods of changing stimulation, without the risk of overdose. A drug that is suitable for intravenous anaesthesia should be rapidly cleared from the body so that changes in plasma concentration, as demanded by the changing clinical situation, can be readily achieved, and so that recovery will be rapid once the infusion is terminated. The drug should be biotransformed to inactive metabolites since these will accumulate during a prolonged infusion and cause either toxic side effects and/or delay recovery.

Fentanyl has a long elimination half-life and would appear to be an unsuitable drug for use by continuous infusion. Nonetheless, there are numerous reports describing fentanyl infusion, in combination with nitrous oxide, for a variety of surgical procedures ranging from superficial operations to scoliosis surgery. In patients undergoing superficial surgery an initial dose of fentanyl 5 μg/kg followed by a constant infusion of fentanyl 3 μg/kg per h provided adequate anaesthesia (Andrews et al., 1982). This regimen resulted in plasma fentanyl concentrations at a steady state of 3—5 ng/ml. Somewhat higher concentrations (4—8 ng/ml) were required to maintain haemodynamic stability in patients undergoing abdominal surgery, anaesthetized with fentanyl and nitrous oxide (McQuay et al., 1979). Fentanyl concentrations of 2—3 ng/ml provide satisfactory analgesia, in the presence of 70% nitrous oxide, for minor surgical procedures (White et al., 1983). Infusions of fentanyl 0.6—3 μg/kg per h, in combination with nitrous oxide, have been successfully used for spinal fusion surgery, allowing a smooth wake-up test without the need for an opioid antagonist (Pathak et al., 1983).

Because of its pharmacokinetic and pharmacodynamic properties, alfentanil is the most appropriate opioid for administration by continuous infusion. The elimination half-life of alfentanil is about 90 min (Bovill et al., 1982b; Bower and Hull, 1982) compared with 185—220 min for fentanyl (McClain and Hug, 1980; Bower and Hull, 1982). The rapid elimination of alfentanil is due to a very small steady-state distribution volume, 27 l, compared to 335 l for fentanyl. The initial distribution volume is also smaller than for fentanyl. Because of differences in distribution and elimination plasma concentrations will decline to subtherapeutic levels faster with alfentanil than with fentanyl. This is reflected in a faster recovery.

All opioids are basic drugs that, with the exception of alfentanil, have $pK_a$ values higher than 7.4. The $pK_a$ of alfentanil (6.5) results in 89% of the free alfentanil molecules in plasma being unionized. This, together with a moderate lipid solubility, is responsible for rapid equilibration between plasma and brain concentration, and thus a fast onset of action. The half-time for plasma/brain equilibration, estimated by using the EEG as an effect parameter, is 1.1 min for alfentanil and 6.4 min for fentanyl (Scott et al., 1985). These properties of rapid onset of action and short elimination half-life allow the anaesthetist to titrate the plasma concentration to desired effect according to patient need.

The pharmacodynamics of alfentanil, i.e. the relationship between plasma concentration and effect, varies with the intensity of stimulation during anaesthesia

TABLE 4.1

$Cp_{50}$ values (the alfentanil plasma concentration for which the probability of no response is 50%) for different events and types of surgery (data from Ausems et al., 1986)

| Event | $Cp_{50}$ (ng/ml) | 95% Confidence limits |
|---|---|---|
| **Single event** | | |
| Intubation | 475 | 418—532 |
| Skin incision | 279 | 238—320 |
| Skin closure | 150 | 103—196 |
| Ventilation[a] | 223 | 197—249 |
| **Intra-operative events** | | |
| Lower abdominal surgery | 309 | 284—334 |
| Upper abdominal surgery | 412 | 319—505 |
| Breast surgery | 270 | 230—310 |

[a]In absence of $N_2O$.

and surgery. These have been defined for a variety of surgical procedures and for different age groups (Ausems et al., 1986; Lemmens et al., 1988). Alfentanil was given as a variable rate infusion with 70% nitrous oxide. Plasma concentrations were measured at frequent intervals and the responses of patients to defined perioperative stimuli recorded. Using logistic regression, curves describing the relationship between concentration and the probability of no response were produced. Each curve is defined by two parameters, a slope parameter and the $Cp_{50}$ (the alfentanil plasma concentration at which the probability of no response to a stimulus is 50%). The $Cp_{50}$ for single events, and for intra-operative events for three types of surgery are presented in Table 4.1. For breast surgery the $Cp_{50}$ values for intra-operative events were similar in younger patients ($<55$ years) and elderly patients ($>55$ years) although the dose of alfentanil needed was less for the elderly patients (Lemmens et al., 1988). Thus the pharmacodynamics of alfentanil are not age related. Age does, however, influence alfentanil pharmacokinetics (Maitre et al., 1987) as does gender (Maitre et al., 1987; Lemmens, 1989).

There are two approaches to the administration of alfentanil infusions for intravenous anaesthesia-fixed rate and variable rate. A common technique using fixed rate infusions involves a loading dose of 50—100 μg/kg followed by an infusion of 0.5—1.5 μg/kg per min (van Leeuwen et al., 1984). The loading dose can be given as a bolus or as a fast infusion. A disadvantage of a single large loading dose is the relatively high incidence of bradycardia, hypotension and muscle rigidity. This can be overcome by giving the loading dose as a fast infusion. A scheme that works well in practice, and furthermore is easy to remember, is 10 μg/kg per min for 10 min followed by 1 μg/kg per min. An infusion of alfentanil 1 μg/kg per min in combination with 60—70% nitrous oxide may be adequate for superficial surgery, but is not so for intra-abdominal operation. Incremental doses of alfentanil, 0.5—1 mg, will be needed for the latter type of surgery.

An alternative approach is to use a variable rate infusion, where necessary supplemented by incremental bolus doses. This is more analogous to the use of inhalational anaesthetics whereby the anaesthetist tries to adjust the plasma concentration of alfentanil to the patients response to the noxious stimulation of surgery and other procedures. Using this technique infusion rates will vary between 0.4 and 2.5 μg/kg per min (Ausems et al., 1983). When using a variable infusion rate technique it is important not only to increase the infusion rate when the patient reacts to noxious stimuli, but perhaps even more important to decrease the rate when no response to stimuli occur during a period of 10—15 min, to avoid unnecessary accumulation of alfentanil and prolonged recovery. Irrespective of whether fixed or variable rate infusions are used it is important to stop the infusion 15—20 min before the anticipated end of surgery to allow prompt recovery of consciousness and return of satisfactory spontaneous ventilation.

A refinement of the variable infusion technique is the use of a computer controlled infusion of alfentanil (Ausems et al., 1985; Lemmens et al., 1988). The computer program is provided with known pharmacokinetic data, and instead of adjusting an infusion rate, anaesthesia is regulated on the basis of predicted plasma concentrations of alfentanil. The accuracy of the predicted concentrations has proved to be reasonably good and is significantly improved when data derived from population kinetics are used (Maitre et al., 1988).

With the availability of rapid and short-acting drugs such as alfentanil and propofol, the possibility of true short-acting non-depolarizing muscle relaxants becoming available in the near future, and on-going developments in infusion pump technology, the application of total intravenous anaesthesia is certain to expand. One must not forget, however, that once a drug is injected intravenously, elimination is almost always dependent on metabolic pathways. Particularly when using opioids one must always be aware of the possibility of delayed respiratory depression. This is especially likely when supplements of i.m. opioids, or sedatives such as benzodiazepines, are given.

## PROBLEMS OF OPIOID ANAESTHESIA

### Respiratory depression

Respiratory depression is a pharmacological effect produced, in a dose-related fashion, by all pure mu-agonist opioids. In most situations it is an undesirable, and potentially fatal, side effect. In others, such as in patients requiring artificial ventilation, respiratory depression is considered a desirable property of these drugs. It is now generally agreed that respiratory depression is the result of activation of the low-affinity $mu_2$-receptor, whereas the high-affinity $mu_1$-receptor subtype is involved in analgesia (Pasternak and Wood, 1986). Pure kappa-receptor agonists have little or no effect on ventilation. This pharmacological separation of analgesia and respiratory depression raises the exciting possibility that, in the future, pure $mu_1$-receptor agonist drugs could be developed that would be potent analgesics without producing respiratory depression. Since the central effects of opioids on gastrointestinal function, and possibly also physical dependence, may also be mediated solely via $mu_2$-receptor (Pasternak, 1988), pure $mu_1$-agonists would offer very considerable clinical and social advantages over conventional drugs.

In addition to retention of carbon dioxide, impaired ventilatory drive caused by opioids may result in patients becoming hypoxic. The CNS has no intrinsic mechanism for detecting and responding to hypoxia, but relies on reflex stimulation that results from activation of peripheral arterial chemoreceptors in the aortic and carotid bodies (McQueen, 1983). The peripheral chemoreceptor response to hypoxia is almost totally abolished by volatile anaesthetic agents (Knill and Gelb, 1978). Although the response to opioids is less marked, they do depress the hypoxic drive to ventilation (Weil et al., 1975), thereby further jeopardizing patient safety. This can be a real problem in patients in whom the nerve or vascular supply to the aorta or carotid bodies has been damaged, e.g. following carotid endarterectomy. In this situation there may be markedly increased sensitivity to the respiratory depressant effects of opioids (Lee et al., 1981).

There have been several reports of delayed, life threatening, respiratory depression following the intra-operative use of opioids, including fentanyl (Becker et al., 1976; Adams and Pybus, 1978) and alfentanil (Lamarche et al., 1984; Sebel et al., 1984). In the case of alfentanil this drug was given by continuous infusion during surgery. Several explanations have been proposed for this delayed effect.

Anaesthesia and surgery may alter both the pharmacokinetics and the pharmacodynamics of drugs given intra-operatively, so that the response observed postoperatively may be different from that predicted from data obtained from volunteers or non-surgical subjects. Hypocapnic hyperventilation to an arterial $PCO_2$ of 2.7—3.3 kPa significantly decreases the whole-body clearance of fentanyl (Cartwright et al., 1983). This level of hypocapnia may occur during, e.g., neurosurgical anaesthesia. When a drug is given by continuous intravenous infusion, as is frequently the case with alfentanil, then the decline in plasma concentrations when the infusion is stopped is less rapid than from a comparable concentration following a single bolus injection. In both cases the initial decline in concentrations results from redistribution of the drug from blood to the tissues. Redistribution following a prolonged infusion is less marked because the tissues are already partially saturated. Indeed if the infusion were to be continued until a true steady state was reached between plasma and all tissue compartment then there would be no distribution phase, and plasma concentration would decline only as a result of the much slower metabolism and elimination of the drug.

Stimulation, and especially pain, is effective in counteracting the depressant effects of opioids. A patient who has received intra-operative opioids may breathe satisfactorily at the end of anaesthesia, when subjected to considerable external stimuli, e.g., removal of the tracheal tube, transfer to bed, etc., but may relapse into respiratory depression some time later when these stimuli are no longer present. Furthermore, the absence of external stimuli, good analgesia and possibly the residual influence of other depressant drugs given during anaesthesia, often results in patients falling asleep. Sleep causes a displacement of the $CO_2$ response curve to the right (Belville et al., 1959; Phillipson, 1978). Opioids and sleep act synergistically leading to impairment of ventilatory control (Catley et al., 1985).

Biphasic respiratory depression has been attributed to a secondary increase in plasma concentration during the elimination phase of fentanyl (McQuay et al., 1979; Stoeckel et al., 1982). It is likely that similar secondary increases in plasma concentration occur with other opioids, including alfentanil. One possible explanation for this phenomenon is enterohepatic recirculation, with sequestration of the drug in the stomach and subsequent reabsorption from the small intestine (Stoeckel et al., 1979). Because of partitioning of fentanyl into gastric juice due to the difference between the gastric pH and the p$K_a$ of fentanyl (8.4), as much as 16% of an administered dose may accumulate in the stomach. However, since the average volume of gastric juice is small (25—100 ml) the amount of fentanyl that will ultimately be presented to the small intestine for reabsorption is likely to be negligible. Furthermore, because of its high 'first-pass' hepatic metabolism, little of the reabsorbed fentanyl will reach the systemic circulation. Direct administration of fentanyl by nasogastric tube resulted in almost undetectable plasma fentanyl concentrations (Lehmann et al., 1982).

The conditions for ion trapping in the stomach are more favourable for alfentanil which has a p$K_a$ of 6.5, compared to 8.4. for fentanyl. Furthermore, alfentanil has only a moderate hepatic extraction so that a higher proportion of the reabsorbed drug can be expected to reach the systemic circulation. However, in animals less than 3% of the total dose of alfentanil is found in the stomach, so that enterohepatic recirculation is unlikely to contribute significantly to recurrent increases in its plasma concentration.

A more likely explanation is that secondary peaks are the result of reuptake from tissue stores, particularly muscle, as blood flow to these tissues increases at the end of surgery. The uptake of fentanyl into muscle is extensive (McClain and Hug, 1980). Because of its lower lipid solubility and smaller volume of distribution, muscle uptake of alfentanil should be much less and clinically significant increases in plasma concentration from redistribution from muscle stores is therefore less likely.

In addition to the parent drug, metabolites may in some circumstances contribute to respiratory depression. The metabolite morphine-6-glucuronide occurs in significant quantities after administrations of morphine. The concentration of morphine-6-glucoronide in plasma exceeds that of morphine within 30 min of intravenous administration (Osborne et al., 1990). This metabolite is pharmacologically active in humans and may be responsible for a considerable proportion of the effects of parenteral morphine (Hand et al., 1987). Morphine-6-glucoronide is a ventilatory depressant with a potency substantially in excess of that of free morphine (Pelligrino et al., 1989). Even allowing for its slower penetration into the brain, it may be that 50% or more of the respiratory depression observed by 1 h following systemic administration of morphine is due to this metabolite, and this contribution will subsequently increase with time (Pelligrino et al., 1989). It makes a significant contribution to morphine intoxication in patients with renal failure (Osborne et al., 1986). Neither fentanyl or alfentanil have metabolites that are pharmacologically active.

One of the metabolites of sufentanil, desmethyl-sufentanil, is pharmacologically active with a potency about one tenth that of sufentanil (Weldron et al., 1985). This metabolite is thus approximately equipotent with fentanyl. Its role in the pharmacological effects of prolonged infusions of sufentanil remains to be elucidated.

## Reversal of respiratory depression

Naloxone, a pure opioid antagonist, is the most commonly chosen drug for reversal of opioid-induced respiratory depression. However, its effects are not selective for ventilatory depression and analgesia will also be antagonized. Particularly when high doses of opioids have been given, this can result in undesirable haemodynamic changes, including tachycardia, hypertension, cardiac arrhythmias and pulmonary oedema (Flacke et al., 1977; Michaelis and Hickey, 1974; Azar and Turndorf, 1979). Sudden death following large doses of naloxone has been reported (Andree, 1980). The antagonism of morphine by naloxone in dogs was associated with 60% increases in coronary blood flow and myocardial oxygen consumption (Patschke et al., 1977). Such changes are potentially detrimental to patients with coronary artery disease. These haemodynamic changes have been attributed to release of catecholamines and sympathetic overactivity resulting from the acute reversal of analgesia (Azar et al., 1981). Potentiation of baroreceptor reflexes following administration of naloxone, so that an exaggerated haemodynamic response to subsequent stimulation occurs, may also contribute to these changes (Montastruc et al., 1981). Fortunately not all administrations of naloxone have such untoward consequences. A recent study suggests that increases in blood pressure and plasma catecholamines after naloxone may be minimized when normocapnia or hypocapnia is established before naloxone is given (Mills et al., 1988).

Because the action of naloxone is of shorter duration than that of most opioids, the chance of recurrence of respiratory depression after single dose administration is real. This can be overcome by giving a continuous infusion of naloxone. An alternative would be an antagonist with a longer duration of action than naloxone. Synthetic analogues of naloxone have been developed, e.g., naltrexone and nalmefene. Nalmefene has an elimination half-life of 8.5 h, compared with 1.5—2.5 h for naloxone, so that its reversal effects are likely to outlast the duration of most opioids, even when given in high doses (Gal and DiFazio, 1986).

An alternative to the use of pure opioid antagonists for reversing opioid action is the use of mixed agonist-antagonist drugs. The most commonly used compound in this class is nalbuphine. It has an elimination half-life of 3.5 h, similar to that of morphine and fentanyl. In contrast to butorphanol and pentazocine it causes few unpleasant psychic reaction and produces fewer haemodynamic changes. Butorphanol has little antagonist activity in man. An additional potential advantage of nalbuphine compared with naloxone is that nalbuphine has analgesic properties, so that the haemodynamic consequences of reversal of analgesia that occur with naloxone may be obtunded. Clinical studies have shown that nalbuphine, in a dose of up to 0.2 mg/kg, is an effective antagonist of opioid-induced respiratory depression (Ramsey et al., 1985; Jaffe et al., 1988). However, its use is associated with a number of side effects including nausea, hypertension, tachycardia and confusion. Larger doses tend to antagonize analgesia so that patients complain of pain (Jaffe et al., 1988). However, by careful titration of small incremental doses of nalbuphine, it is possible to achieve satisfactory reversal of respiratory depression without precipitating pain and haemodynamic side effects.

### Muscle rigidity

Muscle rigidity is a commonly occurring phenomenon associated with the administration of opioids. Rigidity involving the thoracic and abdominal muscles can seriously interfere with ventilation, sometimes to such an extent that manual ventilation is impossible without the use of a muscle relaxant (Scamman, 1983). It is most commonly observed when an opioid is given during induction of anaesthesia, e.g. during high-dose opioid anaesthesia for cardiac surgery, but may manifest itself at other times, including the postoperative period. The incidence of rigidity severely interfering with ventilation when alfentanil is administered rapidly to awake patients varies between 50% and 75% (Nauta et al., 1982). There have been several reports of delayed postoperative rigidity several hours after the end of surgery under high-dose opioid anaesthesia, interfering severely with ventilation (Christian et al., 1983; Goldberg et al., 1985). Muscle rigidity was reversed by intravenous naloxone. Opioid-induced muscle rigidity is totally abolished by neuromuscular blocking drugs (Hill et al., 1981). It is also attenuated by concomitant administration of a barbiturate or a benzodiazepine (Blasco et al., 1986; Sanford et al., 1988). By contrast, the use of nitrous oxide may exacerbate or precipitate muscle rigidity in patients given opioids (Sokoll et al., 1972).

The exact mechanism of opioid-induced muscle rigidity remains to be elucidated. Opioids stimulate the activity of inspiratory neurones in cats (Tabatabai et al., 1989). By causing a continuous and increased efferent traffic to the inspiratory muscles, this could result in sustained inspiration. However, this explanation can be only part of the story. Electromyographic studies in humans, given alfentanil 175 μg/kg during induction of anaesthesia, confirmed a similar pattern of marked rigidity in all muscle groups studied (Benthuysen et al., 1986). These included not only intercostal and abdominal muscles but also forearm flexors and gastrocnemius. That the mechanism of this rigidity had a central rather than peripheral origin was also elegantly demonstrated in this study. A pneumatic tourniquet on one upper arm was inflated to 300 mmHg before administration of alfentanil, thus blocking access of alfentanil and neuromuscular drugs to this limb. Despite this, rigidity in this isolated arm was observed in all patients receiving alfentanil, and persisted when rigidity was abolished in the rest of the body by muscle relaxants. Further evidence for a central mechanism was the observation that rigidity was often markedly accentuated by auditory or tactile stimuli. There is also a difference in the EMG, as measured by power spectral analysis, between voluntary contraction and opioid-induced muscle rigidity (Prutow et al., 1988).

Muscle rigidity is probably a manifestation of the catatonic state, a basic pharmacological property of opioids, which may be related to interactions between opioids and the dopaminergic system, involving inhibition of dopamine release in the striatum. Indeed, the catalepsy observed in rats given large doses of morphine was described originally as analogous to Parkinsonism (Kuschinsky and Hornykiewicz, 1972). Catatonic movements of the limbs are frequently observed in patients given high doses of opioids. Some studies suggest that the rigidity is produced by mu-receptors located on interneurones (most probably GABA-ergic) in the caudate nucleus (Havemann and Kuschinsky, 1981). These are most likely $mu_2$ receptors, since it is these, in conjunction with delta receptors, that are involved in dopamine turnover (Wood and Pasternak, 1983). The ability of preoperative treatment with amantadine, a drug that stimulates release of dopamine within the basal ganglia, to prevent muscle rigidity in a patient given a high dose of fentanyl further emphasizes the similarity between this effect and Parkinsonism (Silbert and Vacanti, 1987).

## Convulsions

There have been several reports in the literature describing alleged seizures associated with administration of fentanyl (e.g. Rao et al., 1982), sufentanil (Brian and Seifen, 1987; Molbegott et al., 1987) and alfentanil (Strong and Matson, 1989). While opioids do produce convulsions in animals, this is usually only at doses considerably in excess of those used in humans. Unfortunately, in few of the reported cases was the EEG recorded during the alleged seizures, and when it was, no electroencephalic seizure activity was detected. In over 1500 high-dose opioid anaesthetics, conducted with continuous EEG monitoring, we have never seen clinical or EEG evidence of convulsive activity (Sebel and Bovill, 1983). Smith et al. (1989) carried out a detailed analysis of EEG recordings of 127 patients anaesthetized with high doses of opioids. They found no evidence of seizure activity and concluded that the available evidence does not support the existence of opioid-induced seizures in the clinical setting. It is likely that the movement observed reflected myoclonic motor activity frequently seen during induction of anaesthesia with an opioid, often in association with muscle rigidity.

## REFERENCES

Adams, A.P. and Pybus, D.A. (1978) Delayed respiratory depression after use of fentanyl during anaesthesia. *Br. Med. J.* 1, 278—279.

Althaus, J.S., von Voigtlander, P.F., DiFazio, C.A. and Miller, E.D. (1987) Effects of U-50488H, a selective kappa-analgesic, on the minimum anesthetic concentration (MAC) of halothane in the rat. *Anesth. Analg.* 66, 391—394.

Althaus, J.S., DiFazio, C.A., Moscicki, J.C. and von Voigtlander, P.F. (1988) Enhancement of anesthetic effect of halothane by spiradoline, a selective kappa-agonist. *Anesth. Analg.* 67, 823—827.

Anand, K.J.S., Sippell, W.G. and Aynsley-Green, A. (1987a) Randomised trial of fentanyl anaesthesia in preterm babies undergoing surgery: Effects on the stress response. *Lancet* 1, 243—248.

Anand, K.J.S., Carr, D.B. and Hickey, P.R. (1987b) Randomised trial of high-dose sufentanil anesthesia in neonates undergoing cardiac surgery: Hormonal and hemodynamic responses. *Anesthesiology* 67, A501.

Andree, R.A. (1980) Sudden death following naloxone administration. *Anesth. Analg.* 59, 782—784.

Andrews, C.J.H., Sinclair, M. and Dye, A. (1982) The additive effect of nitrous oxide on respiratory depression in patients having fentanyl or alfentanil infusions. *Br. J. Anaesth.* 54, 1129.

Arndt, J.O., Mikat, M. and Parasher, C. (1984) Fentanyl's analgesic, respiratory, and cardiovascular actions in relation to dose and plasma concentration in unanesthetized dogs. *Anesthesiology* 61, 335—361.

Ausems, M.E., Hug, C.C. and de Lange, S. (1983) Variable rate infusion of alfentanil as a supplement to nitrous oxide anesthesia for general surgery. *Anesth. Analg.* 62, 982—986.

Ausems M., Hug C.C., Stanski D.R. and Burm A.G.L. (1986) Plasma concentrations of alfentanil required to supplement nitrous oxide anesthesia for general surgery. *Anesthesiology* 65, 362—373.

Ausems, M.E., Stanski, D.R. and Hug, C.C. (1985) An evaluation of the accuracy of pharmacokinetic data for the computer assisted infusion of alfentanil. *Br. J. Anaesth.* 57, 1217—1225.

Ausems, M.E., Vuyk, J., Hug, C.C. and Stanski, D.R. (1988) Comparisons of a computer assisted infusion versus intermittent bolus administration of alfentanil as a supplement to nitrous oxide for lower abdominal surgery. *Anesthesiology* 68, 851—861.

Azar, I. and Turndorf, H. (1979) Severe hypertension and multiple atrial premature contractions following naloxone administration. *Anesth. Analg.* 58, 524—525.

Azar, I., Patel, A.K. and Phau, C.Q. (1981) Cardiovascular responses following naloxone administration during enflurane anesthesia. *Anesth. Analg.* 60, 237.

Becker, L.D., Paulson, B.A., Miller, R.D., Severinghaus, J.W. and Eger, E.I. (1976) Biphasic respiratory depression after fentanyl-droperidal or fentanyl alone used to supplement nitrous oxide anesthesia. *Anesthesiology* 44, 291—296.

Belville, J.W., Howland, W.S., Seed, J.C. and Houde, R.W. (1959) The effect of sleep on the respiratory response to carbon dioxide. *Anesthesiology* 20, 628—634.

Benthuysen, J.C., Smith, N.T., Sanford, T.S., Head, N. and Dec-Silver, H. (1986) Physiology of alfentanil-induced rigidity. *Anesthesiology* 64, 440— 446.

Blasco, T.A., Smith, N.T., Sanford, T.J., Benthuysen, J.C., Dec-Silver, H. and Head, N. (1986) A clinical study of the effects of various pretreatment agents on alfentanil-induced rigidity: EMG data. *Anesthesiology* 63, A380.

Bovill, J.G., Sebel, P.S., Wauquier, A. and Rog, P. (1982a) Electroencephalographic effects of sufentanil anaesthesia in man. *Br. J. Anaesth.* 54, 45—52.

Bovill, J.G., Sebel, P.S., Blackburn, C.L. and Heykants, J. (1982b) The pharmacokinetics of alfentanil (R 39209): A new opioid analgesic. *Anesthesiology* 57, 439—443.

Bovill, J.G., Sebel, P.S. and Stanley, T.H. (1984a) Opioid analgesics in anesthesia: With special reference to their use in cardiovascular anesthesia. *Anesthesiology* 61, 731—755.

Bovill, J.G., Warren, P.J., Schuller, J.C., van Wezel, H.B. and Hoeneveld, M.H. (1984b) Comparison of fentanyl, sufentanil, and alfentanil in patients undergoing valvular heart surgery. *Anesth. Analg.* 63, 1081—1086.

Bower, S. and Hull, C.J. (1982) Comparative pharmacokinetics of fentanyl and alfentanil. *Br. J. Anaesth.* 54, 871—877.

Brian, J.E., Jr. and Seifen, A.B. (1987) Tonic-clonic activity after sufentanil (letter). *Anesth. Analg.* 66, 481—483.

Cahalan, M.K., Prakash, O., Rulf, E.N.R., Cahalan, M.T., Mayala, A.P.G., Lurz, F.C., Rosseel, P., Lachitjaran, E., Siphanto, K., Gussenhoven, E.J. and Roelandt, J.R.T.C. (1987) Addition of nitrous oxide to fentanyl anesthesia does not induce myocardial ischemia in patients with ischemic heart disease. *Anesthesiology* 67, 925—929.

Cartwright, P., Prys-Roberts, C., Gill, K., Dye, A., Stafford, M. and Gray, A (1983) Ventilatory depression related to plasma fentanyl concentrations during and after anesthesia in humans. *Anesth. Analg.* 62, 966—974.

Catley, D.M., Thornton, C., Jordan, C., Lehane, J.R. and Jones, J.G. (1985) Pronounced episodic oxygen desaturation in the postoperative period: Its association with ventilatory pattern and analgesic regimen. *Anesthesiology* 63, 20—28.

Christian, C.M., Waller, J.L. and Moldenhauer, C.C. (1983) Postoperative rigidity following fentanyl anesthesia. *Anesthesiology* 58, 275—277.

Clarke, N.J., Meuleman, I., Liu, W.S., Zwaniken, P., Pace, N.L. and Stanley, T.H. (1987) Comparison of sufentanil-$N_2O$ and fentanyl-$N_2O$ in patients without cardiac disease undergoing general surgery. *Anesthesiology* 66, 130—135.

DiFazio, C.A., Moscicki, J.C. and Magruder, M.R. (1981) Anesthetic potency of nalbuphine and interaction with morphine in rats. *Anesth. Analg.* 60, 629—633.

Dodson, B.A. and Miller, K.W. (1985) Evidence for a dual mechanism in the anesthetic action of an opioid peptide. *Anesthesiology* 62, 615—620.

Flacke, J.W., Flacke, W.E. and Williams, C.D. (1977) Acute pulmonary edema following naloxone reversal of high-dose morphine anesthesia. *Anesthesiology* 47, 376—378.

Gal, T.J. and DiFazio, C.A. (1986) Prolonged antagonism of opioid action with intravenous nalmefene in man. *Anesthesiology* 64, 175—180.

Goldberg, M., Ishak, S., Garcia, C. and McKenna, J. (1985) Postoperative rigidity following sufentanil administration. *Anesthesiology* 63, 199—201.

Hall, R.I., Murphy, M.R. and Hug, C.C., Jr. (1987a) The enflurane-sparing effect of sufentanil in dogs. *Anesthesiology* 67, 518—525.

Hall, R.I., Szlam, F. and Hug, C.C. (1987b) The enflurane-sparing effect of alfentanil in dogs. *Anesth. Analg.* 66, 1287—1291.

Hand, C.W., Blunnie, W.P., Claffey, L.P., McShane, A.J., McQuay, H.J. and Moore, R.A. (1987) Potential analgesic contribution from morphine-6-glucuronide in CSF. *Lancet* ii, 1207—1209.

Havemann, U. and Kuschinsky, K. (1981) Further characterization of opioid receptors in the striatum mediating muscular rigidity in rats. *Naunyn-Schmiedeberg's Arch. Pharmacol.* 317, 321—325.

Hecker, B.R., Lake, C.L., DiFazio, C.A., Moscicki, J.C. and Engle, J.S. (1983) The decrease of the minimum anesthetic concentration produced by sufentanil in rats. *Anesth. Analg.* 62, 987—990.

Heikkilä, H., Jalonan, J., Arola, M., Hovi-Viander, M. and Laaksonen, V. (1987) Low-dose enflurane as adjunct to high-dose fentanyl in patients undergoing coronary artery surgery: Stable hemodynamics and maintained myocardial oxygen balance. *Anesth. Analg.* 66, 111—116.

Hickey, P.R. and Hansen, D.D. (1984) Fentanyl- and sufentanil-oxygen-pancuronium anesthesia for cardiac surgery in infants. *Anesth. Analg.* 63, 117—124.

Hill, A.B., Nahrwold, M.L., de Rosayro, A.M., Knight, P.R., Jones, R.M. and Bolles, R.L. (1981) Prevention of rigidity during fentanyl-oxygen induction of anesthesia. *Anesthesiology* 55, 452—454.

Howie, M.B., McSweeney, T.D., Lingam, R.P. and Maschke, S.P. (1985) A comparison of fentanyl-$O_2$ and sufentanil-$O_2$ for cardiac anesthesia. *Anesth. Analg.* 64, 877—887.

Hug, C.C., Jr., Hall, R.I., Argent, K.C., Reeder, D.A. and Moldenhauer, C.C. (1988) Alfentanil plasma concentration v. effect relationships in cardiac surgical patients. *Br. J. Anaesth.* 61, 435—440.

Jaffe, R.S., Moldenhauer, C.C., Hug, C.C., Jr., Finlayson, D.C., Tobia, V. and Kopel, M.E. (1988) Nalbuphine antagonism of fentanyl-induced ventilatory depression: A randomized trial. *Anesthesiology* 68, 254—260.

Jones, J.G. and Konieczko, K. (1986) Hearing and memory in anaesthetised patients. *Br. Med. J.* 292, 1291—1293.

Knill, R.L. and Gelb, A.W. (1978) Ventilatory responses to hypoxia and hypercapnia during halothane sedation and anesthesia in man. *Anesthesiology* 49, 244—251.

Kuschinsky, K. and Hornykiewicz, O. (1972) Morphine catalepsy in the rat: Relation to striatal dopamine metabolism. *Eur. J. Pharmacol.* 19, 119—122.

Lake, C.L., Duckworth, E.N., DiFazio, C.A., Durbin, C.G. and Magruder, M.R. (1982) Cardiovascular effects of nalbuphine in patients with coronary or valvular heart disease. *Anesthesiology* 57, 498—503.

Lake, C.L., DiFazio, C.A., Moscicki, J.C. and Engle, J.S. (1985) Reduction in halothane MAC: Comparison of morphine and alfentanil. *Anesth. Analg.* 64, 807—810.

Lamarche, Y., Martin, R. and Grenier, Y. (1984) Continuous infusion of alfentanil for surgery. *Can. Anaesth. Soc. J.* 31, 64—65.

Lee, J.K., Hannowell, S., Kim, Y.D. and Macnamara, T.E. (1981) Morphine induced respiratory depression following bilateral carotid endarterectomy. *Anesth. Analg.* 60, 64—65.

Leeuwen van, L., Zuurmond, W.W.A. and Helmers, J.H.J.H. (1984) Alfentanil-dauerinfusion für chirurgische Eingriffe mittlerer und längerer dauer. *Anaesthesist* 33, 173—176.

Lehmann, K.A., Freier, J. and Daub, D. (1982) Fentanyl-Pharmacokinetik und postoperative Atemdepression. *Anaestheist* 31, 111—118.

Lemmens, H.J.M., Bovill, J.G., Burm, A.G.L. and Hennis, P.J. (1988) Alfentanil infusion in the elderly. Prolonged computer-assisted infusion of alfentanil in the elderly surgical patient. *Anaesthesia* 43, 850—856.

Lemmens, H.J.M., Bovill, J.G., Hennis, P.J. and Burm, A.G.L. (1988) Age has no effect on the pharmacodynamics of alfentanil. *Anesth. Analg.* 67, 956—960.

Lemmens, H.J.M., Hennis, P.J., Bovill, J.G., Gladines, M.P.R.R. and Burm, A.G.L. (1989) Effect of gender on the pharmacokinetics of alfentanil. *Anesthesiology* 71, A229.

Lepage, J.-Y.M., Pinaud, M.L., Hélias, J.H., Juge, C.M., Cozian, A.Y., Farinotti, R. and Souron, R.J. (1988) Left ventricular function during propofol and fentanyl anesthesia in patients with coronary artery disease: Assessment with a radionuclide approach. *Anesth. Analg.* 67, 949—955.

Lowenstein, E., Hallowell, P., Levine, F.H., Daggett, W.M., Austen, W.G. and Laver, M.B. (1969) Cardiovascular response to large doses of intravenous morphine in man. *N. Engl. J. Med.* 281, 1389—1393.

Lowenstein, E. (1971) Morphine "anesthesia" — A perspective. *Anesthesiology* 35, 563—565.

Maitre, P.O., Ausems, M.A., Vozeh, S. and Stanski, D.R. (1988) Evaluating the accuracy of using population pharmacokinetic data to predict plasma concentrations of alfentanil. *Anesthesiology* 68, 59—67.

Maitre, P.O., Vozeh, S., Heykants, J. et al. (1987) Population pharmacokinetics of alfentanil. *Anesthesiology* 66, 3—12.

Mainzer, J. (1979) Awareness, muscle relaxants and balanced anaesthesia. *Can. Anaesth. Soc. J.* 26, 386—393.

Mark, J.B. and Greenberg, L.M. (1983) Intraoperative awareness and hypertensive crisis during high-dose fentanyl-diazepam-oxygen anesthesia. *Anesth. Analg.* 62, 698—700.

McClain, D.A. and Hug, C.C. (1980) Intravenous fentanyl kinetics. *Clin. Pharmacol. Ther.* 28, 106—114.

McKay, R.D., Varner, P.D., Hendricks, P.L., Adams, M.L. and Harsh, G.R. (1984) The evaluation of sufentanil-$N_2O$-$O_2$ vs fentanyl-$N_2O$-$O_2$ anesthesia for craniotomy. *Anesth. Analg.* 63, 250.

McQuay, H.J., Moore, R.A., Paterson, G.M. and Adams, A.P. (1979) Plasma fentanyl concentration and clinical observations during and after operation. *Br. J. Anaesth.* 51, 543—550.

McQueen, D.S. (1983) Opioid peptide interactions with respiratory and circulatory systems. *Br. Med. Bull.* 39, 77—82.

Michaelis, L.L. and Hickey, P.R. (1974) Ventricular irritability associated with the use of naloxone hydrochloride. *Ann. Thoracic Surg.* 18, 608—614.

Miller, D.R., Wellwood, M., Teasdale, S.J., Laidley, D., Ivanov, J., Young, P., Madoni, M., McLaughlin, P., Mickle, D.A.G. and Weisel, R.D. (1988) Effects of anaesthetic induction on myocardial function and metabolism: a comparison of fentanyl, sufentanil and alfentanil. *Can. J. Anaesth.* 35, 219—33.

Mills, C.A., Flacke, J.W., Miller, J.D., Davis, L.J., Bloor, B.C. and Flacke, W.E. (1988) Cardiovascular effects of fentanyl reversal by naloxone at varying arterial carbon dioxide tensions in dogs. *Anesth. Analg.* 67, 730—736.

Moffit, E.A., Scovil, J., Barker, R.A., Imrie, D.D., Glenn, J.J., Cousins, C.L., Sullivan, J.A. and Kinley, C.E. (1984) The effects of nitrous oxide on myocardial metabolism and hemodynamics during fentanyl or enflurane anesthesia in patients with coronary disease. *Anesth. Analg.* 63, 1071—1075.

Molbegott, L.P., Flashburg, M.H., Karasic, L. and Karlin, B.L. (1987) Probable seizures with sufentanil. *Anesth. Analg.* 66, 91—93.

Moldenhauer, C.C., Hug, C.C., Nagle, D.M. and Youngberg, J.A. (1981) High-dose butorphanol (Stadol) in anesthesia for aortocoronary bypass surgery. Abstract, *3rd Annual Meeting of the Society of Cardiovascular Anesthesiologists,* San Francisco, pp. 59—60.

Montastruc, J.L., Montastruc, P. and Morales-Olivas, F. (1981) Potentiation by naloxone of pressor responses. *Br. J. Pharmacol.* 74, 105—109.

Moore, R.A., Yang, S.S., McNicholas, K.W., Gallagher, J.D. and Clark, D.L. (1985) Hemodynamic and anesthetic effects of sufentanil as the sole anesthetic for pediatric cardiovascular surgery. *Anesthesiology* 62, 725—731.

Motamura, S., Kissin, I., Aultman, D.F. and Reeves, J.G. (1984) Effects of fentanyl and nitrous oxide on contractility of blood-perfused papillary muscle of the dog. *Anesth. Analg.* 63, 47—50.

Mummaneni, N., Rao, T.L.K. and Montoya, A. (1980) Awareness and recall with high-dose fentanyl-oxygen anesthesia. *Anesth. Analg.* 59, 948—949.

Murphy, M.R. and Hug, C.C., Jr. (1982a) The enflurane sparing effect of morphine, butorphanol, and nalbuphine. *Anesthesiology* 57, 489—492.

Murphy, M.R. and Hug, C.C., Jr. (1982b) The anesthetic potency of fentanyl in terms of its reduction of enflurance MAC. *Anesthesiology* 57, 485—488.

Murphy, M.R. and Hug, C.C. (1983) Efficacy of fentanyl in reducing isoflurane MAC: Antagonism by naloxone and nalbuphine. *Anesthesiology* 59, A338.

Nauta, J., de Lange, S., Koopman, D., Spierdijk, J., van Kleef, J. and Stanley, T.H. (1982) Anesthetic induction with alfentanil: A new short-acting narcotic analgesic. *Anesth. Analg.* 61, 267—272.

Nunn, J.F. (1987) Clinical aspects of the interaction between nitrous oxide and vitamin $B_{12}$. *Br. J. Anaesth.* 59, 3—13.

Osborne, R.J., Joel, S.P. and Slevin, M.L. (1986) Morphine intoxication in renal failure: The role of morphine-6-glucuronide. *Br. Med. J.* 292, 1548—1549.

Osborne, R., Joel, S., Trew, P. and Slevin, M. (1990) Morphine and metabolite behaviour after different routes of morphine administration: Demonstration of the importance of the active metabolite morphine-6-glucuronide. *Clin. Pharmacol. Ther.* 47, 12—19.

Pasternak, G.W. (1988) Multiple morphine and enkephalin receptors and the relief of pain. *J. Am. Med. Assoc.* 259, 1362—1367.

Pasternak, G.W. and Wood, P.L. (1986) Multiple mu receptors. *Life Sci.* 38, 1889—1898.

Pathak, H.S., Brown, R.H., Nash, C.L. and Cascorbi, H.F. (1983) Continuous opioid infusion for scolioisis surgery. *Anesth. Analg.* 62, 841—845.

Patschke, D., Eberlein, H.J., Hess, W., Tarnow, J. and Zimmerman, G. (1977) Antagonism of morphine with naloxone in dogs: Cardiovascular effects with special reference to the coronary circulation. *Br. J. Anaesth.* 49, 525—532.

Pelligrino, D.A., Riegler, F.X. and Albrecht, R.F. (1989) Ventilatory effects of fourth cerebroventricular infusion of morphine-6-glucuronide in the awake dog. *Anesthesiology* 71, 936—940.

Philbin, D.M., Föex, P., Drummond, G., Lowenstein, E., Ryder, W.A. and Jones, L.A. (1985) Postsystolic shortening of canine left ventricle supplied by a stenotic coronary artery when nitrous oxide is added in the presence of narcotics. *Anesthesiology* 62, 166—174

Philbin, D.M., Roscow, C.E., Schneider, R.C., Clark, C. and D'Ambra, M.N. (1986) High dose sufentanil infusions in cardiac patients: Hemodynamic and catecholamine responses. *Anesthesiology* 65, A505.

Phillipson, E.A. (1978) Control of breathing during sleep. *Am. Rev. Respir. Dis.* 118, 909—939.

Prutow, R.J., Head, N. and Smith, N.T. (1988) Power spectral analysis of alfentanil-induced rigidity. *J. Clin. Monit.* 4, 155—156.

Prys-Roberts, C. (1987) Anaesthesia: A practical or impractical construct. *Br. J. Anaesth.* 59, 1341—1345.

Rampil, I.J., Sasse, F.J., Smith, M.T., Hoff, B.H. and Fleming, D.C. (1980) Spectral edge frequency — a new correlate of anesthetic depth. *Anesthesiology* 53, S12.

Ramsay, J.G., Higgs, B.D., Wyands, J.E., Robbins, R. and Townsend, G.E. (1985) Early extubation after high-dose fentanyl anaesthesia for aortocoronary bypass surgery: Reversal of respiratory depression with low-dose nalbuphine. *Can. Anaesth. Soc. J.* 32, 597—606.

Rao, T.L.K., Mummaneni, N. and El-Etr, A.A. (1982) Convulsion: An unusual response to intravenous fentanyl administration. *Anesth. Analg.* 61, 1020—1021.

Raza, S.M.A., Masters, R.W. and Zsigmond, E.K. (1989) Haemodynamic stability with midazolam-ketamine-sufentanil analgesia in cardiac surgical patients. *Can. J. Anaesth.* 36, 617—623.

Reeves, J.G., Kissin, I., Fournier, S.E. and Smith, L.R. (1984) Additive negative inotropic effects of a combination of diazepam and fentanyl. *Anesth. Analg.* 63, 97—100.

Robinson, S. and Gregory, G.A. (1981) Fentanyl-air-$O_2$-anaesthesia for ligation of patent ductus arteriosus in preterm infants. *Anesth. Analg.* 60, 331—334.

Russell, G.N., Wright, E.L., Fox, M.A., Douglas, E.J. and Cockshott, I.D. (1989) Propofol-fentanyl anaesthesia for coronary artery surgery and cardiopulmonary bypass. *Anaesthesia* 44, 205—208.

Safwat, A.M. and Daniel, D. (1983) Grand mal seizure after fentanyl administration (letter). *Anesthesiology* 59, 78.

Sanford, T.J., Smith, N.T., Weinger, M.B., Benthuysen, J.L. and Head, N. (1988) The effect of midazolam pretreatment on alfentanil-induced muscle rigidity. *Anesthesiology* 69, A556.

Scamman, F.L. (1983) Fentanyl-$O_2$-$N_2O$ rigidity and pulmonary compliance. *Anesth. Analg.* 62, 332—334.

Scott, J.C., Ponganis, K.V. and Stanski, D.R. (1985) EEG quantitation of narcotic effect: The comparative pharmacodynamics of fentanyl and alfentanil. *Anesthesiology* 62, 234—241.

Sebel, P.S. and Bovill, J.G. (1983) Fentanyl and convulsions. *Anesth. Analg.* 62, 851—859.

Sebel, P.S. and Bovill, J.G. (1987) Opioid analgesics in cardiac anesthesia. In: *Cardiac Anesthesia*, 2nd Edn., Vol. I, pp. 67—123. Editor: J.A. Kaplan, Grune and Stratton, Orlando.

Sebel, P.S., Bovill, J.G., Wauquier, A. and Rog, P. (1981) Effects of high-dose fentanyl anesthesia on the electroencephalogram. *Anesthesiology* 51, 203—211.

Sebel, P.S., Lalor, J.M., Flynn, P.J. and Simpson, B.A. (1984) Respiratory depression after alfentanil infusion. *Br. Med. J.* 289, 1581—1582.

Shupak, R.C. and Harp, J.R. (1985) Comparison between high-dose sufentanil-oxygen and high-dose fentanyl-oxygen for neuroanaesthesia. *Br. J. Anaesth.* 57, 375—381.

Silbert, B.S. and Vacanti, C.A. (1987) Amantidine in prevention of fentanyl-induced muscle rigidity. *Anesth. Analg.* 66, 3338.

Swenzen, G.O., Chakrabarti, M.K., Sapsed-Byrne, S. and Whitwam, J.G. (1988) Selective depression by alfentanil of group III and IV somatosympathetic reflexes in the dog. *Br. J. Anaesth.* 61, 441—445.

Slogoff, S. and Keats, A.S. (1989) Randomized trial of primary anesthetic agents on outcome of coronary artery bypass operations. *Anesthesiology* 70, 179—188.

Smith, N.T., Dec-Silver, A., Sanford, T.J., Westover, C.J., Quinn, M.L., Klein, F. and Davis, D.A. (1984) EEGs during high-dose fentanyl-, sufentanil-, or morphine-oxygen anesthesia. *Anesth. Analg.* 63, 386—393.

Smith, N.T., Westover, C.J., Quinn, M., Benthuysen, J.L., Dec-Silver, H. and Sanford, T.J. (1985) An electroencephalographic comparison of alfentanil with other narcotics and thiopental. *J. Clin. Monit.* 1, 236—244.

Smith, N.T., Benthuysen, J.L., Bickford, R.G., Sanford, T.J., Blasco, T., Duke, P.C., Head, N. and Dec-Silver, H. (1989) Seizures during opioid anesthetic induction — are they opioid-induced rigidity. *Anesthesiology* 71, 852—862.

Sokoll, M.D., Hoyt, J.L. and Georgis, S.D. (1972) Studies in muscle rigidity, nitrous oxide and narcotic analgesic agents. *Anesth. Analg.* 51, 16—20.

Sprigge, J.S., Wyands, J.E., Whalley, D.G., Bevin, D.R., Townsend, G.E., Nathan, H., Patel, Y.C. and Srikant, C.B. (1982) Fentanyl infusion anesthesia for aortocoronary bypass surgery: Plasma levels and hemodynamic response. *Anesth. Analg.* 61, 972—978.

Stanley T.H. and Liu W-S. (1977) Cardiovascular effects of meperidine/$N_2O$ anesthesia before and after pancuronium. *Anesth. Analg.* 56, 669— 673.

Stanley T.H. and Webster L.R. (1978) Anesthetic requirements and cardiovascular effects of fentanyl-oxygen and fentanyl-diazepam-oxygen anesthesia in man. *Anesth. Analg.* 57, 411—416.

Stanley T.H., Gray N.H., Stanford W. and Armstrong R. (1973) The effects of high-dose morphine on fluid and blood requirements in open-heart operations. *Anesthesiology* 38, 536—541.

Stanley, T.H., Bennett, G.M., Loeser, E.A., Kawamura, R. and Gentker, G.R. (1976) Cardiovascular effects of diazepam and droperidol during morphine anesthesia. *Anesthesiology* 44, 255—258.

Stanley, T.H., Leysen, J., Niemegeers, C.J.E. and Pace, N.L. (1983) Narcotic dosage and central nervous system opiate binding. *Anesth. Analg.* 62, 705—709.

Stanski, D.R., Vuyk, J., Ausems, M., Arts, R., Kramer, S. and Spierdijk, J. (1987) Can the EEG be used to monitor anesthetic depth for alfentanil with $N_2O$? *Anesthesiology* 67, A401.

Stoeckel, H., Hengstmann, J.H. and Schüttler, J. (1979) Pharmacokinetics of fentanyl as a possible explanation for recurrence of respiratory depression. *Br. J. Anaesth.* 51, 741—745.

Stoeckel, H., Schüttler, J., Magnussen, H. and Hengstmann, J.H. (1982) Plasma fentanyl concentrations and the occurrence of respiratory depression in volunteers. *Br. J. Anaesth.* 54, 1087—1095.

Stoelting, R.K., Creasser, C.E. and Gibbs, P.S. (1974) Circulatory effects of halothane added to morphine anesthesia in patients with coronary artery disease. *Anesth. Analg.* 53, 449—455.

Stoelting, R.K. and Gibbs, P.S. (1973) Hemodynamic effects of morphine and morphine-nitrous oxide in valvular heart disease and coronary artery disease. *Anesthesiology* 38, 45—52.

Stolzy, S., Couture, L.J. and Edmonds, H.L. (1986) Evidence of partial recall during general anesthesia. *Anesth. Analg.* 65, S154.

Stone, D.J. and DiFazio, C.A. (1988) Anesthetic action of opiates: Correlations of lipid solubility and spectral edge. *Anesth. Analg.* 67, 663—666.

Strong, W.E. and Matson, M. (1989) Probable seizure after alfentanil. *Anesth. Analg.* 68, 692—693.

Tabatabai, M., Kitahata, L.M. and Collins, J.G. (1989) Disruption of the rhythmic activity of the medullary inspiratory neurons and phrenic nerve by fentanyl and reversal with nalbuphine. *Anesthesiology* 70, 489—495

Thomson, I.R., Bergstrom, R.G., Rosenbloom, M. and Meatherall, R.G. (1988). Premedication and high-dose fentanyl anesthesia for myocardial revascularization: A comparison of lorazepam versus morphine-scopolamine. *Anesthesiology* 68, 194—200.

Tomicheck, R.C., Rosow, C.E., Philbin, D.M., Moss, J., Teplick, R.S. and Schneider, R.C. (1983) Diazepam-fentanyl interaction-hemodynamic and hormonal effects in coronary artery surgery. *Anesth. Analg.* 62, 881—884.

Tuman, K.J., McCarthy, R.J., Spiess, B.D., DaValle, M., Dabir, R. and Ivankovitch, A.D. (1989) Does choice of anesthetic agent significantly affect outcome after coronary artery surgery? *Anesthesiology* 70, 189—198.

Vermeyen, K.M., Erpels, F.A., Janssen, L.A., Beeckman, C.P. and Hanegreefs, G.H. (1987) Propofol-fentanyl anaesthesia for coronary bypass surgery in patients with good left ventricular function. *Br. J. Anaesth.* 59, 1115—1120.

Vermeyen, K.M., Erpels, F.A., Beeckman, C.P., Janssen, L.A. and Adriaensen, H.F. (1989) Low-dose sufentanil-isoflurane anaesthesia for coronary artery surgery. *Br. J. Anaesth.* 63, 44—50.

Weil, J.V., McCullough, R.E., Kline, J.S. and Sodal, I.E. (1975) Diminished ventilatory response to hypoxia and hypercapnia after morphine in normal man. *N. Engl. J. Med.* 292, 1103—1106.

Weldon, S.T., Perry, D.F., Cork, R.C. and Gandolfi, A.J. (1985) Detection of picogram levels of sufentanil by capillary gas chromatography. *Anesthesiology* 63, 684—687.

Welling, E.C. and Donegan, J. (1989) Neuroleptanalgesia using alfentanil for awake craniotomy. *Anesth. Analg.* 68, 57—60.

Welti, R.S., Moldenhauer, C.C., Hug, C.C., Kaplan, J.A. and Holbrook, G.W. (1984) High-dose hydromorphone (Dilandid) for coronary artery bypass surgery. *Anesth. Analg.* 63, 55—59.

White, P.F., Dworsky, W.A., Horai, Y. and Trevor, A.J. (1983) Comparison of continuous infusion fentanyl or ketamine versus thiopental. Determining the mean effective serum concentrations for outpatient surgery. *Anesthesiology* 59, 564—569.

Windsor, J.P.W., Sherry, K., Feneck, R.O. and Sebel, P.S. (1988) Sufentanil and nitrous oxide anaesthesia for cardiac surgery. *Br. J. Anaesth.* 61, 662—668.

Wong, K.C. (1983) Narcotics are not expected to produce unconsciousness and amnesia. *Anesth. Analg.* 62, 625—626

Wood, P.L. and Pasternak, G.W. (1983) Specific $mu_2$ opioid isoreceptor regulation of nigrostriatal neurons: In-vivo evidence with naloxonazine. *Neurosci. Lett.* 37, 291—293.

Wyands, J.E., Wong, P., Townsend, G.E., Sprigge, J.S. and Whalley, D.G. (1984) Narcotic requirements for intravenous anesthesia. *Anesth. Analg.* 63, 101—105.

*B. Kay (ed.) Total Intravenous Anaesthesia*



# 5

# *Opioid supplements in total intravenous anaesthesia (TIVA)*

Brian Kay

## INTRODUCTION AND PHARMACOLOGY

Opioids have been an essential component of most anaesthetic regimens since attempts were first made to dull the pain of surgery. Their primary pharmacological attribute of producing analgesia obviously suggests their use in anaesthesia, but for what purpose? Pain is, definitively, a conscious perception in the human, as it may only be specified to exist in the conscious human. It is not the same thing as a reflex response to noxious stimulation such as may be observed in an unconscious human, or a different animal. Were it so, both pain and analgesia could be measured far more reliably! Thus if a patient is rendered unconscious by a general anaesthetic he can not, by definition, be aware of pain, nor, therefore, of analgesia. Although 'analgesia' has a time-honoured place as a component of 'balanced anaesthesia' since its inception, its use in this context is inappropriate. Rejecting the terminology leads the anaesthetist to consider more carefully the reasons for employing analgesic drugs, including opioids, as a component of his anaesthesia, and to base his use on pharmacological effects that do not include the diminution of perceived pain.

Unlike the volatile anaesthetics, which exert a narcotic effect on cells throughout the body, most obviously on the central nervous system, opioids act at receptors ($\mu$,$K$, etc.). These are situated not only in the central nervous system but in many other tissues and are acted upon by a number of different natural ligands. Thus various opioids may act selectively at dissimilar receptor sites in diverse locations and may also act differently on the receptor, in an agonist, partial agonist or competitive (antagonist) manner. Despite the very large number of permutations of effects that are therefore possible the opioids used in anaesthetic practice are mainly agonists primarily affecting $\mu$ receptors. The main differences in the drugs commonly used are in potency, rate of onset and duration of effect. All have pharmacologic actions that resemble those of morphine.

Morphine-like drugs have their most important effects on the central nervous system, mainly affecting perception. The analgesic effect is not only due to inhibition of transmission in the pain pathways but also due to a change in the way pain is perceived. Consciousness is diminished, ranging from drowsiness to narcosis. There may be euphoria or dysphoria. Metabolism is depressed. Depression of the vasomotor centre and respiratory centre (particularly the responsivness to $CO_2$) occurs but the chemoreceptor zone triggering vomiting is sensitized. Itching is often caused. The Edinger-Westphal nucleus is stimulated, causing meiosis. Massively toxic doses cause convulsions.

Peripherally, an increase in vagal tone causes a decrease in heart rate, otherwise the effects on the myocardium are small except in large dosage when some decreased contractility is apparent. The main effect on the cardiovascular system is that of a decreased systemic vascular resistance. This may be enhanced by those opioids that cause histamine release, which may also cause bronchospasm. The effects on other smooth muscle vary; although activity is generally reduced, e.g. the uterus, sphincter tone is increased leading to constipation and an aggravation of biliary or renal colic. Opioids also may have a tonic effect on voluntary muscle; large doses often cause extensive rigidity throughout the body.

## USES OF OPIOIDS IN ANAESTHESIA

### History

Apart from their use for premedication (see below) opioids are extensively used as a component of anaesthesia to supplement or replace a volatile anaesthetic. Pethidine (demerol) was the first opioid to be used in this context, by Neff et al. (1947). Their methods were observed by Mushin and Rendell-Baker who reported more widely in 1949. They did not specify the use of a muscle relaxant and their somewhat over-optimistic assessment of the technique failed to point out that in the majority of circumstances pethidine was an inferior component of anaesthesia even to the volatile and gaseous anaesthetics then in use. It is not surprising that the technique made little impact at the time, despite observations that patients given pethidine instead of ether woke up faster and were relatively calm and pain-free.

A subsequent limited revival in interest was sparked by the introduction of the use of a combination of pethidine, chlorpromazine and promethazine (Laborit and Huguenard, 1954) which extended the range of efficacy of the opioid at the expense of delaying recovery and potentiating hypotension. It was not until pethidine was replaced as the opioid of choice in another drug combination, with a butyrophenone, that opioids began to offer a widely acceptable alternative to even the new volatile anaesthetics that were appearing. Initially a combination of phenoperidine and haloperidol were used but the introduction of fentanyl and droperidol (DeCastro et al., 1964) ensured the world-wide acceptance of opioid-supplemented anaesthesia and paved the way to TIVA techniques. These were first extensively used and investigated by Savege et al. (1975), who used pethidine and althesin.

## Rationale

### *Premedication*

The concept of premedication was first widely accepted in the 1920s when ether formed the basis of most general anaesthetics and the consequentially essential anti-sialagogue formed the basis of most premedications. Morphine is known to have been used before anaesthesia since 1850, mainly to reduce by its depressant effects the disturbances and difficulties of induction of anaesthesia. Subsequently the use of opioids was justified by three main reasons: to reduce apprehension, to reduce the dose of anaesthetic required and to treat pre-operative pain. Perhaps only the latter has survived as a valid reason.

Reduction of apprehension is the most usual reason given for using an opioid premedication despite the lack of controlled evidence that the drugs are effective in this respect. The assumption is made because the opioids are hypnotic and may induce euphoria; but it has long been known that drowsiness does not necessarily reduce apprehension and that opioids are as likely to induce dysphoria as euphoria in a relatively drug-naive population. In a recent double-blind, controlled survey of the efficacy of routine premedications used in a large hospital, neither of two opioid-containing premedications was any more effective than no premedication (Bowles, personal communication) which is inferior to placebo (Kay, unpublished observation). As the use of opioids at this stage carries with it an incidence of unwanted side-effects such as pre-operative nausea, vomiting, dizziness, sweating, respiratory depression etc., it seems reasonable to use more effective anxiolytics such as benzodiazepines unless there are other strong indications for an opioid, pain being the obvious one. This of course should be treated as quickly as possible and there seems to be little justification for withholding any anxiolytic until 30 or 45 min before anaesthesia and even less for combining it with an antisialogoue that is in any case normally unneccessary at this time.

Opioids may be given as a premedication in order to reduce the dose of anaesthetic required, and most have been shown to be effective in this respect, reducing the induction dose requirement for i.v. anaesthetics and thereby reducing the side-effects of these agents. However, like the use of opioids to prevent tachycardias, dysrhythmias and hypertension at laryngoscopy and tracheal intubation (see below), it is unneccessary to give the drug until immediately before induction of anaesthesia, thereby avoiding unwanted pre-operative side effects.

### *Use during anaesthesia*

One of the main purposes of using opioids in anaesthesia is to diminish reflex responses to noxious anaesthetic or surgical stimulation. These reflex arcs may have efferent pathways involving either somatic or autonomic nerves, but the afferents are usually the same as those involved in the perception of pain, C and delta fibres that may travel in somatic or autonomic nerves, have cell bodies in the posterior root ganglia and synapse in the dorsal horn of the spinal cord. It is at this synapse that opioids have one of their most important actions, combining with pre-synaptic $\mu$ receptors to inhibit transmission, and thereby reduce not only the transmission of painful/noxious stimulation but also the resulting reflex responses. The effectiveness with which the opioid will diminish such responses is primarily dependent on the dose used, although partial agonists and agonist/antagonist drugs have a limited efficacy which may render the drug incapable of suppressing a particular response no matter how much is given. Opioid agonists of high efficacy such as fentanyl, sufentanil or to a lesser extent morphine are capable of blocking the perception of, and almost all responses to, the stimulation of major surgery (see Chapter 4, Opioid Anaesthesia). Some opioid agonists such as pethidine (demerol) cannot be used to this extent because of their inherent toxicity (not opioid activity but such effects as cardiovascular depression) but all are usable to some extent.

The most disruptive reflex response to surgery is the somatic (movement), resulting in withdrawal or less frequently extensor or flexor movements that may be gross even though the patient is totally unconscious of the stimulation. Opioids are frequently used to control such responses during anaesthesia but their usefulness greatly depends on the intensity of stimulation. Movement in response to relatively small stimuli such as dilatation of the uterine cervix, dressing of burns or dental extraction may usually be controlled sufficiently to allow surgery to progress unhindered by a dose of an opioid that still allows adequate spontaneous respiration, especially as the surgery itself may stimulate respiration. This is not always possible with more intense stimulation. Although it may be occasionally possible to render a spontaneously ventilating patient undergoing skin incision immobile by using an opioid, the chances are that the dose required will cause apnoea. This problem may then be compounded by difficulty in artificially ventilating the patient because of opioid-induced muscle rigidity, a life-threatening situation. It is generally easier and safer to diminish the reflex centrally by giving a volatile anaesthetic, if spontaneous ventilation is preferred, or to block the reflex at the neuromuscular junction by using a muscle relaxant.

Autonomic reflex responses to surgery are varied, often widespread and potentially lethal. Catecholamine-induced tachycardias and hypertension are perhaps the most frequently worrying but cholinergic responses such as intense bradycardia may equally cause concern. The extent to which opioids are capable of totally suppressing such reflexes again depends mainly on the intensity of stimulation and even the very high doses used for opioid anaesthesia may fail to suppress the cardiovascular effects of splitting the sternum, for example. In general, the dose of an opioid required to suppress a common stimulus (e.g. laryngoscopy, tracheal intubation) that usually causes a significant autonomic reflex response is similar to that required to suppress movement and therefore not likely to be used in a patient when spontaneous ventilation is preferred. However, adequate diminution of autonomic reflex responses may well be achieved by the use of smaller doses when less severe stimulation occurs or the patient is judged to be fit enough to withstand the responses without any hazard being incurred. Opioids are usually more efficient in controlling autonomic reflex responses and maintaining a stable cardiovascular system than volatile anaesthetics which themselves cause significant cardiovascular effects.

The hypnotic/narcotic effect of opioids is a useful component of anaesthesia at all levels from opioid 'anaesthesia' which produces unconsciousness that persists through even the most intense of stimuli to a small opioid supplement that helps to reduce the dose of intravenous anaesthetic or benzodiazepine being used to keep a patient unaware of surgery. There appears to be some differences in the ratio of hypnotic to analgesic effects between the opioids that are commonly used; nalbuphine and buprenorphine, for instance, have been assessed as being more hypnotic than an equi-analgesic dose of morphine. This is hardly surprising, as the hypnotic effect of opioids is primarily due to their action at $K$ receptors and different opioids do have relatively different intensities of effect at $K$ and $\mu$ receptors. However, the differences are not marked and little account has been taken of them in the selection of an opioid to use as a component of anaesthesia. Indeed, the hypnotic effect is rarely taken into account when assessing which opioid and what dose to use in any situation. The major indications of reflex response suppression and duration of effect usually determine these things. More investigation is undoubtedly required to assess and compare the intensity of hypnotic effect of the commonly used drugs over a range of dosage and to determine how it can be reliably used as a component of anaesthesia.

The analgesic effect of opioids should theoretically never become a reason for using the drugs during anaesthesia. Nevertheless, mistakes do occur and there is a great deal of difference between a paralysed patient who is aware of surgery and intense pain and one who is aware but pain-free. The latter situation has occurred not infrequently during the course of major cardiac surgery conducted under opioid 'anaesthesia' and almost invariably the patient has been prepared to accept the situation after due apology and explanation. The analgesic effect of opioids is particularly relevant in relation to TIVA, where monitoring of consciousness may be extremely difficult in the paralysed patient. Prevention of severe pain should the patient unwittingly be aware thus becomes a significant reason for using a sufficient dose of an opioid as a component of anaesthesia.

When the use of an opioid during anaesthesia is being considered, the usual alternative available is that of a volatile anaesthetic but this is not the situation during TIVA. Nevertheless, one should never undertake TIVA if the use of a volatile anaesthetic would be better. Reasons for using TIVA are considered in Chapters 1 and 2 but it is still appropriate to make an assessment at this stage. One difficulty in conducting a true comparison is that all anaesthetists are well practised at using volatile anaesthetics whereas this is not true for TIVA or even the use of opioids in the place of volatile agents. All practising anaesthetists become very well aware of the considerable problems associated with the use of volatile agents and become expert in avoiding or at least minimising their dangerous or unwanted effects. It may be salutory, however, to enumerate some of these.

(1) All reduce vasomotor tone, cardiac output and myocardial contractility, also tissue blood perfusion. They increase cardiac irritability and dysrhythmias and potentiate arrest.

(2) All diminish lung function and depress respiration. They inhibit ciliary function and predispose to pulmonary infection.

(3) All diminish hepatic blood flow and liver function. Most may cause liver damage, occasionally fatal.

(4) All diminish renal blood flow and urine output. Some may cause renal damage that may be lethal.

(5) All increase cerebral blood flow and intra-cranial tension. Some cause convulsions.

(6) All may trigger malignant hyperpyrexia.

(7) All interact with muscle relaxants and may be dangerous in myasthenia.

(8) All inhibit pulmonary arterial hypoxic vasoconstriction.

(9) All pollute the atmosphere and may decrease the attentiveness of operating room staff.

(10) Some are explosive. Some are anti-analgesic, patients may wake in severe pain. Some may be teratogenic.

In addition, recovery after opioid-supplemented anaesthesia is usually faster, calmer and less painful than that after the use of volatile anaesthetics. The specific advantages of the use of opioids are due to the fact that unlike the volatile agents the opioids are highly selective in their actions and may therefore be used for specific requirements indicated by their pharmacological effects without producing the widespread general effects of the volatile agents listed above. The problems associated with the use of opioids in anaesthesia are considered below.

In any consideration of whether to use an opioid as a supplement to an intravenous hypnotic or anaesthetic for TIVA two main questions must be asked: can a satisfactory anaesthetic be given without the opioid and will the use of an opioid improve the anaesthetic that is given? The answer to these questions depends on the pharmacology of the i.v. anaesthetics available, considered in Chapter 2. Virtually all those used are lacking an 'analgesic' effect. Although they have rarely been assessed as analgesics, what is meant is that they have little capacity to suppress autonomic or somatic reflex responses to noxious stimulation. This is hardly surprising as, like all hypnotics, they have evolved from processes designed to manufacture drugs that act on the cerebral cortex in a highly selective manner rather than causing wide-spread central nervous system depression with all its problems. Thus they can not be expected to depress spinal cord reflexes in the dosage necessary to produce unconsciousness. Although some practitioners use them for this purpose in situations where only mild surgical stimulation is likely to occur, virtually every study comparing the use of almost any i.v. anaesthetic alone or with an opioid has found that the incorporation of an opioid reduces the dose of i.v. anaesthetic required, provides better operating conditions and allows faster recovery with fewer side effects at all stages of anaesthesia. The use of selective drugs for specific purposes in minimal dosage is clearly supported. The one i.v. anaesthetic that is an exception to this rule is ketamine, although most anaesthetists rarely assess ketamine anaesthesia as satisfactory, compared to other agents. Even in this case, however, some anaesthetists still use opioids in conjunction with ketamine in order to reduce the dose of ketamine and its side effects.

**Problems of using opioids**

Undoubtedly the major problem associated with the use of opioids in TIVA is respiratory depression.

In spontaneously ventilating patients, opioid-induced respiratory depression limits the dose that may be used and thereby limits the applicability of the technique to surgery that does not produce major stimuli. However, the surgical stimulation will itself counteract to some extent the respiratory depression caused so that this becomes variable in degree and generally most obvious and important in the period between giving the opioid and the start of surgery.

In ventilated patients opioid-induced respiratory depression causes problems when spontaneous ventilation is being restored after reversal of muscle relaxation and in the postoperative period. In the former situation the difficulties are frequently aggravated because of the level of ventilation that has been maintained during surgery. In order to maintain a normal pattern and level of spontaneous ventilation in a patient who is still subject to a significant opioid effect the patient must have a raised $PaCO_2$, due to reduced sensitivity of the ventilatory centre to $CO_2$. Thus it is important to induce a raised level (say 5.5 kPa) to help to initiate a rapid return to spontaneous ventilation. Spontaneous ventilation may, however, return at a $CO_2$ level that is lower than that required for an adequate maintained volume, particularly if the patient is stimulated as is common at the end of anaesthesia and on initial entry to a recovery ward. Then the pattern of ventilation may well be abnormal, usually periodic, with apnoeic episodes during which the patient may become acutely hypoxic. Such a situation is undoubtedly the cause of some of the problems that have incorrectly been attributed to 'secondary peaks' that may occur during a falling opioid plasma concentration. In the postoperative period respiratory depression is likely after opioid supplementation of TIVA. When it is of a degree that is comparable to that which would be induced by a dose of opioid given to the patient for pain relief it may be of little consequence. The greatest danger lies in the occurrence of hypoxia, which may be associated with apnoea due to the reason given above or due to a persistent level of opioid effect that is incompatible with adequate ventilation in a resting patient, but that may have not have been apparent whilst the patient was being stimulated. A 'secondary peak' of plasma concentration is another possible cause, but a more frequently encountered one is an interaction with another respiratory depressant drug given without due appreciation that it may cause this problem. Benzodiazepines are most often implicated in this respect. A patient with an adequate level of ventilation may well have a raised $PaCO_2$. This does not usually cause problems although it may be associated with throbbing headache, but in some cases it is entirely unacceptable. Patients with raised intracranial pressure or with significant pulmonary disease, particularly hypoxic respiratory drive, are obvious examples. These problems are best avoided by using an opioid with an appropriate duration of effect and a choice of dosage and method of application that ensures that no unwanted level of effect persists into the postoperative period. The use of a suitable reversal agent or a partial reversal technique to ensure a level of opioid effect that gives adequate postoperative analgesia with a sufficient level of ventilation is another acceptable approach to this problem (see below). But in every case it is best to ensure that all patients given TIVA, especially with opioids, have adequate monitoring of ventilation in the postoperative period. Use of a pulse oximeter is convenient and is recommended.

The other side effects of the opioids may also cause problems. Post-operative nausea and vomiting may be seen, but this may be no worse than that encountered after other methods of anaesthesia or induced by the treatment of postoperative pain. Again the choice and dose of drug used is important; any emetic effect of alfentanil, for instance, may have disappeared before the patient regains consciousness. Also important in reducing the incidence not only of nausea and vomiting but also other side effects such as dizziness, postural hypotension, sweating etc. is to ensure that the patient is allowed to rest quietly, preferably with eyes closed, until the effects of the opioid have diminished. Asking the patient to move quickly and particularly to rise or sit up is inviting trouble.

Other effects of the opioids may also occasionally cause problems. Meiosis and drowsiness may be particularly unwelcome after neurosurgery as they may hinder proper assessment, and the situation should be avoided or reversed as above.

## CHOICE OF OPIOID

As intimated above, the main factors indicating the choice of opioid to be used as a component of TIVA in a particular circumstance are the rate of onset and duration of effect. Other major factors are pharmacokinetic parameters (see Chapter 4, Opioid Anaesthesia, and Chapter 2), efficacy, specificity (potency, incidence of side effects) and availability.

### Duration of effect

The opioids may be grouped according to their duration of effect. The most commonly used opioids fall into the following categories.

*Long acting*

These drugs are rarely used for TIVA, having a duration of effect that is far longer than most anaesthetics. Some may occasionally be used to provide a low-level of opioid effect that may be initiated before induction of anaesthesia as a premedication, act throughout anaesthesia, supplemented as necessary, and remain to provide some degree of postoperative pain relief. Sustained-release morphine, lofentanil, levorphanol and buprenorphine are examples of long-acting opioids.

*Medium acting*

These drugs may be used for surgery of long duration (4—6 h), sometimes to establish a basal level of opioid effect which may be supplemented by use of other opioids with a shorter duration of effect, particularly towards the end of surgery.

Morphine is the major drug in this group; papaveretum has similar actions. Dextromoramide is less commonly used. Nalbuphine has a similar duration of effect.

Morphine has been compared double-blind with other opioids frequently used for TIVA. In a comparison with fentanyl and sufentanil, morphine 0.4 mg/kg was shown to have a significantly longer initial duration of effect (87 min) than equipotent doses of the other drugs (37 and 40 min, respectively) (Kay and Rolly, 1977). Other comparisons using different dose ratios did not expose a different duration of initial effect, but demonstrated that the effect of morphine persisted longer into the postoperative period than that of the other drugs (Ghoneim et al., 1984; Flacke et al., 1985). These studies also indicated that morphine supplementation of $N_2O$ was frequently incapable of suppressing autonomic reflex responses to anaesthesia and surgery; this was probably due as much to the relatively slow onset of effect of an i.v. dose of morphine as to lack of efficacy. In addition, morphine has long been known to release histamine in some patients (probably about 10%) causing hypotension, tachycardia and bronchospasm and this has been measured during anaesthesia (Flacke et al., 1987). These factors indicate that morphine has severe limitations for use as an opioid component of TIVA. The slow onset and relatively long duration of effect make it inflexible to use and the high dosage that may be necessary to suppress autonomic reflex responses in some cases means that one may frequently encounter significant postoperative depression or dangerous conditions due to histamine release. The same criticisms must apply to papaveretum which derives almost all its activity from its morphine content.

Nalbuphine has a very limited efficacy. It is a suitable component of TIVA for minor surgery such as cystoscopy or D & C where it will allow a reduction in the dose of i.v. anaesthetic required and thereby allow better operating conditions, fewer side effects and faster recovery (Kay et al., 1984); but it is not capable of suppressing autonomic reflex responses to greater stimuli such as laryngoscopy and intubation, or intra-abdominal surgery (Kay et al., 1985). Other workers purporting to demonstrate the efficacy of nalbuphine in general anaesthesia have co-administered other drugs so that the effect of nalbuphine alone could not be detected. It has, however, the great advantage of causing a limited, almost negligible degree of respiratory depression.

*Medium-short acting drugs*

The most commonly used drug in this category is pethidine (demerol). Others that have been extensively used are phenoperidine and pentazocine. Tramadol, butorphanol and meptazinol have had limited applications.

Pethidine, although the first drug to be used as a component of anaesthesia and of TIVA (see History, above) is undoubtedly the worst commonly used opioid supplement. It is the most toxic (De Castro et al., 1979), causes most side effects (Flacke et al., 1985, 1987) and is amongst the least efficacious (Ghoneim et al., 1984; Flacke at al., 1985). It cannot be used in high doses as for opioid 'anaesthesia' because of its toxicity to the cardiovascular system and high incidence of significant release of histamine. A claim that it is spasmolytic is not supported by evidence (Virtue, 1980) and indeed it can cause biliary spasm (Pickering et al., 1949). Its use is not recommended.

Phenoperidine has none of these disadvantages, but its use and availability have been curtailed by the advent of shorter acting drugs. Pentazocine is also now becoming obsolete, mainly due to the high incidence of sigma receptor mediated dysphoria and hallucinations when high doses are given, when it may also cause convulsions. Like nalbuphine, it has a limited efficacy at $\mu$ receptors indicated by a limited, but not negligible, capacity for inducing respiratory depression and like nalbuphine may be used as an effective component of TIVA for surgery causing limited but not major stimulation. Experience with butorphanol and meptazinol has reached similar conclusions; both cause a generally unacceptable incidence of side effects. Early optimistic reports that tramadol was highly efficacious but did not cause respiratory depression were, not surprisingly, unsubstantiated by later investigations.

*Short-acting drugs: fentanyl and sufentanil*

Early experience with fentanyl rapidly raised it to the position of the most extensively used opioid component of anaesthesia. In single, small to moderate doses it is shorter acting than any of the drugs previously available and is also more efficacious and less toxic, with fewer side effects. Its arrival made opioid 'anaesthesia', previously attempted using morphine, a viable technique. It is largely predictable in effect. Problems associated with its use have mainly been due to lack of understanding of its pharmacokinetics and particularly of its capacity to cumulate, also the importance of its residual effects after redistribution has caused an initial rapid decline in plasma concentration. Its use for TIVA was first described in 1977 (Kay, 1977) and it is still the opioid of choice as a component of TIVA in many situations.

Sufentanil is a more potent derivative of fentanyl and as such has been shown to be less toxic (De Castro et al., 1979). However, at the doses of these drugs used in clinical practice this difference is irrelevant. Some of the findings of early comparisons between the drugs such as a faster onset of effect and greater efficacy of sufentanil, together with greater cardiovascular depressant effects, were due to the use of a relatively greater dose ($\times$ 0.2) of sufentanil than fentanyl and may be inaccurate. Investigation of equipotencies has reinforced the original conclusions that sufentanil is approximately 10 times as potent as fentanyl (Flacke et al., 1985; Welchew and Herbert, 1985). In this dosage it has an onset of effect similar to that of fentanyl (Scott et al., 1991). However, it is more rapidly eliminated from the body and is less cumulative than fentanyl. This seems to be its major advantage of clinical importance over the older drug, to which it is pharmacologically otherwise virtually indistinguishable in normal clinical practice (Kay and Rolly, 1977)

These short acting drugs have proved to exert an appropriate duration of effect in most circumstances where TIVA has been used in paralysed patients, short enough for postoperative depression to be at an acceptable level when dosage has been adequate to suppress autonomic responses to anaesthetic and surgical stimulation even for surgery as brief as 40 min. Yet both have been regularly used for surgery exceeding 12 h without problems; indeed, they are still drugs of choice even in long cases because levels of effect can be adjusted rapidly and flexibly to meet different levels of stimulation and a high level of effect can be obtained even toward the end of surgery, yet still allow rapid recovery as plasma levels fall due to redistribution of the drug (cf. Chapter 2). Sufentanil has the advantage of being less cumulative when used for long cases. Flexibility of use of both drugs is enhanced by their very rapid onset of effect, shorter than that of morphine or pethidine.

In addition to possessing excellent times to onset and for duration of effect, these drugs are the most potent and specific opioids available, with the least toxicity and fewest side effects. One or other should be first choice as an opioid component of any TIVA expected to last for more than 45 min.

*Ultra-short acting: alfentanil*

Alfentanil is unique in having the fastest onset and shortest duration of effect of any opioid. More than 50% of maximum effect is usually apparent 1 min after i.v. injection and the effect of a clinically useful dose has usually declined to less than 50% maximum within 10 min. An obvious application for such a short-acting drug is as a component of anaesthesia for brief surgical procedures such as D & C. Its use with althesin in a TIVA technique in this context was compared with althesin alone (Kay and Cohen, 1981) where it was shown to decrease the dose of althesin required, decrease recovery time, decrease the incidence of side effects and improve the quality of anaesthesia. Subsequent work has generally confirmed these findings. In this context alfentanil is also better than fentanyl, allowing faster recovery not only of consciousness but also of perception, reaction and manipulative skills, with fewer side effects (Kay and Venkateraman, 1983).

In paralysed patients, the advantage of alfentanil over fentanyl has only been demonstrated in cases of relatively short duration (up to 30 min approximately). In patients undergoing laparoscopy it allowed faster recovery with less respiratory depression (Kay et al., 1982), and it is better than fentanyl in suppressing autonomic reflex responses to laryngoscopy and intubation in patients where rapid recovery of spontaneous ventilation is required (Black et al., 1984)

Alfentanil infusion as a component of TIVA for major surgery of a duration in excess of 1 h has been well documented and shown to be an effective method of obtaining an opioid effect. For cases of this length it is obviously appropriate to use an infusion rather than the intermittent dosage that would be required to maintain an effect. The problem is, should alfentanil be used in these longer anaesthetics in preference to fentanyl or sufentanil? Increased cost is an obvious reason not to use alfentanil, but is that increased cost outweighed by better results? In the case of opioid 'anaesthesia' for major surgery the answer appears to be clear; virtually all practitioners of this technique use fentanyl or sufentanil; but in these cases very rapid recovery is rarely required and in addition the less potent alfentanil tends to cause more side effects when extremely high doses are used.

The theoretical reasons for preferring to use alfentanil infusions in long anaesthetics are that it should be possible to obtain faster recovery and it is also possible to obtain greater flexibility of control. However, in order to elicit these advantages it is necessary to infuse the alfentanil in minimal dosage maintaining a constant manipulation of infusion to anticipate or react to surgical situations which cause greater or lesser degrees of stimulation (which is surely the best way of giving the drug). But it is difficult to write a research protocol to examine such an approach and this, together with a degree of fixation on the maintenance of theoretical 'therapeutic' blood levels using mean pharmacokinetic data, means that no proper assessment has been made as to whether alfentanil can provide better anaesthesia and recovery than fentanyl or sufentanil in long cases.

It is therefore only clear that alfentanil is the opioid of choice for TIVA lasting up to about 45 min. When properly applied in these circumstances it is capable of giving surprisingly excellent results (especially when used with propofol), particularly in the speed and quality of recovery. Even typical opioid effects such as nausea or vomiting and dizziness can be eliminated from the postoperative period if the administration of the drug is stopped 10 min or so before the end of surgery. It may be that these side effects are less apparent with alfentanil than other opioids as they have rarely been observed in volunteer studies of the drug.

A further option is available for the use of alfentanil in anaesthesia of longer duration. As the drug has essentially the same effects as the opioids that may be preferred for long anaesthetics, it may be substituted for these agents towards the anticipated end of anaesthesia (say during the last half hour) if additional opioid effect is required, thereby gaining the advantage of a rapid diminution of the opioid effect, corresponding to the end of anaesthesia. Such a technique may be particularly useful when a severe stimulus of brief duration (such as traction on the peritoneum) occurs towards the end of surgery.

## TECHNIQUES OF ADMINISTRATION

### Predetermined

Much has been written about techniques of administration that are designed to rapidly achieve a so-called 'therapeutic' blood concentration of the opioid concerned, then to maintain it at a constant level. Many complex mathematical equations often figure in papers dealing with this subject and the 'problem' has been raised to a level where computer programmes and even computerized equipment has been produced to achieve these ends. The average anaesthetist thinking of undertaking TIVA may well wonder how he might manage without a great deal of knowledge about the pharmacokinetics of all the drugs, a degree in mathematics and equipment that he cannot afford. But what is the validity of these aims?

First, the question of individual variability must be considered. Any formula based on 'mean' pharmacokinetics, often derived from a small group inevitably selected by protocol limitations and exclusions, must produce a wide range of blood concentrations (usually approximately 10-fold) when applied to the diverse population that constitutes the patients an anaesthetist usually has to deal with. But the aim is to produce an effect, not a blood concentration, so to this unpredictability due to variable pharmacokinetics one must add another range of unpredictability, again approximately 10-fold in extent, that of pharmacodynamic response. Even if the resulting combination of variability was small in extent, which it is not, it would still be illogical to base therapy of this importance on mean values which imply that 50% of patients are under-dosed and 50% overdosed. Also, to give a dose that would adequately treat the 'resistant' patient would grossly overdose the 'sensitive' patient. In clinical practice the results of such an approach are generally poor.

Secondly, the idea that a constant level of plasma concentration or even effect is a desirable aim is a false one. Consideration of the reasons for using the opioid make it clear that one is usually treating a continually variable level of anaesthetic and surgical stimulation. It is necessary to have a level of effect that is adequate to deal with the most intense stimuli at the times when they occur. To maintain this level of effect throughout anaesthesia is to give an overdose. Does this matter? The opioids recommended may generally be given in massive dosage to ventilated patients without causing significant toxic effects. But sustained, high concentrations of these lipophilic drugs will cause a continual slow transfer into poorly perfused fatty tissues from which they will subsequently, in the postoperative period, return to the plasma from where they may exert unwanted effects; also transfer from this lipid compartment will slow down the reduction of the final plasma concentration that occurs when administration is stopped.

**Alternative approaches**

So what alternative approaches may be used? The simplest is to deal with opioid administration in the same clinical way that anaesthetists deal with other drugs that they use, such as volatile anaesthetics or muscle relaxants. Taking the latter example, the requirements for effect are usually very similar to those for an opioid, i.e. an intense action early in the anaesthetic, then a variable requirement through the course of surgery when the effect is allowed to decline until stimulation is anticipated or occurs, then a frequent need for a peak effect toward the end of surgery. Using a muscle relaxant it is usual for the anaesthetist to give an initial estimated dose that will produce an effect that is more than adequate for most patients (although occasionally a supplement may be required). This intentional overdosage of most patients produces anticipated and acceptable effects as it does also with opioids. It also allows a period of stability early in the course of anaesthesia when the anaesthetist has many other things to attend to. Monitoring of returning responses then guides the anaesthetist to subsequent control at an appropriate level of effect. The patient's response to the large, arbitrary dose given initially (duration of action, whether a sufficient effect is obtained or whether a supplementary dose is immediately needed) helps the anaesthetist to select a suitable dose to maintain the effect required for the length of time desired. Only rarely is neuromuscular blockade maintained at 100% throughout surgery, which is the equivalent to maintaining a constant level of maximum required effect for an opioid. When an increased intensity of effect is required toward the end of surgery, e.g. for closure of the peritoneum, the anaesthetist will anticipate the need and give the minimum effective dose, often using the shortest-acting drug available that is compatible with the agent that has been used throughout maintenance of anaesthesia. Opioids are frequently required in exactly the same situation and may be applied in exactly the same way. The only significant difficulty in using this approach with opioids is that of monitoring their effects, which is more difficult than measuring neuromuscular transmission.

Such an approach is easily understood and used by any anaesthetist. It also brings into question the necessity to give opioids for TIVA by infusion, which is always time-consuming to set up, needs continual attention, consideration and adjustment, and undoubtedly puts off many anaesthetists who would otherwise use the technique. In Chapter 2 Dr Sear outlines many infusion techniques that are designed to achieve a certain level of effect rapidly and then maintain it. This approach is not essential for either opioids or muscle relaxants, and is not the method that most anaesthetists use when giving these drugs, which is to give an initial large bolus and subsequent small intermittent injections as required. As fentanyl and sufentanil have a similar duration of effect to many muscle relaxants that are commonly employed, it is entirely reasonable to use them in the same way, when the patient is to be paralysed; because of induced muscle rigidity large doses of opioids should not be given to unparalysed patients. Just as many anaesthetists choose to infuse the shorter-acting muscle relaxants should they choose to use one for a long case, so they may choose to infuse alfentanil in similar circumstances. But even alfentanil may be conveniently used by intermittent dosing for anaesthesia of up to 45 min duration.

Another alternative approach to achieving a desired effect is to give the drug slowly until the required effect is obtained. Again, this is a method of administration that all anaesthetists understand and are well practised in, being frequently the method of induction of anaesthesia using i.v. anaesthetics or benzodiazepines. It is, however, unsuitable for the administration of a large dose of opioid in order to obtain an intense effect. Not only is it unnecessarily and unacceptably time-consuming for this purpose, but it sets the problem of when to give the muscle relaxant (and subsequently intubate the trachea to ensure ventilation) that will be required to prevent rigidity. The problems that may result from an unnecessarily large dose of i.v. anaesthetic caused by giving it too quickly are likely to be much greater than those posed by an 'overdose' of opioid given to a paralysed patient, so in the latter case it is not necessary to titrate to effect.

This is not the case in unparalysed patients however. In this situation it is best to give the necessarily small dose of opioids slowly until the required level of effect is obtained. As with i.v. anaesthetics this will also tend to minimize side effects and the respiratory depressant effect by avoiding the impact of a high concentration and by allowing a build up of $PaCO_2$ to combat the depression. In this situation it is obviously best to use an opioid with a rapid onset of effect and as most of the cases where small doses of opioid and spontaneous ventilation are required are likely to be short ones the use of alfentanil is appropriate. Indeed, it may be dangerous to give alfentanil very rapidly. Muscle rigidity, apnoea and difficulty in maintaining artificial ventilation have been observed personally after a dose of as little as 0.25 mg given to an adult.

The partial, or agonist/antagonist, opioids are easier to give. All have limited efficacy and none cause acute apnoea and muscle rigidity even when given rapidly. In addition they have relatively flat dose-response curves which ensure that even if a misjudged dose is given the effect is not likely to be far from that required. Overdosage causes few acute problems, but may precipitate dysphoria and hallucinations in the cases of pentazocine and butorphanol, severe emesis in the case of meptazinol and important respiratory depression in the case of buprenorphine, particularly as in TIVA it is combined with an i.v.anaesthetic or benzodiazepine.

**Supplementary dosage**

The difficulties in assessing when a supplementary dose of opioid is required during TIVA, and deciding what dose to give, have already been alluded to. As the main reason for using an opioid is usually to prevent or diminish a reflex response to stimulation, the anticipation or occurrence of such an unwanted response is the major indication for giving another dose.

Whilst it is often easy to anticipate that the surgeon will stimulate the patient to an extent that will frequently cause an unwanted response (e.g. when traction is about to be applied to the uterus or peritoneum) it may be less easy to assess whether the effects of the opioid medication already given to the patient are sufficient to suppress the responses that might occur. Before giving a supplementary dose many factors must be considered, such as whether it is essential to prevent *any* response, how much residual opioid effect exists (this is often very difficult to assess if there has been little recent stimulation), the duration of effect of preceding supplementary doses, the expected duration of surgery, etc. Such a complex assessment is frequently difficult to make and apparently sure indications may be misleading. One has personally seen pin-point pupils dilate widely and very slow heart rates double in immediate response to stimulation.

Dosing in response to the occurrence of unwanted reflex responses is also far from straightforward, and again may require an element of prediction. The problem is that most opioids take several minutes to exert a high proportion of their effect but the stimulation, and the response to it, may only be momentary. Thus the anaesthetist must be able to assess whether such stimulation is likely to re-occur before deciding whether to react to a reflex response by giving a supplementary dose of opioid. It is not surprising that experience not only in the use of opioids during anaesthesia but also of anaesthesia in general allows better use of this technique.

The usual reflex responses that give rise to concern are increases in heart rate or arterial blood pressure, or movement. Sweating and lachrymation are other common indices of inadequate opioid effect. Several of these indications are more apparent in patients who have not received anticholinergic medication; $\alpha$ or $\beta$ adrenergic blockers also tend to conceal these indications.

Another major indication for the use of an opioid during TIVA is its hypnotic effect and any indication that the patient may be becoming aware (see Chapter 10) may also be an indication for supplementary opioid medication. Again, one of the main problems about this use is the relatively slow onset of effect of most opioids compared to that of the i.v. induction agents. The importance of maintaining unconsciousness is so great that any indication that the patient may become aware should be treated initially by use of an i.v. anaesthetic rather than an opioid, although it may be perfectly reasonable to use the fast-acting alfentanil in this circumstance.

Indeed, the availability of alfentanil has made the use of opioids in TIVA very much easier. Its onset of effect is so fast that should one have unwittingly allowed an unwanted reflex response to stimulation occur, it may be suppressed within the minute by use of i.v. alfentanil, which is compatible with any opioid chosen as the main analgesic component of anaesthesia. This allows a great deal more flexibility in the level of opioid effect to be maintained and in particular allows the effect to be run down to an acceptable level towards the end of anaesthesia despite the anticipation of later stimulation.

**Ending opioid supplementation**

It is usually desirable to give the final dose of opioid during anaesthesia at a time when its effects will persist into the postoperative period only to an acceptable level. This is normally a degree of effect that allows adequate respiration, reflexes and awareness yet still provides the necessary level of analgesia. It is obviously extremely difficult to be able to predict this time, particularly as the time when surgery will end is always unpredictable. In general one would usually prefer not to give another dose of one of the short-acting opioids (fentanyl or sufentanil) within 1/2 h of the anticipated end of surgery but this preference may have to be ignored if the level of opioid effect after this time is inadequate or a major stimulus (e.g. closing the peritoneum) is expected between this time and the end of surgery. As mentioned above, however, the availability of alfentanil has virtually removed problems in this area. A small dose (e.g. 7 μg/kg) may be given either to prevent or diminish an unwanted reflex response within minutes of the end of surgery without having a significant effect on the postoperative condition, so short is its duration of effect.

Should the level of opioid effect be too great when surgery is complete, the question of reversal must be addressed (see below).

## DOSAGE

Only an approximation of dose requirement can be offerred, but the methods of use advocated above are meant to cope with the problems of individual variation of response and neither is dependent on the accurate selection of dosage. Both allow treatment to be adjusted not only to the patient's responses but also the varying demands of stimulation.

**Initial dosage for patients to be paralysed and ventilated**

The first intense stimulus to be seen in these patients is that of laryngoscopy and tracheal intubation. The means of attenuating or preventing the autonomic reflex responses to this readily reproducable stimulus have been extensively studied. That some of the results obtained are not the same is usually due to the fact that the study conditions have rarely been the same, e.g. anaesthetics used, type of patient studied, degree of suppression required. Nevertheless there is a remarkable similarity in the means of the doses quoted as being effective, but beware of relying on a mean value when complete suppression of the response is necessary! Generally speaking, the dose required to suppress these reflexes will also be adequate to suppress responses to subsequent skin incision, opening of peritoneum etc., if the drug has a persistent enough effect. However, unless there is a specific concern about the effects of a larger dose or the anaesthetic might turn out to be a short one, there is no reason why the initial dose of the opioid given need be limited to that necessary to attenuate cardiovascular responses to intubation. A dose of double that size may usually be given safely and this will have the advantage of ensuring suppression of the response and allowing a variably long period after administration before signs of recovery from the effects begin to appear.

Here are some recorded dose requirements for attenuation of reflex responses to intubation, together with suggestions for initial large doses to be used and approximate times for which these will continue to exert a sufficient effect to suppress autonomic reflex responses to intra-abdominal surgery. Note that major stimulation such as traction on the lower oesophagus or uterus may well cause responses well before these times.

*Fentanyl* 5 μg/kg abolished increases in the means of heart rate and arterial blood pressure (Black et al., 1984); 15 μg/kg may be required to block all increases in heart rate (Iver and Russell, 1988) An initial dose of 10 μg/kg is appropriate for an effect lasting 45—60 min.

*Sufentanil* 0.5 μg/kg blocked increases in mean values; 1 μg/kg suppressed increases in heart rate and arterial pressure in all patients (Kay et al., 1987). An initial dose of 1 μg/kg will be effective for approximately 45 min.

*Alfentanil* 15 μg/kg blocked rises in means of all arterial pressures, but not heart rate, which was suppressed by 30 μg/kg (Black et al., 1984). An initial dose of 30 μg/kg will be effective for approximately 20 min.

*Morphine* is not a good drug to use in an attempt to block responses to intubation. It is frequently ineffective even in relatively high doses (Flacke et al., 1985). An initial dose of 0.5 mg/kg is therefore inadequate for this purpose but may control responses to subsequent moderate stimulation for 30—60 min. Larger doses should be used with great caution because of haemodynamic effects that are significantly greater in some patients than those of the other opioids above.

### *Partial and agonist/antagonist drugs*

These drugs are only partially effective in blocking responses to intubation. Although some suppression of increases in arterial pressure may be obtained they are less efficacious in preventing an increase in cardiac rate (Kay et al., 1985; Kay, 1986). Agonist opioids should generally be used for suppression of responses during maintenance of anaesthesia but buprenorphine, the most efficacious partial agonist is reasonably effective, and also long-acting (Kay, 1980).

## Dosage for spontaneously breathing patients

Working on the principle of starting with a small dose and building to a desired effect the following doses may be used initially and for increments. Intravenous injection should be over at least 20 s. Spontaneous ventilation is likely to be significantly depressed by the time a dose of twice the initial dose has been given, unless the patient is being stimulated. Fentanyl, 1.5 μg/kg followed by 0.8 μg/kg; sufentanil, 0.15 μg/kg followed by 0.08 μg/kg; alfentanil, 4 μg/kg followed by 2 μg/kg; morphine, 0.1 mg/kg followed by 0.05 mg/kg; buprenorphine, 0.15 μg/kg repeated; butorphanol, 30 μg/kg followed by 15 μg/kg; meptazinol, 1 mg/kg repeated; nalbuphine, 0.2 mg/kg followed by 0.1 mg/kg; pentazocine, 0.5 mg/kg followed by 0.25 mg/kg.

It is important to allow time for the effects of a dose to be apparent before repeating; in this respect remember the slow onset of effect of morphine and that buprenorphine is even slower.

## REVERSAL OF OPIOID EFFECT

The principal reason for wishing to reverse the effects of an opioid used as a component of TIVA is to reduce respiratory depression in the postoperative period. There are a number of ways in which the respiratory effects of opioid may be reduced, but most anaesthetists prefer to use a specific opioid antagonist rather than rely on non-specific measures. Unfortunately, this method also reduces the analgesic effect of the opioid, which may have unpleasant consequences for the patient. The decision to reverse the effects of the opioid should therefore never be taken lightly, whether a specific or non-specific method is used.

Before deciding to take active therapeutic measures to treat respiratory depression an attempt should be made to determine exactly the cause of the depression. It is of course easy to reason that the administration of a specific opioid antagonist will assist with that determination and also, in many cases, reverse the depression adequately at the same time. This coarse method may not, however, produce the best result for the patient.

One common cause of respiratory depression after administration of an opioid during anaesthesia is a relative hypocarbia. A degree of hyperventilation is readily caused by unmonitored mechanical ventilation, especially during TIVA when the metabolism of the patient may be significantly reduced by several of the drugs used. Opioids in particular may also depress the sensitivity of the respiratory centre to carbon dioxide so that adequate ventilatory volumes and pattern will depend on an increased $PaCO_2$. Treatment of apparent respiratory depression should therefore be deferred until this has been established (say to 5.5—6 kPa) whilst maintaining full oxygenation of the blood.

The other drugs used in TIVA may also cause respiratory depression. Inadequate ventilation due to persistent neuromuscular blockade is usually readily recognized by the experienced anaesthetist but must always be excluded before therapy to reverse opioid effects is given. The respiratory effects of other drugs commonly used in TIVA such as benzodiazepines or i.v. anaesthetics are not so easily differentiated from opioid-induced respiratory depression. It may be appropriate to test the cause of the depression by use of a specific opioid antagonist but this could lead to problems; if the main factor causing depression is not the opioid one could still be left with significant depression but also with a patient with an unwanted increase in cardiac rate and arterial blood pressure due to the elimination of the analgesic effect of the opioid. This can be catastrophic in some patients and this consequence of specific opioid reversal, also the possibility of severe perceived pain must always be remembered when the use of an opioid antagonist is being considered. There are three approaches that may be used to minimise problems. The first is simply to wait, whilst continuing ventilation, preferably at a slow rate, to maintain a $PaCO_2$ that is higher than the patient's normal and a high $PaO_2$. Conversation with the patient should be maintained at a normal level. Unfortunately this is an option that is rarely available but if the depression is primarily due to a short-acting i.v. anaesthetic it is indubitably the best method.

A second approach is to give a specific opioid antagonist by titrating its effect against the patient's respiration. Small doses, e.g. naloxone 1.5 $\mu$g/kg should be used, giving each dose full time to work before repeating it. If the depression is opioid-induced an improvement will very rapidly become apparent and dosing may continue until the desired level of effect (adequate ventilation with pain control) has been achieved. If no improvement is apparent after two or three doses, administration should stop as the depression probably has another cause. If naloxone is used its short duration of effect must be remembered and it may be necessary to continue treatment by infusion of i.m. injection.

The third approach is to give an opioid agonist/antagonist or partial agonist. This method, described as 'sequential analgesia' allows the displacement of the opioid agonist used during anaesthesia by an opioid that has a lesser effect at the receptors that it occupies. All the agonist/antagonist or partial agonist opioids may be used in this way; although pentazocine was initially employed its side effects make its use less desirable than some of the newer drugs. The less efficacious the drug is in producing analgesia and respiratory depression, the more effective it is as a reversal agent. Thus nalbuphine will be most effective in restoring respiratory drive but it will also leave least analgesia and there have been several reports of patients being left in severe pain after its injudicious use. If chosen, it should be titrated slowly to effect in the same way as an antagonist. Buprenorphine is at the opposite end of the scale, being least efficacious as an antagonist but leaving the patient with the greatest degree of analgesia. Again, one should not be too heavy-handed in giving the drug lest the patient is left with an unacceptable degree of buprenorphine-induced respiratory depression.

Should the second or third approaches not prove satisfactory one is still left with the option of using a non-specific respiratory stimulant. Whilst these drugs have the considerable advantage of improving respiratory drive without diminishing analgesia they have disadvantages that leads one not to recommend their use ahead of the other reversal agents. The first is the problem of dosage; in the case of nikethamide and doxapram there is a fairly small interval between an effective and a toxic dose. Whilst frank convulsions are rare, lesser degrees of central stimulatory effects are not. Doxapram is perhaps the most efficacious but usually causes the patient to feel distinctly dysphoric and it may specifically interact to produce toxic effects with morphine (Khanna and Pleuvry, 1978) and with alfentanil (Smith and Kay, 1985). It is short-acting and must usually be given by infusion when treating the effects of the longer-acting opioids; the infusion rate must be carefully controlled. Almitrine may be the drug of choice as its effects are mainly peripheral rather than central, but it too has a disappointingly short duration of effect (Kay and Pollard, 1988).

See also Chapter 5.

## ADJUVANT DRUGS

It would be inappropriate to end a discussion of the use of opioids as a component of TIVA without considering the use of adjuvant and so-called 'potentiating' drugs. Mixtures of drugs that include opioids have been extensively advocated for anaesthetic use over many years. Important examples include combinations used for premedication, the 'lytic cocktail' and 'hibernation therapy' of Laborit and Huguenard (1954) and 'neuroleptanaesthesia' (De Castro et al., 1964); but there is virtually no evidence to indicate that any of the drugs suggested 'potentiate' by a synergistic rather than a simple additive effect of a common action.

There is, however, surely no place in rational anaesthetic practice for the use of routine (i.e., given without thinking) fixed-ratio drug combinations. This principle applies as firmly to the use of a standard premedication such as morphine and atropine as to such preparations as Thalamonal (Innovar), except for convenience when the particular combination is deemed, after consideration, to be best.

A very large number of drugs have been suggested as being appropriate for use with an opioid in such combinations, mainly phenothiazines, butyrophenones and benzodiazepines, and it would be inappropriate as well as unneccessary to consider them here. There are in many instances clear indications for the use of such adjuvants, e.g. the use of a butyrophenone to diminish opioid-induced nausea and vomiting or vasoconstriction induced by a noxious stimulus; but not only must the reason for the adjuvant drug be clear but the dose and time of administration must be considered, as must the consequences of the other effects of the adjuvant drug. In this respect the interaction of the effects on respiration of opioids and benzodiazepines is too often overlooked.

See also Chapter 15.

## REFERENCES

Black, T.E., Kay, B. and Healy, T.E.J. (1984) Reducing the haemodynamic responses to laryngoscopy and intubation. A comparison of alfentanil with fentanyl. *Anaesthesia* 39, 883—887.

De Castro, J., Mundeleer, P. and Bauduin, T. (1964) Critical evaluation of ventilation and acid-base balance during neuroleptanalgesia. *Ann. Anaesthesiol. Fr.* 5, 425—436.

De Castro, J., Van de Water, A., Wouters, L., Xhonneux, R., Reneman, R. and Kay, B. (1979) Comparitive study of cardiovascular, neurological and metabolic side-effects of 8 narcotics in dogs. *Acta Anaesthesiol. Belg.* 30, 5—99.

Flacke, J.W., Bloor, B.C., Kripke, B.J., Flacke, W.E., Warneck, C.M., Van Etten, A.P., Wong, D.H. and Katz, R.L. (1985) Comparison of morphine, meperidine, fentanyl and sufentanil in balanced anesthesia. *Anesth. Analg.* 64, 897—910.

Flacke, J.W., Flacke, W.E., Bloor, B.C., Van Etten, A.P. and Kripke, B.J. (1987) Histamine release by four narcotics *Anesth. Analg.* 66, 723—730.

Ghoneim, M.M., Dhanaraj, J. and Choi, W.W. (1984) Comparison of four opioid analgesics as supplements to nitrous oxide anesthesia. *Anesth. Analg.* 63, 405—412.

Kay, B. (1977) Total intravenous anaesthesia with etomidate I. *Acta Anaesthesiol. Belg.* 28, 107—113.

Kay, B. (1980) A double-blind comparison between fentanyl and buprenorphine in analgesic-supplemented anaesthesia. *Br. J. Anaesth.* 52, 453—457.

Kay, B. (1986) Reduktion der Kreislaufreaction auf trachealintubation die wirkung von meptazinol. *Anaesthesist* 35, 500—503.

Kay, B. and Cohen, A.T. (1981) Althesin and alfentanil for minor surgery In: *Proceedings of the European Academy of Anaesthesiology*. Editor: M. Vickers, Springer, Berlin, p. 104.

Kay, B. and Pollard, B. (1988) L'almitrine supprime temporairement la dépression respiratoire causée par la buprenorphine. *Ann. Fr. Anesth. Reanim.* 7, 176—177.

Kay, B. and Rolly, G. (1977) Duration of action of analgesic supplements to anaesthesia. A double-blind comparison between morphine, fentanyl and sufentanil. *Acta Anaesthesiol. Belg.* 28, 25—32.

Kay, B. and Venkateraman, P. (1983) Recovery after fentanyl and alfentanil in anaesthesia for minor surgery. *Br. J. Anaesth.* 55, 169S—172S.

Kay, B., Cohen, A.T., Shaw, J. and Healy, T.E.J. (1982) Anaesthesia for laparoscopy; alfentanil and fentanyl compared. *Ann. R. Coll. Surg.* 65, 316—317.

Kay, B., Hargreaves, J. and Healy, T.E.J. (1984) Nalbuphine and althesin anaesthesia. *Anaesthesia* 39, 666—669.

Kay, B., Healy, T.E.J. and Bolder, P.M. (1985) Blocking the circulatory responses to trachel intubation; a comparison of fentanyl and nalbuphine. *Anaesthesia* 40, 960—963.

Kay, B., Nolan, D., Mayall, R. and Healy, T.E.J. (1987) The effect of sufentanil on the cardiovascular responses to tracheal intubation. *Anaesthesia* 42, 382—386.

Khanna, V.K. and Pleuvry, B.J. (1978) A study of naloxone and doxapram as agents for the reversal of neuroleptanalgesic respiratory depression in the conscious rabbit. *Br. J. Anaesth.* 50, 905—909.

Laborit, H. and Huguenard, P. (1954) *Pratique de l'Hibernotherapie en Chirurgie et Medicine.* Masson, Paris.

Mushin, W.W., Rendell and Baker, L. (1949) Pethidine as an adjunct to nitrous oxide anaesthesia. *Br. Med. J.* 2, 472.

Neff, W., Mayer, E.C. and Perales, M.L. (1947) Nitrous oxide and oxygen anesthesia with curare relaxation. *Calif. Med.* 66, 67.

Pickering, R.W., Abreu, B.E., Bohr, D.F. and Reynolds, W.F. (1949) Some effects of meperidine on gastro-enteritic, extrahepatic biliary and cardiovascular activity. *J. Am. Pharmacol. Soc.* 38, 188.

Savege, T.M., Ramsay, M.A.E., Curran, J.P.J., Cotter, J., Walling, P.T. and Simpson, B.R. (1975) Intravenous anaesthesia by infusion. *Anaesthesia* 30, 757.

Scott, J.C., Cooke, J.E. and Stanski, D.R. (1991) Electroencephalographic quantitation of opioid effect: comparative pharmacodynamics of fentanyl and sufentanil. *Anesthesiology* 74, 34—42.

Smith, P. and Kay, B. (1985) The analgesic and respiratory effects of alfentanil and doxapram in the mouse. In: *Alfentanil; Experimental and Clinical Studies,* Section 2B. Thesis for D.Med.Sci, B. Kay, University of Gent, pp. 16—17.

Sugioka, K., Boniface, K.J. and Davis, D.A. (1957) Influence of meperidine on myocardial contractility of the intact dog. *Anesthesiology* 18, 623.

Virtue, R.W. (1980) In: *Trends in Intravenous Anesthesia.* Editors: J.A. Aldrete and T.H. Stanley, Symposia Specialists Inc., Miami, p. 386.

Welchew, E.A. and Herbert, P. (1985) Effects of sufentanil on respiration and heart rate during nitrous oxide and halothane anaesthesia. *Br. J. Anaesth.* 58, 120P.

B. Kay (ed.) Total Intravenous Anaesthesia



# 6

# Ketamine

Brian Kay

## INTRODUCTION

Ketamine was the first drug designed and used extensively for total intravenous anaesthesia (TIVA) and it may still be the drug most widely used for this purpose.

Ketamine differs chemically from all other anaesthetics, being derived from the psychotropic drug phencyclidine. Its effects also differ markedly from other anaesthetics, so that it has been said to produce 'dissociation' and analgesia rather than the usual pattern of anaesthesia. As an anaesthetic it has serious disadvantages that make its use in sophisticated surroundings rare, but it also possesses unique pharmacological properties which make it indispensible in some unusual circumstances so that it is to found in the armamentarium of most anaesthetists. It is also unusual in that it has been used extensively to produce anaesthesia without the concomitant use of any other drugs.

## PHARMACOLOGY

Ketamine hydrochloride dissolves in water to produce a clear, colourless, acid (pH 3.5—5.5) solution available as 10, 50 or 100 mg base/ml. The latter concentrations contain a benzethonium preservative and are adequately stable in solution for use over many hours. Ketamine may be given by either i.m. or i.v. injection. The former is usually painful; local pain occasionally occurs after the latter and this may be accompanied by reddening of the vein, which may progress to thrombosis, especially after infusion.

Loss of consciousness occurs more slowly after i.v. injection of ketamine than after most other i.v. anaesthetics, usually taking 2—3 min. Slow i.v. administration (over 1 min) is recommended in order to reduce the respiratory depressant effect of the drug, which is dose-dependent. However, loss of consciousness may be achieved using ketamine with less respiratory depression than will normally result from the use of a barbiturate or propofol. Because of their markedly differing effects it is impossible to compare dosage of ketamine with that of other anaesthetics; 1 mg/kg i.v. is usually used to induce anaesthesia but loss of consciousness may occur after much smaller doses; 2 mg/kg will produce a period of 'anaesthesia' (little reaction to surgical stimulation) lasting for about 10 min with loss of consciousness for about twice that time. It is not possible to obtain very short periods of unconsciousness (1 or 2 min) reliably by the use of a small dose of ketamine.

Induction of anaesthesia by ketamine produces unusual cardiovascular effects. An increase in both cardiac rate and arterial blood pressure normally results, a rise of 20—25% can be expected following a dose of 1—2 mg/kg, persisting for 15—20 min. Cardiac dysrhythmias may be precipitated, especially in nervous patients. These effects appear to be mainly due to an effect of ketamine on the central nervous system which increases sympathetic nervous system activity but the myocardium may be sensitized to exo- and endogenous catechol amines and there also seems to be inhibition of re-uptake of catecholamines. The direct effect of ketamine on the myocardium is, however, depressant and hypotension or bradycardia may occur, especially in patients receiving $\alpha$- or $\beta$-adrenergic blockers, or receiving volatile anaesthetics (Stanley, 1973). Blood pressure may also fall unexpectedly in critically ill patients (Waxman et al., 1980). Although variable effects on peripheral resistance have been reported, pulmonary arterial resistance and pressure are usually significantly increased as is right cardiac work (Tarnow et al., 1979).

A rise in cerebrospinal fluid pressure and intra-ocular pressure may also occur as a result of ketamine induction of anaesthesia. Respiratory depression occurs in a dose-related manner and may be clinically important after large doses or concomitant depressant medication. Fast injection or infusion of the drug is also likely to cause respiratory depression. Like opioids, the curve of the respiratory response to $CO_2$ is shifted to the right by ketamine (Bourke et al., 1987). Ketamine also usually has a bronchodilator effect which seems to be mainly due to increased $\beta$-adrenergic activity. Hypoxic pulmonary vasoconstriction may not be diminished (Lumb et al., 1979).

Ketamine-induced anaesthesia is accompanied by manifestations not regularly produced by other anaesthetics. Movement is common; not only in response to stimulation when anaesthesia is inadequate, but also spontaneous movements seen even when large doses have been given. These may be tonic, clonic, or athetoid and often involve ocular or laryngeal muscles so that nystagmus or phonation occurs. Such movements may persist through the recovery period, even after consciousness has been regained. The eyes frequently remain open throughout anaesthesia.

Unlike most anaesthetics, ketamine anaesthesia is not characterized by a reduction in muscle tone, which may increase. This may increase the difficulty of some types of surgery, even simple reduction of a fractured bone. Despite this, ketamine increases the effect of most of all muscle relaxants although this increase is not of great importance clinically. These effects are probably due to interference with the calcium flux mechanisms. Ketamine anaesthesia increases the tone of the uterus at term (Marx et al., 1979).

One surprising and useful feature is that laryngeal and pharyngeal reflexes are frequently well maintained, so that the patient may be capable of maintaining an airway, swallowing, coughing and even ejecting vomit during a state of anaesthesia where surgery is possible. Whilst it would be totally irresponsible to rely on these facts to the extent of waiving normal safety restrictions on the use of anaesthesia, ketamine has been widely used safely and successfully in circumstances where these restrictions cannot be complied with. Gross aspiration may not occur even in circumstances where it would seem likely under other anaesthetics. Laryngeal sensitivity and activity mean that laryngospasm may readily occur especially as salivation is often excessive during ketamine anaesthesia.

Recovery from ketamine anaesthesia is slow and gradual and is also accompanied by unusual manifestations. Foremost amongst the unwanted effects is the very frequent occurrence of vivid dreams which the patient often remembers as unpleasant. These are also often accompanied by the purposeless movements and phonation that are sometimes observed during maintenance, so that the patient may appear to be grossly disturbed. Such phenomena are most often encountered in young adults. Post-operative nausea and vomiting occur more commonly after ketamine than after many methods of general anaesthesia.

Ketamine is usually said to be a powerful analgesic, but there is little firm evidence for this if a strict definition of analgesia is applied, e.g., that pain is diminished without a change in conscious perception. It indubitably has an anti-nociceptive effect in animals in doses insufficient to produce 'anaesthesia', but in humans it seems to be difficult to relieve pain without causing some dissociation from the surroundings, at the very least. Attempts have been made to treat pain by the infusion of ketamine in low dosage but the technique has not proved to be popular because of the high incidence of side-effects, particularly changes in perception.

## PHARMACOKINETICS (See also Chapter 2)

Ketamine is almost entirely metabolized in the body, very little is excreted unchanged. Renal inadequacy has little effect on the action of ketamine. Most of the metabolism takes place in the liver, the two main mechanisms of breakdown being N-demethylation and ring hydroxylation but several other mechanisms are postulated and numerous metabolic products have been identified, some with similar but less potent pharmacodynamic effects to ketamine.

Ketamine is highly lipophilic and after i.v. injection it is rapidly distributed and metabolised, with a clearance rate of 18 ml/kg per min. If the declining plasma concentration is analysed using a three-term exponential model the initial distribution phase, $t_{1/2}\pi$ has a mean value of only 24 s, redistribution, $t_{1/2}\alpha$ is 4.68 min and the elimination half-life, $t_{1/2}\beta$ is 2.17 h (Domino et al., 1984). The effects of ketamine are increased and prolonged by the simultaneous use of diazepam, not only because of some similar pharmacodynamic effects of diazepam but also because it increases ketamine plasma levels and inhibits the hepatic metabolism of the drug, prolonging $t_{1/2}\alpha$ and $t_{1/2}\beta$ (Atiba et al., 1988). During continuous infusion of ketamine a $t_{1/2}\beta$ of 79 min was established (Idvall et al., 1979).

It seems therefore that redistribution of the drug, rather than metabolism, is the cause of the decrease in brain tissues that limits the action of ketamine. What is surprising is that this highly lipophilic drug, with a $pK_a$ of 7.5 and a plasma concentration profile after i.v. injection that resembles that of most i.v. induction agents should have such a slow onset and relatively long duration of effect. It seems apparent that either its transfer to its final site of action, or the process by which it mediates its effects are relatively slow.

## MECHANISMS OF ACTION

The reasons why ketamine produces the effects that it does are uncertain. Its actions are however almost certainly due to interference with normal ligand/receptor interactions in many parts of the central nervous system rather than to a direct narcotic or cell-membrane effect. It is therefore very possible that its two main actions, analgesia and dissociative 'anaesthesia', are mediated in different ways.

The analgesic effect may well be at least partially due to an interaction between ketamine and some opioid receptors, which has been demonstrated in vitro (Finck and Ngai, 1982). That this is the mechanism of analgesic effect is still uncertain, however, mainly due to the lack of conclusive evidence that naloxone antagonises the analgesic effect of ketamine. The poor clinical experience of the analgesic effect of epidural ketamine also casts doubt on this theory.

Another point at which some opioids act is the $\sigma$ receptor, which may induce blockade of spinal nociceptive reflexes. One subgroup of this category may be activated by *N*-methyl aspartate, an excitatory amine, and these receptors are blocked by ketamine (Thomson et al., 1985). This may also be the cause of the dysphoria and hallucinations associated with the use of ketamine. The anti-nociceptive effects of ketamine may also be explained by an action on noradrenaline and 5-hydroxytryptamine receptors since blocks of these receptors attenuate this effect (Pekoe and Smith, 1982).

In addition ketamine acts at cholinergic (muscarinic) receptors in the central nervous system (Wachtel, 1988), this may contribute to its 'anaesthetic' effect and also be related to its interactions with muscle relaxants.

## INDICATIONS FOR USE

The main indications for the use of ketamine occur when anaesthesia is urgently required and the circumstances or the condition of the patient would make the use of any other anaesthetic agent dangerous. The most common conditions are when the patient has a full stomach or is significantly hypovolaemic, particularly when emergency surgery is required in field conditions, e.g., at the site of a major accident. Relative risks of the use of ketamine anaesthesia, which is not invariably safe in these conditions, and delay of surgery to improve the condition of the patient must of course be carefully calculated. It has also proved to be safe and useful when anaesthesia has had to be provided for a patient who is remote from the anaesthetist (but under continuous observation), e.g., a child requiring radiotherapy; but again, its safety under these conditions should not be assumed.

Another major indication is where no anaesthetist is available and anaesthesia must be conducted or supervised by the surgeon. Ketamine may be the anaesthetic of choice where the availability of other agents, particularly gases, is restricted. It has proved useful in the paediatric wards where it is desired to protect a child from the unpleasant experience of some medical or surgical procedures such as lumbar puncture or dressing of burns, especially when these are required repeatedly. As with every anaesthetic, apparatus for resuscitation must invariably be available for use before ketamine anaesthesia is undertaken.

Ketamine may be indicated in situations where the fall in arterial blood pressure normally seen after i.v. induction of anaesthesia by other agents would be inadvisable. Hypovolaemia and cardiogenic shock are perhaps most frequently encountered indications but other critical conditions where ketamine may be the anaesthetic of choice are constrictive pericarditis and pericardial tamponade. The bronchodilator effect should be remembered when it is necessary to anaesthetize a patient during an asthmatic attack or even when one is feared.

Ketamine may be particularly useful for the induction of anaesthesia for Caesarian section or forceps delivery; a small dose will have little respiratory depressant effect on the baby, will maintain blood pressure and uterine contractility, and unconsciousness may be readily maintained by further doses whilst allowing the administration of 100% oxygen to the mother. The use of TIVA by ketamine and muscle relaxant alone throughout the obstetric surgery is not recommended because of side-effects and the difficulty of assessment of dosage (see below), but induction by ketamine and muscle relaxant can minimize the possibility of an aware, conscious patient in the time up to the delivery of the baby, when other, more depressant, drugs such as opioids, benzodiazepines or i.v. anaesthetics may be introduced to complete the period of anaesthesia. Under the effect of these other agents any unpleasant phenomena often associated with recovery from ketamine will not be apparent and all the effects of ketamine may have passed by the time anaesthesia is complete. Ketamine is particularly indicated in obstetric practice when emergency surgery is required to save the baby yet the mother is unfit for conventional anaesthesia, for instance after an acute, severe haemorrhage or due to a severe asthmatic attack.

## CONTRAINDICATIONS FOR USE

The most common contraindication to the use of ketamine is when the condition of the patient is such that an elevation in blood pressure or heart rate would constitute a serious risk to life. Tachycardia is particularly dangerous in patients with ischaemic or other myocardial disease, also inadequately controlled hyperthyroidism. Hypertension caused by ketamine may be lethal not only in these conditions but also in patients with cerebral vascular disease or with hypertensive disease. This includes pregnant women with eclampsia or pre-eclampsia. The use of ketamine in patients where an increased cerebrospinal fluid or intra-ocular pressure would constitute a significant hazard, e.g., head injury, raised intracranial pressure or penetrating eye injury, is also contraindicated.

Apart from the cardiovascular effects, ketamine is not, however, a perilous drug to use, having a wide margin of safety, but its use has been associated with the occurrence of malignant hyperpyrexia. Otherwise the main contra-indications for use are the relative ones of movement, phonation, etc. during maintenance which many surgeons (and others) find distressing, and the unpleasant emergence phenomena. One personally would hesitate to use it in a patient with a psychiatric disease or addicted to psychotropic drugs. Although it has frequently been used for dental surgery, particularly in children, care must be taken if any surgery around the mouth, nose or pharynx might involve stimulation of the vocal cords and thereby precipitate spasm .

## TECHNIQUES OF USE FOR TIVA

The relatively long duration of action of ketamine means that intermittent dosing can readily be used to maintain a fairly consistent level of effect. An induction dose of about 1 mg/kg can be followed by doses of approximately 0.5 mg/kg whenever anaesthesia is becoming inadequate. The first supplementary dose may be required after only 5—10 min but thereafter the intervals between doses are likely to become longer; all will depend on the intensity of stimulation, however.

The pharmacokinetic data, particularly the fairly short elimination half-life, indicate that ketamine may very reasonably be infused in order to maintain a more constant level of effect. Many papers have described different techniques that are summarised by White et al. (1982). An induction dose of 1—2 mg/kg has been usual, followed by infusions given at widely varying rates ranging from 8—110 μg/kg per min. The difficulty in assessing the dose requirement for ketamine (see below) is apparent in these figures. Much will depend on what other drugs are given at the same time. The use of a reasonable dose of diazepam, e.g., 0.25 mg/kg at the same time will allow the use of a reasonable dose of ketamine, e.g., 10—25 μg/kg per min whether given by infusion or intermittant injection.

The great problem about TIVA using ketamine is the difficulty in deciding when anaesthesia is becoming inadequate. It is extremely difficult to predict when the next dose will be required during an average surgical procedure; it is usually given in response to patient reaction to surgery, a generally unsatisfactory method of working. The problem is due to the inherent effects of ketamine, which are the same as those which will normally warn the anaesthetist the anaesthesia is becoming inadequate; tachycardia, increased blood pressure and movement. It may be extremely difficult to decide whether movement of the patient is due to the effect of the drug wearing off, although this is supposedly purposive, or due to the neuromuscular effects which may be seen even during deep ketamine anaesthesia. It matters little to the surgeon who only requires an immobile patient.

As with all agents used for TIVA, it is wrong to base the dose requirement solely on mean pharmacokinetics; whether giving the drug by intermittent injection or infusion, dosage must be based essentially on the patient's responses to the drug and to the surgery; when these responses are so similar, adjustment of dosage to preclude uneven adequacy of anaesthesia is difficult. Use of ketamine by infusion may produce a more consistent level of effect but the advantage over intermittent dosage is not marked and it is much easier to overdose; in addition, the level of stimulation during surgery and therefore the requirement for ketamine is rarely constant and infusion is technically much more demanding than intermittent dosage.

Because of the hypertonic effect, the need to use a muscle relaxant is often greater during ketamine anaesthesia than with other agents. This of course gets rid of the problem of movement, both due to or due to the lack of ketamine. However, as with TIVA using any other agent, it deprives the anaesthetist of perhaps the most important indicator of inadequate anaesthesia, so that he may not be certain that his paralysed patient is unconscious. Whilst consciousness during ketamine anaesthesia is unlikely, (slow recovery is more usual), the two other important signs that may indicate it (tachycardia and hypertension) are almost always apparent, due to the ketamine. In this situation, it is easy for the cautious anaesthetist to overdose.

Because of the other important side-effects of ketamine, it is often necesary to use additional concomitant medication in order to achieve satisfactory anaesthesia. But almost every additional drug given may cause a problem as difficult as that it cures. Some recommendations are:

### Premedication

The tachycardia caused by ketamine may be increased if the patient is nervous before induction. The use of an anxiolytic or vagotonic premedication is therefore often to be recommended. A benzodiazepine or opioid may be given long enough before induction to ensure that the patient is well sedated before induction. The use of such drugs may not always be effective, however, but will invariably increase the respiratory depressant effect of the dose of ketamine used. This may not be acceptable, although the premedication may allow a reduction in the dose of ketamine required. It is essential that the anaesthetist takes time to talk to the patient and ensure that he is as calm and tranquil as possible. For short anaesthetics it may be possible to give any drugs required to modify recovery problems (e.g. benzodiazepines) as part of the premedication.

In patients who are to breathe spontaneously during ketamine anaesthesia, salivation may be a problem. In these cases, it may be advisable to give an anti-sialogogue premedication such as atropine, hyoscine or glycopyrrholate. But these drugs, especially the former, may not only increase the incidence of unpleasant dreams (Morgan et al., 1971) but also enhance the tachycardia caused by ketamine by increasing the anxiety of the patient and by their vagolytic effect. They must therefore be given a sufficient time before induction to allow the patient time to get used to their effects, which of course must be explained by the anaesthetist beforehand.

Ketamine is best avoided in cases where tachycardia would constitute a significant hazard, but if its use is otherwise indicated the cardiovascular effects of ketamine may be reduced by the judicious use of $\alpha$ or $\beta$ adrenergic blockers as premedication, whilst remembering that in the absence of its adrenergic effects, ketamine is a myocardial depressant. Labetolol, which has both actions, may be the drug of choice; it may be given by slow i.v. injection in a dose of 0.5—1 mg/kg just before induction.

### Induction

The usual induction dose quoted for ketamine is 0.5—2 mg/kg. Loss of consciousness almost invariably follows the use of the lower end of this range, but satisfactory conditions for a surgical incision a few minutes later may not, so maintenance of anaesthesia must be started shortly after induction by this dose. This is a method of use that is personally recommended as it avoids the more marked cardiovascular and respiratory effects associated with rapid administration of a larger dose of ketamine.

The effects of induction may be further attenuated by combined use of another i.v. agent which will also help by reducing the dose of ketamine required, but this may lose the advantage of ketamine for which the drug was chosen (see below). A benzodiazepine is usually preferred because of its additional effect of ameliorating emergence phenomena. Given shortly before the ketamine, a benzodiazepine will also greatly increase the rate of induction of unconsciousness from even a small dose of ketamine. A technique has been described (Sher, 1980) that is particularly suitable for the use of ketamine in high-risk patients; diazepam 2—5 mg i.v. is followed by ketamine 2—4 mg/min until satisfactory conditions are obtained. The use of an opioid instead of diazepam (e.g. fentanyl 2 $\mu$g/kg) is similarly effective and is personally recommended in patients who will also receive a muscle relaxant and ventilation, as the respiratory depression caused by the combination may be considerable. The fentanyl helps to reduce the cardiovascular responses to laryngoscopy and tracheal intubation. Combinations of ketamine with i.v. induction agents are not personally recommended.

### Maintenance

Whilst it is pefectly possible to given an anaesthetic using ketamine alone, the movements, rigidity, salivation, phonation, cardiovascular effects etc. that are so frequently encountered make it always inelegant and frequently unacceptable. It is virtually impossible to peform intra-abdominal surgery under ketamine alone and the movements and rigidity may make any surgery difficult. In most cases therefore, ketamine is best used in combination with a muscle relaxant. The choice of this drug may be influenced by many factors but it is usually advisable to consider a relaxant with cardiovascular effects that minimize those of ketamine. In particular those relaxants that induce tachycardia such as pancuronium or gallamine are best avoided if possible. For a discussion of the choice of relaxants for TIVA see Chapter 7.

Simultaneous use of a muscle relaxant removes most of the objective problems associated with the use of ketamine during maintenance of TIVA. The subjective responses and the conditions when a relaxant is not used may be improved to some extent by a reduction in the dose of ketamine required. This is perhaps best achieved by the simultaneous administration of another 'anaesthetic' but the choice of additional agent available for use during TIVA is limited and published experience about combinations is limited.

The concurrent use of a benzodiazepine is perhaps best documented, although there are few published reports of the continuous use of a benzodiazepine (whether by infusion or intermittent injection) with ketamine throughout maintenance of anaesthesia. The benzodiazepine most suited for this use in terms of similarity of onset and duration of effect, water solubility and pharmacokinetics, is midazolam, and Restall et al. (1988) have published a report on the combined administration of ketamine, midazolam and vecuronium for TIVA (the drugs were mixed). Personal experience confirms that this method will usually produce acceptable results. The rate of administration used was midazolam, 50 μg/kg per h; ketamine 2 mg/kg per h; vecuronium 120 μg/kg per h. Although the dose of ketamine used was lower than most other quoted rates (see above) it is not surprising that, together with the amnesic/hypnotic effect of midazolam, there was no report of awareness during surgery. It would be of interest to those who are concerned about the phenomenon to assess the incidence of subconscious awareness after ketamine or ketamine/benzodiazepine anaesthesia.

One would expect that the combined use of ketamine and another i.v. agent such as a benzodiazepine, an opioid or an i.v. anaesthetic would allow a significant reduction in the dose of ketamine required and this is normally the case. Whilst such combinations may influence favourably the conditions of anaesthesia produced in most respects, they almost invariably increase the respiratory depression caused, compared with ketamine alone, and also reduce the safety factors such as the ability to maintain an airway which were probably the basis of the choice of ketamine in the first place. It is not therefore surprising that such combinations are not widely used.

**Recovery**

The dreams and movements that often trouble recovery are said to be diminished by keeping the patient in quiet, peaceful surroundings and minimizing tactile contact. Medications are a more certain way of preventing or treating these problems. The dreams are best inhibited by use of hypnotic drugs and of these the benzodiazepines are to be preferred both for their efficacy and also because they cause fewer side-effects. Nevertheless, they will invariably cause additional respiratory depression, and further delay recovery of consciousness. Drugs with a sufficient duration of effect may be given as an anxiolytic premedication and continue to work to reduce dreaming (but increase respiratory depression) throughout anaesthesia and recovery. Lorazepam is widely recommended, being highly effective and long acting. But other hypnotics are also effective. If ketamine is particularly indicated as an induction agent, say for obstetric anaesthesia, but TIVA may be continued later by other agents, the dreaming that occurs as the effects of the ketamine are diminishing will be inhibited by the subsequent anaesthetics and the patient may recover without the usual effects seen after ketamine.

The movements that occur both during ketamine anaesthesia and particularly during recovery may be diminished by the use of a butyrophenone or, less effectively, a phenothiazine. Both have the additional advantages of reducing postoperative nausea and vomiting and also the hypertensive response to ketamine. Droperidol 2—5 mg. i.v. is recommended, but one personally is wary of the possible ill effects of unpleasant dreams on someone medicated with droperidol and would always use the drug in combination with a benzodiazepine in these circumstances. In the absence of antiemetic medication the incidence of nausea and vomiting after ketamine is higher than after most anaesthetics.

Although slow recovery is usually associated with the use of ketamine, waking can be advanced if the use of the drug is discontinued before the end of surgery, which is really possible only in paralysed patients. Using this technique Bailie et al. (1989) were able to attain faster recovery of consciousness after using TIVA with ketamine, midazolam and vecuronium than after propofol, alfentanil and vecuronium infused to the end of surgery. This method introduces the danger of allowing a paralysed patient to recover consciousness during surgery however, and tests of functions associated with later stages of recovery have not been performed. Nevertheless, it does allow an early discharge of a fit patient from the recovery room.

## SUMMARY

Ketamine has remained in the drug cupboards of most anaesthetists because of its unique effects which make it the drug of choice in some unusual circumstances. Other unusual effects ensure that it is not widely used. It was the first drug to provide relatively safe and effective TIVA and its continued use in this context is assured in some circumstances. Although it has been available for many years its use as an agent for TIVA is continually being improved, partly by advances in techniques of administration but mainly because of the development of new drugs which improve the quality of ketamine anaesthesia. Much research is still required to evaluate not only the safety and efficacy of combinations of ketamine with existing drugs; anaesthetics, hypnotics, psychotropics and those affecting the cardiovascular system, but also new drugs as they appear.

## REFERENCES

Amiot, J.F., Bouju, P. and Palacci, J.H. (1985) Effect of naloxone on loss of conscioiusness induced by i.v. ketamine. *Br. J. Anaesth.* 57, 930.

Bailie, R., Craig, G. and Restall, J. (1989) Total intravenous anaesthesia for laparoscopy. *Anaesthesia* 44, 60—63.

Bourke, D.L., Malit, L.A. and Smith, T.c. (1987) Respiratory interactions of ketamine and morphine. *Anesthesiology* 66, 153—156.

Domino, E.F., Domino, S.E. and Smith, R.E. (1984) Ketamine kinetics in unmedicated and diazepam premedicated subjects. *Clin. Pharmacol. Ther.* 36, 645—653.

Finck, A.D. and Ngai, S.H. (1982) Opiate receptor mediation of ketamine analgesia. *Anesthesiology* 56, 291—297.

Idvall, J., Ahlgren, I., Aronson, K.F. et al. (1979) Ketamine infusions; pharmacokinetics and clinical effects. *Br. J. Anaesth.* 51, 1167—1172.

Lumb, P.D., Silvay, G., Weinreich, A.I. and Shiang, H. (1979) A comparison of the effects of continuous ketamine infusion and halothane on oxygenation during one-lung anaesthesia in dogs. *Can. Anaesth. Soc. J.* 26, 394—401.

Marx, G.F., Hwang, H.S. and Chandra, P. (1979) Postpartum uterine pressures with different doses of ketamine. *Anesthesiology* 50, 163—166.

Morgan, M., Loh, L. and Singer, L. (1979) Ketamine as the sole anaesthetic for minor surgical procedures. *Anaesthesia* 26, 158—165.

Pekoe, G.M. and Smith, D.J. (1982) The involvement of opiate and monoaminergic neuronal systems in the analgesic effects of ketamine. *Pain* 12, 57—73.

Restall, J., Tully, A.M., Ward, P.J. and Kidd, A.G. (1988) Total intravenous anaesthesia for military surgery. A technique using ketamine, midazolam and vecuronium. *Anaesthesia* 43, 46—49.

Sher, M.H. (1980) Slow-dose ketamine; a new technique. *Anaesth. Intensive Care J.* 8, 359—361.

Stanley, T.H. (1973) Blood pressure and pulse rate responses to ketamine during general anesthesia. *Anesthesiology* 39, 648—649.

Tarnow, J., Hess, W., Schmidt, D. et al. (1979) Narcoseeinleitung bei patienten mit koronar herzkrankheit; Flunitrazepam, diazepam, ketamine, fentanyl. *Anesthesist* 28, 9—11.

Thomson, A.M., West, D.C. and Lodge, D. (1985) An N-methylaspartate receptor-mediated synapse in rat cerebral cortex; a site of action of ketamine? *Nature* 313, 479—481.

Wachtel, R.E. (1988) Ketamine decreases the open time of single-channel currents activated by acetylcholine. *Anesthesiology* 68, 563—570.

Waxman, K., Shoemaker, W.C. and Lippman, M. (1989) Cardiovascular effects of anaesthetic induction with ketamine. *Anesth. Analg.* 59, 355—358.

White, P.F., Way, W.L. and Trevor, A.J. (1982) Ketamine; its pharmacology and therapeutic uses. *Anesthesiology* 56, 119—136.

# 7

# *Relaxants for total intravenous anaesthesia*

Brian J. Pollard

## INTRODUCTION

Total intravenous anaesthesia by definition implies that the entire process of anaesthesia is managed by drugs administered intravenously as opposed to any other route. Not only the drugs which maintain anaesthesia but also all adjuncts to anaesthesia should also be administered by the intravenous route, and this includes the neuromuscular blocking agents. It is usual to administer the neuromuscular blocking agents intravenously and so the normal use of these agents should retain the integrity of the technique. It is, however, appropriate to note here that it is possible to administer a neuromuscular blocking agent by a different route under certain circumstances. Suxamethonium may be given intramuscularly, as may tubocurarine or gallamine, (Atkinson et al., 1982). The non-depolarising neuromuscular blocking agents may also be given by the transtracheal route (Simionescu and Bandila, 1979), although their onset is very much slower (10—15 min) when given in this way. The principal route of administration, however, remains intravenous. There are two aspects to the use of a neuromuscular blocking agent in anaesthesia: the first is to secure paralysis and the second to maintain paralysis. The same or a different drug may be used in either of these two circumstances.

## THE ONSET OF NEUROMUSCULAR BLOCKADE

At the induction of anaesthesia, tracheal intubation requires virtually complete paralysis, which is generally secured by the administration of an intubating dose of a neuromuscular blocking agent. How much is an intubating dose? Following the administration of a dose of neuromuscular blocking agent, sufficient to just produce 95% neuromuscular blockade ($ED_{95}$), there is a short delay caused by the circulation and distribution of the drug. This is followed by the progressive onset of neuromuscular blockade.

Once the muscle relaxant has been administered intravenously the concentration within the blood will be determined by the volume injected, the dose injected and the blood volume. The rate at which it is dispersed will be dependent upon the blood circulation time. It is the amount of free drug present within the blood which dictates quantity of relaxant which eventually reaches the neuromuscular junction. Most of the neuromuscular blocking agents are bound to plasma-proteins, leaving only a limited amount free to diffuse out of the capillaries and into the extra-cellular fluids surrounding the neuromuscular junction. It is the amount of free neuromuscular blocking agent present at the neuromuscular junction which ultimately determines the degree of paralysis.

Neuromuscular blockade does not progress very rapidly following the $ED_{95}$ bolus dose and maximum neuromuscular blockade is not reached for some 5—6 min, (Kreig et al., 1980). Most people would regard this as too slow. Where is the rate-limiting step and can it be manipulated in order to accelerate the onset of paralysis? The neuromuscular junction appears to be better perfused with blood than the muscle as a whole and drug access to the junction requires only distribution within the extra-cellular space without crossing any membranes (Miller, 1984). The rate at which drug diffuses from plasma into extra-cellular fluid will be determined therefore principally by the concentration difference of free drug between these two compartments. The delivery of drug-laden plasma will in turn be determined by the circulation time of the blood. There are thus two principal factors governing the onset of neuromuscular blockade. The first is the plasma concentration and the second the circulation time. For the purpose of simplicity, metabolism, excretion and binding to other extra-junctional sites have not been taken into account in this discussion. Although it might theoretically be of value, it is not practical to manipulate the blood circulation time. Indeed, the anaesthetic induction agent may lower cardiac output and thus prolong circulation time (Grounds et al., 1985; Thomas et al., 1989). It is possible, however, to increase the plasma concentration by administering a larger bolus dose. The larger the dose, the faster should be the onset time, although a limit will logically be reached due to the need for at least one circulation time to occur. This acceleration in onset with increasing dose can be readily demonstrated (Agoston et al., 1980; Bencini and Newton, 1984). If the $ED_{95}$ and the manufacturers recommended dose are compared (Table 7.1) it can be seen that the manufacturers have taken this route only with atracurium and vecuronium, recommending intubating doses which are about twice the $ED_{95}$. The intubating doses, therefore, do not give the fastest rate of onset but are a compromise between a dose sufficiently large to increase the rate of onset to an acceptable figure, one which produces reliable intubating conditions in the great majority of patients, and one which avoids too many unwanted side effects.

It is appropriate to consider these three points further. Firstly, what is an acceptable rate of onset? In the case of the urgency patient requiring a rapid sequence

TABLE 7.1.

| Relaxant | $ED_{95}$[a] (mg/kg) | Recommended[b] intubating dose (mg/kg) | Infusion rate for steady state blockade (mg/kg per h) |
|---|---|---|---|
| Alcuronium | 0.22 | 0.25 | 0.076 |
| Atracurium | 0.21 | 0.3—0.6 | 0.25 |
| Pancuronium | 0.067 | 0.05—0.08 | 0.032 |
| Tubocurarine | 0.48 | 0.5 | 0.12 |
| Vecuronium | 0.043 | 0.08—0.1 | 0.078 |

[a]Data from Shanks (1986).
[b]Data from manufacturers product information.

induction of anaesthesia the answer must be as short a time as possible. In the elective patient who is not at risk from regurgitation such speed is not essential. But in these latter patients, what is acceptable? This is clearly difficult to define and somewhat subjective. The constraints of a busy operating list may make a minute seem like a long time. It is a not uncommon fault, therefore, for tracheal intubation to be attempted too early, which may lead to problems with cord spasm and resistance to opening the mouth. The patient may even be subsequently labelled as a difficult intubation solely for this reason. Despite these points, most anaesthetists expect satisfactory intubating conditions after approximately 2 or 2.5 min. This time scale is only possible when using atracurium or vecuronium which can be administered in doses 2—3 times the $ED_{95}$.

The neuromuscular blocking agent with the fastest rate of onset is suxamethonium, and if this agent is used in the recommended dose then profound blockade is produced rapidly in under 60 s in most patients. The duration of effect of suxamethonium is short, assuming normal plasma cholinesterase concentrations. If the recommended intubating dose (1 to 1.5 mg/kg) and the $ED_{95}$ (0.3 to 0.5 mg/kg) (Smith et al., 1988; Chestnut et al., 1989) are inspected, however, it can be seen that in this case also the intubating dose is approximately two to three times the $ED_{95}$.

There is, in a normal population, a scatter about the mean and the onset and degree of paralysis resulting from the administration of a dose of a neuromuscular blocking agent are no exception. Giving an $ED_{95}$ dose to each of a group of patients will produce a range of degrees of neuromuscular blockade from 100% in some patients to possibly less than 50% (hopelessly inadequate) in others. Chestnut et al. (1987) found that the degree of paralysis resulting from the administration of suxamethonium 0.3 mg/kg varied from 28% to 98%. It is impossible to predict who is going to fall into which group. Furthermore, circumstances may make the same patient more or less sensitive to the same agent on more than one occasion, e.g. interactions with other drugs, electrolyte disorders. The administration of a larger dose will, therefore, serve also to reduce the interpatient variability and to make the use of the agent more predictable.

TABLE 7.2

Onset and duration of action of vecuronium

| Dose (mg/kg) | Onset time as injection to peak effort (s)[a] | Time (min) to return to 10% of control of first twitch of train of four[b] | Time (min) to return to 25% of control of first twitch of train of four[a] |
|---|---|---|---|
| 0.1 | 164 | 28.4 | 42 |
| 0.15 | — | 40.9 | — |
| 0.2 | 120 | 54.2 | 68 |
| 0.25 | — | 72.4 | — |
| 0.3 | 88 | — | 111 |
| 0.4 | 78 | — | 115 |

[a]Tullock et al. (1990).
[b]Feldman and Liban (1987).

To consider the third point, side effects are principally dose-related. Atracurium and vecuronium are the relaxants with the least side effects and so it is safe to recommend their use in larger doses for intubation. It might be possible, however, to accelerate the onset still further by giving even larger doses and this possibility was tested out using vecuronium. Bencini and Newton (1984) showed that the onset could be reduced from 3 min with 0.1 mg/kg to 2 min by increasing the intubating dose to 0.2 mg/kg. Tullock et al. (1990) have recently confirmed these findings and also shown that further reductions in onset time can be achieved by increasing the dose still further, to 0.3 and 0.4 mg/kg (Table 7.2). Clearly this technique is not appropriate to most of the neuromuscular blocking agents because of their side effects. A larger dose will also increase the duration of action, and so the technique is only appropriate if this extended duration is matched by the expected length of the surgery. There is a second method, in addition to the 'larger dose' method, for accelerating the onset of the neuromuscular blocking agents. This is the priming principle. The priming principle has been the subject of some debate and controversy (Jones, 1989). In this technique, a small dose of non-depolarising neuromuscular blocking agent is administered, which is not sufficient by itself to cause measurable neuromuscular blockade. This sub-paralysing dose is typically of the order of 3 mg of tubocurarine or 20 mg of gallamine or their equivalent. This sub-paralysing dose occupies the majority of the spare receptors, thus reducing the margin of safety of neuromuscular transmission (Paton and Waud, 1967). A second (intubating) dose then acts more rapidly because little of the second dose is needed to saturate the spare receptors before neuromuscular blockade begins. There is a fundamental problem with the priming technique, however, which is inherent in the priming dose itself. The priming dose has to be administered some 3—5 min before the intubating dose and it may produce an uncomfortable degree of weakness in a number of patients. The exact timing of the doses and their ratio is of great importance in order to get a reliable reduction in onset time without any unwanted problems (Jones, 1989). It is probably for these reasons that it has never really caught on for routine clinical use.

## MAINTENANCE OF NEUROMUSCULAR BLOCKADE

Neuromuscular blockade having been secured and the trachea intubated, the maintenance of paralysis is the next consideration. If a long-acting neuromuscular blocking agent, such as tubocurarine or pancuronium, has been used then adequate neuromuscular blockade lasting some 45 to 60 min can be expected in most patients. If surgery lasts longer, further increments can be given. If surgery is brief, however, difficulties may occasionally be encountered with reversal. Despite these drawbacks, the longer-acting agents are frequently used for longer procedures and many would recommend that this continues. Problems may be minimised by the use of one of the intermediate acting agents atracurium or vecuronium. Either is usually readily reversible after about 15 to 20 min when given in a normal intubating dose and neuromuscular blockade may be extended in a number of ways. These include the use of a large initial bolus, the use of a continuous infusion or the use of incremental boluses. These three methods will be taken in order.

### Large initial bolus

This technique has already been considered with respect to the rate of onset of the neuromuscular blocking agents. If a large initial bolus is administered, the duration of action is extended as well as the rate of onset being increased. Provided that it is safe to give initial bolus doses which are larger than those normally used to allow tracheal intubation, then an increased duration of action can be achieved with ease. Of the drugs in current clinical use, vecuronium is the safest for this approach in that cardiovascular side effects and histamine release are minimal (Tullock et al., 1990). The duration of action of a series of doses of vecuronium were determined by Feldman and Liban in 1987 and these are shown in Table 7.2. Table 7.2 also includes the more recent data from Tullock et al. (1990), and it is evident that a quite predictable duration of effect can be achieved with a carefully selected dose of vecuronium. One potential difficulty with this technique is that although the average patient will be catered for admirably, those with either an unusual sensitivity or reduced clearance will have an extended block which may be extremely difficult to antagonise. Furthermore, it is often difficult to anticipate the exact length of the operation.

### Infusions

When it is desired to maintain a constant level of effect of an agent, the most logical approach is to administer it in such a way that there remains a constant activity at the receptor site. Such activity is usually synonymous with concentration at the receptor site, except where there is an alteration in the receptor or in the drug receptor complex. This may result in the appearance of tachyphylaxis or increased sensitivity. In the context of the use of the non-depolarising neuromuscular blocking agents in clinical practice there is no evidence of the development of such a phenomenon. The action of suxamethonium is the exception to this point because its interaction with the receptor changes with time. Making the assumption, therefore, that concentration at the neuromuscular junction is the important factor, maintenance of a constant degree of neuromuscular blockade should be possible if that concentration is held constant. The neuromuscular blocking agents are all polar water-soluble substances which diffuse freely throughout the extracelluar fluid and it would therefore be expected that the concentration at the neuromuscular junction would be reflected by the plasma concentration. Maintenance of a constant plasma concentration should therefore produce a constant degree of neuromuscular blockade and this is borne out in practice (Shanks, 1985). There are certain drugs which it may be appropriate to administer on a bolus basis, e.g. an antibiotic, where a profound bactericidal action is produced by the peak concentration. The neuromuscular blocking agents are, however, given for an effect where it is most convenient and of assistance to the surgeon that a constant degree of neuromuscular blockade is maintained through the majority of the procedure. It is also useful if this degree of blockade can be attained without delay, altered relatively easily and be reversible without problems at the end of surgery.

In order to maintain a constant plasma level (and therefore a constant effect) the most appropriate technique of administration would seem to be to administer a constant infusion of the drug. If the rate of delivery of the drug is equal to its rate of clearance from the plasma at steady-state then this will be achieved. In order to use this technique it is of course necessary to know certain basic facts with respect to the drug, namely the plasma concentration which produces the desired degree of neuromuscular blockade and also the rate of clearance from the plasma. On the assumption that clearance remains constant (which it may not do in the early stages until steady state is reached) then the desired rate of drug delivery can be calculated mathematically from the following formula (Mitenko and Ogilvie, 1972):

$$\text{Infusion rate} = \text{plasma concentration} \times \text{clearance}$$

If an infusion is started at time zero the plasma concentration will rise until it ultimately reaches the desired level, where it will remain. The problem is that this takes some time (approximately 15—20 min) to achieve. Taking vecuronium as an example, the clearance is approximately 300 ml/kg per h (Shanks, 1985). If we assume that the target plasma concentration to achieve 95% neuromuscular blockade is 0.2 mg/ml (van der Veen and Bencini, 1980), then the infusion delivery rate to achieve this will be 0.06 mg/kg per h. A more practical way than simply to begin an infusion is to first administer a bolus which is calculated to bring the plasma concentrations to the desired level and then to begin the infusion in order to maintain it at that level. It is necessary now to know an additional pharmacokinetic parameter, namely the volume of distribution. One can then mathematically calculate the bolus required for the following formula (Mitenko and Ogilvie, 1972):

Bolus dose = volume of distribution × plasma concentration

Using vecuronium as an example again, the distribution volume is approximately 0.25 l/kg (Shanks, 1985) and so the bolus dose in the patient would be 0.05 mg/kg. This figure agrees well with previously published $ED_{95}$ values for vecuronium, which lie between 0.037 and 0.059 mg/kg (Shanks, 1986).

The bolus/infusion approach is in practical terms a great improvement over the simple infusion technique. In practice a delay of some 3—4 min is required before neuromuscular blockade has reached its maximum. It is, however, a useable technique and is in common use by many anaesthetists. In fact, because tracheal intubation requires a greater degree of neuromuscular blockade than does surgery, it is usual to administer a larger bolus loading dose, wait for recovery to the desired level and then to begin an infusion.

Returning to vecuronium again, the recommended intubating dose is 0.01 mg/kg. This is greater than our calculated $ED_{95}$ and should therefore produce a degree of neuromuscular blockade adequate for intubation and in a reasonable length of time in the great majority of patients. Recovery to a suitable level for surgery is awaited and at that point an infusion of vecuronium 0.06 mg/kg per h (clearance × desired plasma concentration) is then begun. From the foregoing arguments, this might be expected to produce the desired effect. The difficulty now is that the exact effect of the neuromuscular blocker may not be completely dependent upon plasma concentration. In addition, working on a milligram per kilogram bodyweight basis is a reasonable predictor but is not completely accurate. Lean body mass is probably the more correct. Other agents administered during the course of the operation or previously might also affect neuromuscular blockade. A method is therefore needed of predicting the infusion rate in each patient.

It was shown by Harrison (1990a,b) that it is possible to predict the rate of infusion in any given patient by observing the duration of action of a small bolus of the agent in the presence of a partial block from that agent. When using this technique, an intubating dose is given in the usual way. When recovery has reached the desired point a second small bolus is given, Harrison recommends 4 mg for vecuronium, and recovery to the same point is again awaited. The infusion rate to maintain this desired degree of neuromuscular blockade can then be determined from the duration of action of this second bolus dose (Fig. 7.1). The method has the distinct advantage that it is unique to that particular patient under those particular circumstances. There is presumably no reason why it should not be possible to apply this approach to all neuromuscular blocking agents and not just to vecuronium, the relaxant which was the subject of the original work.

It is thus logical to employ a continuous infusion of neuromuscular blocking agent in order to secure a constant degree of neuromuscular blockade. It may not be possible to always use Harrison's bolus technique and so it is useful to know

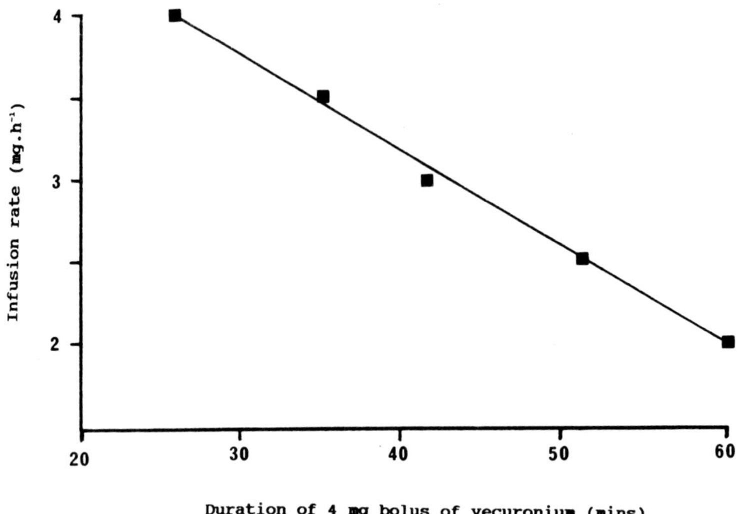


Fig. 7.1. Calculation of infusion rate from duration of action of a 4-mg bolus dose of vecuronium. Graph drawn from data of Harrison (1990b).

the approximate rates of usage of each neuromuscular blocking agent when given by infusion. These are shown in Table 7.1, together with the manufacturers recommended intubating dose and the $ED_{95}$. If an infusion is started at the rate recommended in Table 7.1 the desired level of neuromuscular blockade should be maintained in most patients, although minor adjustments will be necessary to allow for patient variability.

An alternative approach to this problem of selection of correct infusion rate is to use an automatic microprocessor controlled system. A nerve stimulator and recording system monitor neuromuscular blockade and these in turn control a syringe driver of relaxant, usually through the medium of a small microprocessor. This has a number of clear theoretical advantages in that the operator can dial up whatever degree of neuromuscular blockade he requires and leave the machine to sort it out. It is not always as easy as that, however. The systems are expensive and complicated and require an accurate reliable EMG signal to allow reliable feedback. Most of the systems to date have used the Datex Relaxograph as the centrepiece and have claimed very satisfactory results with a high degree of accuracy (Clutton-Brock et al., 1987; Webster and Cohen, 1987). At present they remain a research tool and are not really of practical use to everyday clinical anaesthesia.

## Incremental boluses

The administration of a drug by continuous infusion necessitates a certain degree of preparation and availability of equipment, e.g. syringe drivers. It is also necessary

TABLE 7.3

Increments to maintain 90% neuromuscular blockade

| Relaxant | Increment size (mg) | Approximate duration (min) |
|---|---|---|
| Alcuronium | 1 | 14 |
| Atracurium | 1 | 4 |
| Pancuronium | 0.5 | 15 |
| Tubocararine | 1 | 10 |
| Vecuronium | 1 | 10 |

to use a dedicated intravenous line if possible in order to ensure the constancy of the infusion rate and to make sure that there is no incompatibility problem with other drugs or fluids which may be administered through the main infusion lines. It is possible to obtain operating conditions which are almost as constant as those by infusion by the use of repeated small incremental boluses and this is the technique employed by many clinical anaesthetists. As in the bolus/infusion technique, an initial intubating dose is required to secure neuromuscular blockade. When recovery has reached the desired level, repeated small increments are given in order to maintain neuromuscular blockade at this level or greater. If infusion administration possesses the disadvantages of equipment availability and preparation, this technique possesses what many might regard as a greater disadvantage, namely that of a fluctuating block, which may become inadequate for surgery if recovery is allowed to proceed too far. In the context of a complicated anaesthetic where there are many calls on the anaesthetist's attention, this is a definite problem. Constant vigilance and regular monitoring are therefore essential. This can be circumvented to a limited degree by watching the duration of action of the first increment and then administering the same increment on a rigid timescale, possibly using a timer for assistance. This might be regarded as a manual variation to Harrison's infusion technique. Once again, every patient is different, but it is useful to know the approximate size of increment which will result in a sensible extension of neuromuscular blockade under average circumstances. These are outlined in Table 7.3. There is a certain degree of predictability within these figures in that twice the dose should produce approximately (but not exactly) twice the duration of effect. It must be remembered that patient variability and other drugs which are administered intra-operatively are likely to affect these data.

## MONITORING, AND THE DEGREE OF PARALYSIS

If an anaesthetic textbook dating from before the introduction of muscle relaxants is consulted, it is clear that muscular relaxation could be secured by the use of an increased depth of anaesthesia alone. In Guedel's classification, stage 3, plane 3 is described as providing adequate muscular relaxation for most abdominal procedures. The introduction of muscle relaxants into anaesthetic practice by

Griffiths and Johnson (1942) was therefore a revolution. It was no longer necessary to resort to increasing the depth in order to increase the muscular relaxation.

The amount of neuromuscular blockade required will depend on the nature of the surgical stimulus. It will also depend on the depth of anaesthesia and on many other factors which might modify reflex responses. There is therefore theoretically a continuous spectrum of neuromuscular blockade, ranging from zero paralysis to 100% (full) paralysis with every different procedure requiring a different level. For the sake of simplicity it is possible generally to reduce these to two approximate levels in the clinical situation. The first of these is 100% paralysis, which is required at the induction of anaesthesia for the purpose of atraumatic tracheal intubation. The second is the maintenance degree of paralysis required for that surgery. This latter degree of paralysis will, of course, depend upon the nature and site of surgery. Thoracic and upper abdominal procedures require a greater degree of paralysis than do pelvic and limb surgery. Lee and Katz (1980) proposed that a minimum of 80% blockade was appropriate for most types of abdominal surgery.

In order to maintain a constant, defined degree of paralysis it is necessary to use some form of monitoring system. If an automatic infusion system is in use, then the monitoring system clearly has to be suited to that purpose and will be included. In most cases, however, a simple hand-held stimulator is adequate. Monitoring systems all consist of two parts, the stimulator and the detector. The stimulator should be capable of delivering square wave pulses of approximately 0.2 ms width at a strength of up to about 300 volts at a current of not more than 70 mamps in order that supramaximal stimulation may be achieved. Most of those available for clinical purposes, whether handheld or automatic, fulfil these basic criteria. The most common recording system used by anaesthetists is the simple tactile or visual movement of the thumb after stimulation of the ulnar nerve at the wrist (Viby-Mogenson et al., 1985). Quantifying that movement with respect to the degree of movement before the administration of a relaxant is extremely difficult (probably impossible) without the use of a force transducer or EMG detection and recording apparatus. It was for that reason that the technique of train of four stimulation was introduced. In this technique a train of four stimuli, each separated from each other by 0.5 s are delivered to a nerve and the response is noted (Ali et al., 1970). The number of twitches can be correlated with the degree of neuromuscular blockade as follows (Ali, 1985):

| | |
|---|---|
| 4 twitches present | — <75% blockade |
| 3 twitches present | — 75% to 80% blockade |
| 2 twitches present | — 80% to 90% blockade |
| 1 twitch present | — 90% to 95% blockade |
| no twitches present | — >95% blockade |

It is thus possible to estimate the degree of blockade with a surprising degree of accuracy from simply counting the number of twitches without having to resort to measuring their intensity. Many anaesthetists refine the technique still further by grading the twitch as strong or weak.

# "Match the Molecule" Answer Sheet

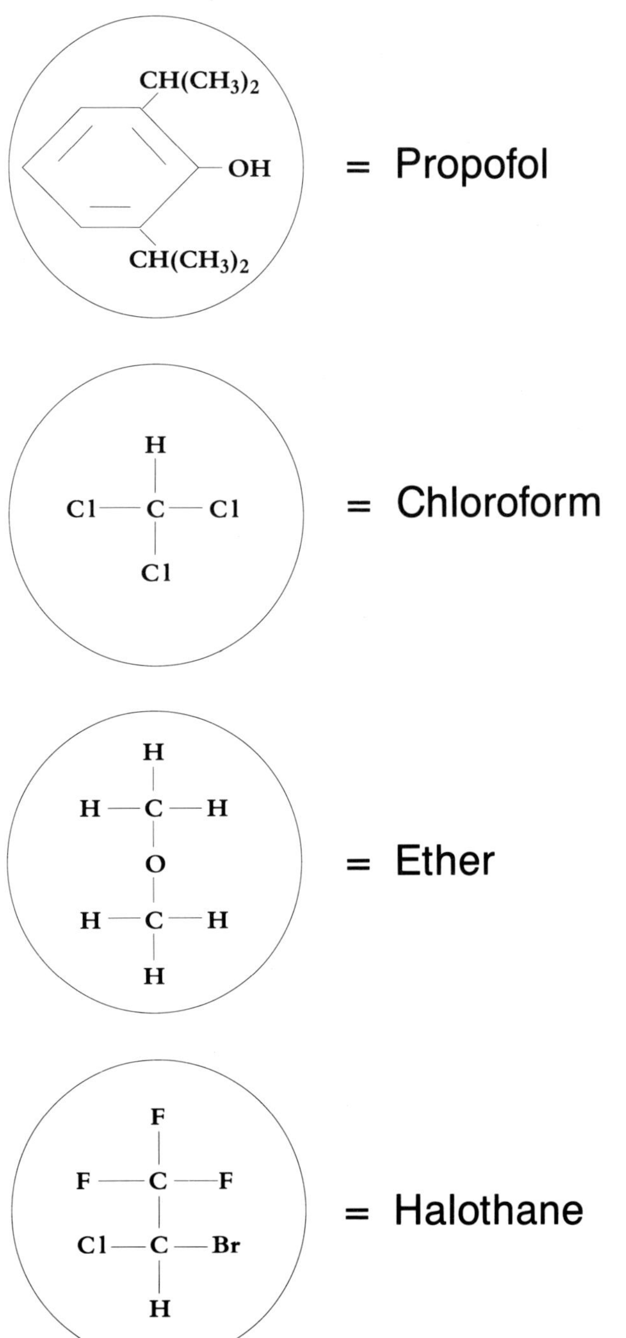

A similar technique has recently been introduced, that of double-burst stimulation. In this technique, three supramaximal stimuli, each separated from the next by 20 ms (50 Hz) are given, followed 0.75 s later by a second identical burst of three stimuli (Drenck et al., 1989; Engbaek et al., 1989). It has been suggested that this technique allows better quantification of fade patterns, particularly during recovery from neuromuscular blockade (Drenck et al., 1989). It is unlikely that this will replace the train of four pattern for the measurement of intra-operative blockade.

The use of tetanic trains (e.g., 50 Hz for 5 s) and post-tetanic count are principally for the quantification of profound degrees of neuromuscular block (greater than 95%) when there is no response to the train of four. It is unlikely that it will be necessary to maintain this level of block frequently for surgery.

## CHOICE OF NEUROMUSCULAR BLOCKING AGENT

For reasons advanced earlier, if a constant effect is desired (neuromuscular blockade in this case) it is logical to administer the drug in a manner which will achieve that constant effect, i.e. by continuous infusion. The available neuromuscular blocking agents essentially fall into three categories — long acting (tubocurarine, pancuronium, alcuronium, doxacurium, pipecuronium); intermediate acting (atracurium, vecuronium); short acting (suxamethonium, mivacurium, Org 9426). The long duration of action and relatively slow elimination of the first group makes them unsuitable for infusion administration in all but the longest of procedures. Their use is therefore principally confined to administration by initial bolus, followed by repeated small increments if required. It is those agents in the intermediate and short categories which have a rapid clearance from the plasma, and therefore a rapid recovery of effect which are most suitable for administration by infusion.

Atracurium is a bisquaternary compound. It is a complicated molecule, containing an ester linkage which is susceptible both to hydrolysis and also to spontaneous degradation by Hofmann elimination reaction (Stenlake et al., 1983). These features give it an elimination half-life of approximately 20 min (Ward et al., 1983) and it appears to be unaffected by renal or hepatic dysfunction (Ward and Neill, 1983). Is is thus very suited to administration by continuous infusion. Indeed, many would suggest that it is unsuited to use by incremental bolus technique because of the frequency with which repeated doses are necessary in order to maintain a reasonable level of neuromuscular blockade.

Vecuronium is clinically very similar to atracurium in many respects. It has a short duration of action, with recovery of adductor pollicis response to 90% of control values within 20 min following an $ED_{90}$ dose (Robertson et al., 1983). This might initially be thought to be surprising in view of its long elimination half-life of approximately 60 min (Shanks, 1986). It is, however, very rapidly redistributed and so its short pharmacological action is probably the result of redistribution rather than metabolism (Sohn et al., 1986). If a continuous infusion is administered for long enough then it should theoretically be possible to saturate all of the distribution volume, at which point vecuronium will exhibit a prolonged duration of action. This is borne out in practice but is only significant after a large dose of vecuronium has been administered to patients with renal impairment (Slater, 1989).

Suxamethonium is the shortest acting of the whole group, assuming normal plasma cholinsterase activity. It has a half-life of approximately 4 min (Cook et al., 1976). It might be thought that this very short half-life would make suxamethonium even more suited to infusion administration. Unfortunately, in the continued presence of suxamethonium molecules the acetylcholine receptors at the neuromuscular junction appear to undergo a 'desensitization' phenomenon which produces tachyphylaxis to the neuromuscular blocking action of the suxamethonium. The characteristics of the block also change with the gradual appearance of a 'phase 2' block which is dependent upon the dose of suxamethonium, the time for which it has been administered and the choice of anaesthetic agent, and is rather unpredictable (Hilgenberg and Stoelting, 1981; Donati and Bevan, 1983; Futter et al., 1983). It may also be difficult to antagonise. Profound bradycardia may also result from the continued use of suxamethonium. It is for these reasons that most anaesthetists regard it as unsuitable for administration by infusion.

The two newest agents, mivacurium and Org. 9426 are both short acting and undergoing clinical trials at present. The published work on these two agents is scanty, but it is likely that their short duration of action will make them eminently suited to administration by continuous infusion.

## CONCLUDING REMARKS

When considering muscle relaxants for use in a total intravenous anaesthetic technique then it is clear that the choice is wide and the agent should be tailored to both the patient and to the proposed duration of surgery. Either of the two intermediate acting agents, atracurium or vecuronium, are the most appropriate for use by continuous infusion and are sufficiently versatile to cater for procedures from 20 min to several hours. Whichever agent is in use, neuromuscular monitoring should be undertaken so that the degree of neuromuscular blockade can be maintained at the level required for surgery. Degrees of blockade which are excessive and possibly difficult to reverse, or otherwise inadequate for surgery, are thus avoided. The use of a continuous infusion to maintain a continuous effect is recommended.

## REFERENCES

Agoston, S., Salt, P., Newton, D., Bencini, A., Boomsma, P. and Erdmann, W. (1980) The neuromuscular blocking action of Org. NC45, a new pancuronium derivative in anaesthetized patients. *Br. J. Anaesth.* 52, 53S—59S.

Ali, H.H. (1985) Monitoring of neuromuscular function and clinical interaction. *Clin. Anaesthesiol.* 3, 447—465.

Ali, H.H., Utting, J.E. and Gray, T.C. (1970) Stimulus frequency in the detection of neuromuscular block in humans. *Br. J. Anaesth.* 42, 967—978.

Atkinson, R.S., Rushman, G.B. and Lee, J.A. (1982) *A Synopsis of Anaesthesia*, 9th. Edn. John Wright and Sons Ltd., Bristol, pp. 280—321.

Bencini, A. and Newton, D.E.F. (1984) Rate of onset of good intubating conditions, respiratory depression and hand muscle paralysis after vecuronium. *Br. J. Anaesth.* 56, 959—965.

Chestnut, R., Jr, Healy, T.E.J. and Harper, N.J.N. (1987) Suxamethonium — the relation between dose and response. *Br. J. Anaesth.* 59, 1322P—1323P.

Clutton-Brock, R., Hutton, P. and Black, A.M.S. (1987) Simple feedback control of neuromuscular block. *Br. J. Anaesth.* 59, 135P.

Cook, D.R., Wingard, L.B. and Taylor, F.H. (1976) Pharmacokinetics of succinylcholine in infants, children and adults. *Clin. Pharmacol. Ther.* 20, 493—498.

Donati, F. and Bevan, D.R. (1983) Potentiation of succinylcholine phase II block with isoflurane. *Anesthesiology* 58, 552—555.

Drenck, N.E., Ueda, N., Olsen, N.V., Engbaek, J., Jansen, E., Skovgaard, L.T. and Viby-Mogenson, J. (1989) Manual evaluation of residual curarization using double burst stimulation: A comparison with train of four. *Anesthesiology* 70, 578—581.

Engbaek, J., Ostergaard, D. and Viby-Mogenson, J. (1989) Double burst stimulation (DBS). A new pattern of nerve stimulation to identify residual curarization. *Br. J. Anaesth.* 62, 274—278.

Feldman, S.A. and Liban, J.B. (1987) Vecuronium — A variable dose technique. *Anaesthesia* 42, 199—201.

Futter, M.E., Donati, F., Sadikot, A.S. (1983) Neostigmine antagonism of succinylcholine phase II block: A comparison with pancuronium. *Can. Anaesth. Soc. J.* 30, 575—580.

Griffiths, H.R. and Johnson, G.E. (1942) The use of curare in general anaesthesia. *Anesthesiology* 3, 418—420.

Grounds, R.M., Twigley, A.J., Carli, F., Whitwam, J.G. and Morgan, M. (1985) The haemodynamic effects of intravenous induction. Comparison of the effects of thiopentone and propofol. *Anaesthesia* 40, 735—740.

Harrison, M.J. (1990a) Prediction of infusion rates: a computer study. *Br. J. Anaesth.* 64, 283—286.

Harrison, M.J. (1990b) Prediction of infusion rates: validation of a computer simulation using vecuronium. *Br. J. Anaesth.* 64, 287—293.

Hilgenberg, J.C. and Stoelting, R.K. (1981) Characteristics of succinylcholine produced phase II neuromuscular block during enflurane, halothane and fentanyl anaesthesia. *Anesth. Analg.* 60, 192—196.

Jones, R.M. (1989) The priming principle: How does it work and should we be using it? *Br. J. Anaesth.* 63, 1—3.

Kreig, N., Crul, J.F. and Booij, L.H.D.J. (1980) Relative potency of Org. NC45, pancuronium, alcuronium and tubocurarine in anaesthetised man. *Br. J. Anaesth.* 52, 783—787.

Lee, C. and Katz, R.L. (1980) Neuromuscular pharmacology. A clinical update and commentary. *Br. J. Anaesth.* 52, 173—188.

Miller, R.D. (1984) In: *Pharmacokinetics of Anaesthesia.* Editors: C. Prys Roberts and C.C. Hug Jr., Blackwell Scientific Publications, Oxford, pp. 246—269.

Mitenko, P.A. and Ogilvie, R.I. (1972) Rapidly achieved plasma concentration plateaus, with observation on theophylline kinetics. *Clin. Pharmacol. Ther.* 13, 329—335.

Paton, W.D. and Waud, D.R. (1967) The margin of safety of neuromuscular transmission. *J. Physiol.* 191, 59—90.

Robertson, E.N., Booij, L.H.D. and Fragen, R.J. (1983) Clinical comparison of atracurium and vecuronium (Org. NC45). *Br. J. Anaesth.* 55, 125—129.

Shanks, C.A. (1985) Design of therapeutic regimens. *Clin. Anaesthesiol.* 3, 283—291.

Shanks, C.A. (1986) Pharmacokinetics of the nondepolarizing neuromuscular relaxants applied to calculation of bolus and infusion dosage regimens. *Anesthesiology* 64, 72—86.

Simionescu, R. and Bandila, T. (1989) Intratracheal muscle relaxant — a possible route. *Anaesthesia* 44, 264.

Slater, R.M., Pollard, B.J. and Doran, B.R.H. (1988) Prolonged neuromuscular blockade with vecuronium in renal failure. *Anaesthesia* 43, 250.

Smith, C.E., Donati, F. and Bevan, D.R. (1988) Dose-response curves for succinylcholine. Single versus cumulative techniques. *Anesthesiology* 69, 338—342.

Sohn, J.J., Bencini, A.F. and Scaf, A.H.J. (1986) Comparative pharmacokinetics and dynamics of vecuronium and pancuronium in anaesthetized patients. *Anesth. Analg.* 65, 233—239.

Stenlake, J.B., Waigh, R.B., Urwin, J., Dewar, G.H. and Coker, G.G. (1983) Atracurium: Conception and inception. *Br. J. Anaesth.* 55, 3S—10S

Thomas, A.N., Pollard, B.J., Ratcliff, A. and Ryan, J.P. (1989) Haemodynamic responses to induction with thiopentone and propofol measured using impedance cardiography. *Br. J. Anaesth.* 63, 228P—229P.

Tullock, W.C., Diana, P., Cook, D.R., Wilks, D.H., Brandrom, B.W., Stiller, R.L. and Beach, C.A. (1990) Neuromuscular and cardiovascular effects of high dose vecuronium. *Anesth. Analg.* 70, 86—90.

Van der Veen, F. and Bencini, A. (1980) Pharmacokinetics and pharmacodynamics of Org. NC45 in man. *Br. J. Anaesth.* 52, 37S—41S.

Viby-Mogenson, J., Jensen, N.H., Engbaek, J., Ording, H., Skovgaard, L.T. and Chrasmer-Jorgensen, B. (1985). Tactile and visual evaluation of the response to train of four nerve stimulation. *Anesthesiology* 63, 440—443.

Ward, S. and Neill, E.A.M. (1983) Pharmacokinetics of atracurium in acute hepatic failure (with acute renal failure). *Br. J. Anaesth.* 55, 1169—1172.

Ward, S., Neill, E.A.M. and Weatherly, B.C. (1983) Pharmacokinetics of atracurium besylate in healthy patients after a single intravenous bolus dose. *Br. J. Anaesth.* 55, 113—118.

Webster, N.R. and Cohen, A.T. (1987) Closed loop administration of atracurium. *Anaesthesia* 42, 1085—1091.

B. Kay (ed.) Total Intravenous Anaesthesia



# 8

# *Haemodynamic effects of continuous infusion anaesthesia and sedation*

M. Rucquoi and F. Camu

## INTRODUCTION

The development of new short-acting intravenous (i.v.) anaesthetics made the management of i.v. anaesthesia easier than was heretofore possible. Although i.v. anaesthesia offers some advantages compared with inhalation anaesthesia, it is in itself not devoid of drawbacks which every clinical anaesthesiologist should know. The main disadvantages of intravenous anaesthesia remain the lack of clear clinical signs in relation to depth of anaesthesia and relatively poor controllability of the level of anaesthesia. There are many reasons for this.

Depth and duration of effects depend amongst others on the amount of drug injected, the affinity of the drug for its receptors, the pharmacokinetic parameters of the drug, speed of distribution to and removal from the target organs, the large intersubject variability of the pharmacokinetic data and the influence of pathophysiological conditions such as changes in cardiac output or metabolism and excretion on the general pharmacokinetic behavior of the drug.

### Stable anaesthesia for cardiovascular stability?

The use of short-acting anaesthetic drugs has been advocated in order to maintain a tight control on the clinical effects with a flexible dosage. Is this correct reasoning? We know that in the multivariate situation of anaesthesia, consciousness impairment, pain, haemodynamics and respiration are interrelated. For instance, painful stimuli can trigger the autonomic nervous system and induce blood pressure and heart rate changes while the generated cortical impulses will influence both the state of vigilance and respiratory control mechanisms. Therefore, might it not be more logical to use long-acting drugs for certain goals of the intravenous anaesthesia technique?

Another problem of i.v. anaesthesia is related to the administration strategy of the drugs. In many clinical situations, perhaps even most surgical cases, the drugs are administered by intermittent injections. This implies the occurrence of high peak plasma levels with possible side effects and unstable plasma concentrations with peaks and troughs influencing the kinetics of the drug at the receptor sites. Although a direct relationship between drug effect and its plasma concentration is not evident for all drugs used in i.v. anaesthesia, it remains true that if the receptor-drug association and dissociation rates are rapid, such as is the case for alfentanil (Leysen et al., 1983) and fentanyl (Hermans et al., 1983), frequent changes in plasma concentration will preclude the maintenance of a stable level of anaesthesia. The pharmacodynamic relation between concentration and effect can be expected to be significant and reliable only when a state of dynamic equilibrium between the different tissue compartments has been reached. This implies that the drug plasma concentration required for the desired effect be kept within a narrow range by the administration regimen. A constant i.v. infusion is more adequate for this purpose than discrete i.v. boli (Norman, 1983) and should therefore afford the best degree of precision, reliability and predictability of effect in everyday clinical practice. The importance of constant plasma concentrations has recently been enlightened by the evidence of a definite hysteresis associated with changing fentanyl and alfentanil plasma concentrations, as assessed by the effect of rapid i.v. infusions on EEG waveforms (Scott et al., 1985).

Stable anaesthetic conditions will, however, not be quickly achieved by using constant infusion rates of a drug unless a loading dose is administered before the start of the continuous infusion. Indeed, steady-state plasma concentrations during infusion are reached only after four to five elimination half-times. Therefore, anaesthesiologists must choose not only a suitable infusion rate for maintenance of steady-state but also an adequate loading dose in order to attain the drug concentration equilibrium quickly in the blood and at the sites of action. Other strategies have been devised, aiming at a balance between the rate of administration and the rate of loss from the circulation: manually switched two-stepped constant flow schemes, with or without prior loading bolus, or three-stepped continuous infusions, computer-generated exponentially declining regimens either relying on previously defined elimination-based pharmacokinetic parameters (Alvis et al., 1985; Crankshaw et al., 1985), or iteratively improved by estimating the plasma drug efflux (Crankshaw et al., 1987). However, even with such strategies, other unwanted effects, such as haemodynamic and respiratory side effects may still appear, also toxic effects may arise due to cumulation of the used drugs (e.g. thiopentone) in some body compartments. Continuous infusions of drugs in principle provide more cardiovascular stability by reducing the haemodynamic side effects due to boli injections or to inadequate plasma concentrations in regard to the surgical stimulation.

# CARDIOVASCULAR EFFECTS OF ANAESTHESIA

## Hypnotic agents

### *Thiopentone*

The pharmacokinetic profile of thiopentone is characterized by a low initial hepatic extraction index of 0.15, constantly increasing with time to about 0.30 after 1 h so that thiopentone elimination is not affected by alterations in hepatic blood flow and depends more on the degree of plasma protein binding. Thiopentone has furthermore a relatively low clearance value of 1.6—4.3 ml/kg per min (Hudson et al., 1983) and a moderately large apparent volume of distribution at steady state of 1.45—3.3 l/kg (Morgan et al., 1981), resulting from the extensive distribution of thiopentone into muscle and fat tissues. This suggests that redistribution to muscle and fat is more important than metabolism for termination of the effect of thiopentone. Therefore, it should be borne in mind that after thiopentone infusions, high plasma concentrations may remain after completion of drug distribution to peripheral tissues, leading to a prolonged anaesthetic effect. Indeed, thiopentone elimination kinetics become non-linear at high doses with steady-state clearance decreasing with increasing plasma concentrations of thiopentone, probably related to saturation of hepatic enzymatic metabolism (Turcant et al., 1985).

Thiopentone is the only hypnotic agent which maintains the relation between myocardial oxygen supply and demand (Reiz et al., 1981). Although this property was demonstrated following bolus dosing of the drug, it might be the best rationale for the use of thiopentone by continuous infusion. There is a wide inter-individual variation in thiopentone serum concentrations needed to obtund the eyelash reflex: the published mean values vary from 20 to 40 μg/ml in the presence of nitrous oxide 67% after narcotic premedication (Becker, 1978; Christensen et al., 1980; Turcant et al., 1985). Such levels were reached with infusion rates between 0.15 and 3 mg/kg per min. At these plasma concentrations, non-invasive cardiac measurements indicated a slight decrease in stroke volume with an estimated 15% decrease in myocardial contractility (Becker and Tonnesen, 1978). As thiopentone decreases the tone of systemic capacitance vessels a reduction in preload was probably the major determinant of the observed changes in cardiac function. Using computer assisted exponentially decreasing infusions generating plasma levels of 15—20 μg/ml, other authors did not observe significant changes in blood pressure or heart rate in the presence of nitrous oxide and fentanyl (Carbon et al., 1978; Crankshaw et al., 1985).

Even the administration of large doses of thiopentone at a rate of 1.25 mg/kg per min under controlled normocapnic ventilation with air-oxygen had insignificant effects on the vascular pressures (mean arterial blood pressure (MAP) −13%) and resistances (systemic vascular resistance (SVR) −16%) if preload was well maintained. Venodilatation was important and required volume loading up to 1.5 l. Most remarkably, a direct myocardial depressant effect shown by a decrease of stroke volume by 14% was compensated by an increase in heart rate (+16%) thus maintaining cardiac output (Todd et al., 1982). Afterload also remained unaffected by these high doses of thiopentone.

Long-term thiopentone infusion (3—5 mg/kg per h during 4—8 days) used for post-traumatic brain protection purposes, producing average steady-state plasma concentrations ranging between 30 and 50 μg/ml, was reported not to have been associated with cardiovascular instability in a study aimed at pharmacokinetic and neurologic determinations in which no details were given as to the haemodynamic status of the patients or the corrective measures taken (Turcant et al., 1985).

*Methohexitone*

Though methohexitone and thiopentone have remarkably similar distribution kinetics, some differences are of major clinical importance. The hepatic extraction ratio of methohexitone is as high as 0.5. Also hepatic blood flow variations can affect methohexitone clearance which is grossly three times greater than the clearance of thiopentone (7.8—12.5 mg/kg per min) (Hudson et al., 1983). Methohexitone has an apparent volume of distribution at steady-state (2.2 l/kg) similar to thiopentone — but its elimination half-life is three times shorter because of the greater clearance, making recovery from methohexitone faster than recovery from thiopentone. Therefore, methohexitone appears preferable whenever a more rapid recovery is desired at the end of a continuous infusion of barbiturate.

A minimum infusion rate (MIR), the infusion rate which will prevent movement to surgical incision in 50% of patients was assessed as 49—66 μg/kg per min following an initial bolus of 1 mg/kg in the presence of nitrous oxide, depending on the type of premedication used (Sear et al., 1983). This infusion rate yielded a steady-state plasma concentration of 4.5 μg/ml. Plasma concentrations associated with sleep and EEG burst suppression varied from 3.4 to 10.7 μg/ml (Lauven et al., 1987).

Infusions of small doses of methohexitone (49—97 μg/kg per min) at constant or variable rate in opioid premedicated patients scheduled for outpatient surgery were associated with significant increases in heart rate but no changes in blood pressure (Doze et al., 1986).

Infusions of large doses of methohexitone at a rate of 400 μg/kg per min during controlled normocapnic ventilation with air-oxygen caused significant peripheral vasodilatation. Large fluid volumes had to be given to maintain cardiac filling pressures. Peripheral resistance decreased with a concomitant mild decrease in blood pressure. Also myocardial function was depressed by 20% but the decrease of stroke volume was compensated by a mild tachycardia sufficient to keep cardiac index within normal limits (Todd et al., 1984).

Concomitant administration of nitrous oxide and allowance for a slight degree of hypercapnia during spontaneous ventilation altered the cardiovascular response to methohexitone as central venous pressure increased significantly, suggesting

TABLE 8.1

Cardiovascular effects of continuous infusion of methohexitone

| Infusion rate μg/kg per min | Heart rate | Blood pressure | CVP | Cardiac output | Stroke volume | SVR | Comment[a] |
|---|---|---|---|---|---|---|---|
| 50 | | | | | | | |
| 60—65 | +11% | −22% | +70% | −26% | −31% | +5% | SV, premedication morphine, atropine nitrous oxide 67% |
| 60—65 | +3% | −13% | +100% | −38% | −39% | +37% | CV, same conditions as above |
| 120 | +14% | −21% | +59% | −34% | −41% | +27% | same conditions as above |
| 400 | +31% | −16% | +25% | +13% | −13% | −25% | CV, premedication diazepam, morphine air-oxygen 50% |

[a]SV = spontaneous ventilation; CV = controlled ventilation.

TABLE 8.2

Haemodynamic effects induced by propofol infusions expressed as percent change from control values

| Authors/technique | PCWP (%) | HR (%) | SAP (%) | CO (%) | SVR (%) | CVP (%) | Infusion rate (mg/kg per h) | Comment |
|---|---|---|---|---|---|---|---|---|
| **SV-air/$O_2$** | | | | | | | | |
| Claeys et al. (1988) | −12 | −2 | −30* | −2 | −30* | −13 | 6 | No surgery |
| Stephan et al. (1986) | −20* | +12 | −18* | −19 | ±2 | −16* | 12 | No surgery |
| Jessop et al. (1985) | — | −22* | −17* | — | — | — | 6.2 | Locoregional block |
| **SV-$N_2O/O_2$** | | | | | | | | |
| Coates et al. (1987) | — | −11 | −28* | −36* | +6 | +45 | 3.2 | Surgery |
| Monk et al. (1987) | — | −14 | −47* | −31* | −11 | — | 3.2—3.9 | Surgery |
| Coates et al. (1987) | — | −4 | −36* | −31* | −3 | −2 | 6.5 | Surgery |
| **CV-$N_2O/O_2$** | | | | | | | | |
| Coates et al. (1987) | — | −14* | −20 | −52* | +48* | +36 | 3.2 | Surgery |
| Coates et al. (1987) | — | −8 | −36* | −53* | +30* | +2 | 6.5 | Surgery |

*$P < 0.05$.

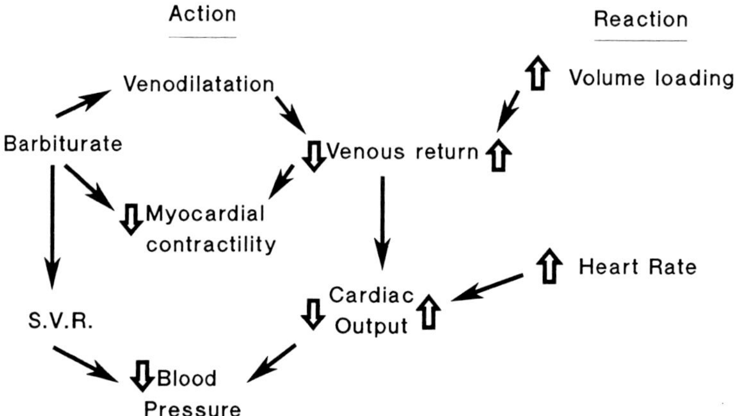


Fig. 8.1. Cardiovascular effects and compensatory mechanisms during continuous infusions of barbiturates.

venodilatation was suppressed (Prys-Roberts et al., 1983). Cardiac output and stroke volume decreased but the rise of peripheral resistance was insufficient to prevent a further decrease of blood pressure. These changes were even more pronounced when the patients were artificially ventilated (Table 8.1).

Therefore, continuous i.v. administration of barbiturates required careful volume monitoring to allow compensatory changes to exert their effects and maintain the haemodynamic status within narrow limits (Fig. 8.1). Combinations with nitrous oxide, hypercapnia and opioids may cause profound cardiovascular changes in patients with reduced cardiac reserve or hypovolaemia.

In the elderly the clinical pharmacology of barbiturates indicates an increased sensitivity and an age-related prolongation of postoperative recovery (Sear et al., 1983a). These changes may result from pharmacokinetic modifications induced by ageing, such as differences in distribution volumes, but the plasma clearance is not affected by age (Christensen et al., 1980). No studies however are available which assess the sensitivity of the nervous system to a given concentration of barbiturate or the haemodynamic effects in geriatric patients.

*Etomidate*

In contrast to barbiturates, this drug has a high safety margin in cardiac patients. However, because etomidate suppresses the normal cortisol response to anaesthesia and surgery, some doubts have been cast on the wisdom of using etomidate for long-term infusion. Its fundamental pharmacokinetic profile is profoundly influenced by the administration strategy: a single bolus (Van Hamme et al., 1978) induces a rapid onset of action and a rapid recovery, consistent with the drug being rapidly distributed to both central and peripheral compartments, whereas prolonged infusions lead to a lower clearance, longer recovery times and slower intercompartmental transfer rates (Hebron et al., 1983). The simultaneous administration of fentanyl may decrease the hepatic clearance of etomidate. Furthermore, there is an age-related pharmacokinetic variation for etomidate, the elderly showing a smaller initial distribution volume leading to higher initial blood concentrations after a given dose (Arden et al., 1986). Plasma concentrations associated with hypnotic activity vary between 0.3 and 1 μg/ml (Schüttler et al., 1985).

When given by infusion at rates between 1 and 25 μg/kg per min, as for sedative purposes in the intensive care unit, cardiovascular indices remained stable (Edbrooke et al., 1982). For maintenance of hypnosis during anaesthesia with fentanyl and air-oxygen ventilation (Fragen et al., 1983a), the plasma concentration of etomidate must remain above 300 ng/ml. This required rates of 20—50 μg/kg per min at which mean arterial pressure decreased by 10% while heart rate increased to the same extent (Dearden and McDowall, 1985). Such an etomidate plasma concentration can be reached more quickly with the administration of an initial fast constant-rate infusion (8 mg/min for 10 min) followed by a slower infusion (0.8 mg/min), with the drawback of a short (10 min) initial overshoot up to 2 μg/ml. Only slight circulatory effects are reported to occur using such a technique with a mild increase in heart rate during the initial fast infusion without variation in blood pressure. At an infusion rate of 2.4 mg/kg per min administered to geriatric patients artificially ventilated, a decrease of mean arterial blood pressure, heart rate and cardiac index was observed. In parallel to the reduction in myocardial work, myocardial blood flow and oxygen consumption decreased, but no myocardial lactate production, a sign indicative of local ischaemia, occurred (Larsen et al., 1988).

More detailed haemodynamic studies in dogs, however, showed serious cardiovascular effects of etomidate given at a rate of 70 μg/kg per min in the presence of nitrous oxide (Van Lambalgen et al., 1982). A negative inotropic effect appeared, decreasing stroke volume, left ventricular contractility and cardiac output while systemic vascular resistance increased, probably through baroreceptor control. This compensatory mechanism allowed mean arterial pressure to remain stable. No changes in heart rate were observed. These cardiac effects were accompanied by a redistribution of cardiac output, in particular a 50% reduction of splanchnic and hepatic artery blood flows, which may impair the metabolism of the drug in the liver (Heykants et al., 1975).

*Benzodiazepines*

Amongst the many benzodiazepine molecules used in clinical anaesthesiology applications, midazolam is the most useful for anaesthetic purposes because of its water-solubility, its good vascular tolerance, its short elimination half-life and the absence of long acting metabolites of any clinical relevance. Furthermore, it is the only benzodiazepine for which the use of continuous infusion regimens makes sense.

Very few data are available on the pharmacokinetics of midazolam infusions. Midazolam clearance values between 200 and 700 ml/min have been reported, indicating a wide inter-patient variability (Lauven et al., 1985; Nilsson et al., 1986; Oldenhof et al., 1988). The pharmacokinetics of midazolam seem not to be influenced by the simultaneous use of alfentanil or fentanyl.

Clinical investigations initially suggested a minimal effective plasma concentration of midazolam of at least 0.2 $\mu$g/ml (Brown et al., 1979). More recently, in a thoroughly designed pharmacokinetic study using computer-driven variable flow continuous midazolam infusions, the minimum plasma level producing a reliable hypnotic effect was defined as 0.5 $\mu$g/ml (Lauven et al., 1982) in volunteers spontaneously breathing room air. In the presence of opiods 0.3 $\mu$g/ml was considered to be the target concentration for hypnosis during lower abdominal surgery.

The haemodynamic effects of midazolam given by continuous infusion in combination with alfentanil, fentanyl or spinal anaesthesia show a mild decrease in blood pressure and heart rate for infusion rates varying between 0.05 and 0.25 mg/kg per h (Nilsson et al., 1986; Blake et al., 1988; Nilsson et al., 1988; Bursztein, 1989).

Peroperative three-step midazolam infusions (bolus 0.15—0.20 mg/kg, 700 $\mu$g/min for 20 min, 300 $\mu$g/min afterwards) used in combination with nitrous oxide during upper abdominal surgery induced few significant haemodynamic changes. Continuous infusions of midazolam at rates up to 0.2 mg/kg per min have been used in postoperative care for sedative purposes. Under these circumstances, adequate volume loading was mandatory to maintain systemic blood pressure within normal limits. Such treatments may thus be particularly dangerous in patients with impaired myocardial oxygen delivery capacity (Ex, 1987).

The detailed mechanism of the cardiovascular and haemodynamic effects of midazolam was investigated in clinical studies with bolus dosing using invasive measurements.

Although midazolam, like other benzodiazepines, is devoid of any important direct inotropic effect (List and Ponhold, 1983), it exerts its major haemodynamic effects at the peripheral level with a small decrease in systemic vascular resistance but marked venodilatation (Samuelson et al., 1981; Reves et al., 1985), much like nitroglycerine. By decreasing the venous return, preload is reduced which contributes to a fall in cardiac output and blood pressure. Maintenance of the cardiac output greatly depends on compensatory mechanisms such as increased baroreceptor activity, blood mobilization from the splanchic area and increased sympathetic outflow. In patients with hypovolaemia, hypertension and beta-adrenergic blockade, impairment of these compensatory mechanisms is reported to induce serious hypotensive episodes (Adams et al., 1985), which are also described in patients with severe non-cardiac systemic illness, in whom midazolam reduces not only the systemic vascular resistance and the mean arterial pressure, but also cardiac output, heart rate and stroke volume (Lebowitz et al., 1983). On the other hand, midazolam causes only minor haemodynamic changes in surgical patients without concomitant debilitating affections (Fragen et al., 1978) and has been called 'safe' in heart disease: its nitroglycerin-like vasodilating effect is beneficial both in case of pulmonary hypertension (Murday et al., 1985) and congestive heart failure, while cardiac output is unaffected in patients with ischaemic heart disease (Reves et al., 1979).

On theoretical grounds, midazolam could be contra-indicated in case of aortic stenosis, but definitive evidence is lacking (Murday et al., 1985; Schulte-Sasse and Tarnow, 1984). Furthermore, interactions with other anaesthetic agents, such as nitrous oxide and ketamine are obvious but poorly documented.

*Propofol*

Onset and disappearance of the hypnotic effect of propofol are conditioned by the specific pharmacokinetic profile of this drug. The onset of unconsciousness occurs at plasma concentrations between 1.07 and 10.5 mg/l depending upon the rate of administration of propofol. Surgical anaesthesia required plasma levels ranging from 7 to 10 mg/l (Hazeaux et al., 1987). The disappearance of the hypnotic effect of propofol results from its rapid and extensive redistribution and high clearance from plasma. As more than 70% of the administered dose is eliminated during the first and second exponential phases, most of the amount administered by continuous infusion will have to compensate for both this elimination and redistribution of the drug (Gepts et al., 1987). The good concentration-effect relationship with low individual variability and the easy adaptability of infusion rate to desired effect makes propofol very suitable for intravenous infusion regimens. The infusion rates of propofol reported in the literature vary from 13 μg/kg per min (Grounds et al., 1987) for sedation in intensive care to 100—150 μg/kg per min to supplement nitrous oxide or fentanyl in surgical conditions (de Grood et al., 1985; Rolly et al., 1985; Coates et al., 1987). The amount of propofol required to maintain a steady-state level of unconsciousness decreased with age, opiate premedication or simultaneous use of narcotics and nitrous oxide.

When administered by continuous infusion for sedation or for maintenance of anaesthesia at a rate of 100 μg/kg per min in the absence of nitrous oxide, large decreases (30%) in arterial pressure were observed (Claeys et al., 1988). This was related to a 30% reduction of systemic vascular resistance, while preload decreased by 12%. Cardiac output was not affected at any time nor was stroke volume or heart rate. Thus the arterial hypotension was mainly due to the reduction of arterial impedance not compensated by a reflex increase in heart rate or cardiac output. As such propofol may be regarded as exerting a central depression of sympathetic outflow. When used as a sedative for supplementation of regional anaesthesia techniques, at infusion rates of 100—150 μg/kg per min, propofol significantly reduced heart rate and arterial blood pressure (Jessop et al., 1985). This effect appeared despite the chemical vasodilatation already induced by the regional blockade. Recently, it has been suggested that propofol induced a negative inotropic effect (Larsen et al., 1988; Van Aken et al., 1988) and depressed regional myocardial contractility and left ventricular afterload in a dose-dependent fashion (Coetzee et al., 1989).

Quite different haemodynamic changes have been recorded in patients scheduled for coronary bypass surgery receiving beta-adrenergic or slow calcium channel blocking agents (Stephan et al., 1986). Following heavy premedication and an initial bolus of 2 mg/kg propofol, a continuous infusion of 200 μg/kg per min propofol elicited a significant tachycardia, a lesser fall in systemic blood pressure (15%), cardiac index and stroke volume index (by 19% and 25%, respectively); systemic vascular resistance did not change significantly (Table 8.2). Myocardial blood flow and myocardial oxygen consumption fell, resulting in decreased lactate uptake and extraction; lactate release was however noted in one patient in whom mean arterial pressure fell by 20%.

Sedation of mechanically ventilated patients with long-term low-dose propofol infusions (1—3 mg/kg per h for 8 h) elicited a slight decrease in heart rate only during the first infusion hour, with a decrease in systolic, mean and diastolic blood pressures (Newman et al., 1987). Hypotension appeared roughly dose-related and was marked following bolus dosing, was often associated with a deep level of sedation, and responded to a reduction in infusion rate. With mean propofol blood levels ranging between 0.6 and 1 μg/ml, the patients remained asleep while undisturbed, yet rousable on verbal command. Similar but poorly documented haemodynamic changes occurred after a three-stage propofol infusion aiming at linearly increasing (0.15 μg/ml per min) propofol blood levels (Schüttler et al., 1985b) in healthy volunteers. The hypnotic effect was attained with propofol blood levels of 1.07 ± 0.08 μg/ml.

With concurrent administration of nitrous oxide, stroke volume decreased by 11—20% and cardiac output by 20—31%. These effects seemed unrelated to the rate of administration of propofol as they occurred to a similar extent with either 60 or 120 μg/kg per min (Coates et al., 1987; Monk et al., 1987). Also, marked resetting of the baroreceptor reflex was observed allowing lower arterial pressures without tachycardia. As systemic vascular resistance remained unaffected despite respiratory acidosis in these spontaneously breathing patients, the observed haemodynamic changes could result from a direct myocardial depressant effect of nitrous oxide.

The combination of propofol and fentanyl (7.5 μg/kg per h) or alfentanil infusions (0.7 μg/kg per min) did not produce marked haemodynamic effects, although all these agents are centrally acting vagotonic drugs (de Grood et al., 1985; Kay, 1986). In normal patients heart rate was usually unaffected while blood pressures decreased slightly. Surgical stimulation induced no change of this cardiovascular status indicating that the narcotic-propofol combination was more able to block the autonomic sympathetic responses than propofol alone. In patients with heart disease, the surgical stimulation raised blood pressure and systemic vascular resistance despite the presence of fentanyl, but a further decrease of cardiac index was noted. Fentanyl had no effect on the increase of coronary vascular resistance induced by propofol. These authors concluded that, despite the maintenance of an adequate supply-demand relationship for myocardial oxygen, propofol-fentanyl anaesthesia may induce regional inbalance of coronary blood flow in myocardial areas supplied by stenotic arteries (Stephan et al., 1986).

## Opioids

Continuous infusions of opioids should provide better cardiovascular stability during anaesthesia than doses of the same opioids injected at discrete intervals (White, 1983), which may induce prolonged respiratory depression and provide shorter postoperative analgesia (Pathak et al., 1983). This review covers only fentanyl and its newer homologues alfentanil and sufentanil, which have gained great popularity in current anaesthetic practice. Discussion of continuous infusion of 'older' opioids, such as morphine or pethidine, is nowadays only of historical interest.

It has been suggested that endogeneous opiates may play a role in cardiovascular regulation under both physiological and pathological conditions (Holaday, 1983). In the rat (Gautret and Schmitt, 1985) fentanyl acts at three different levels on cardiovascular regulation: (a) immediate activation of the opioid receptors located at vagal nerve endings with an immediate and short-lasting hypotension and bradycardia, suppressed by bilateral vagotomy and reduced in extent by previous atropine, an effect also demonstrated in man (Reitan et al., 1978); (b) direct cerebral stimulation of sympathetic out-flow leading to hypertensive episodes only evidenced after vagotomy and suppressed by alpha-receptor blocking drugs but not by adrenalectomy; (c) direct stimulation of cardiac opioid receptors on the sino-atrial node inducing bradycardia; this latter effect exists also in man.

*Fentanyl*

In adult patients scheduled for intra-abdominal surgery, fentanyl plasma levels of 4—8 ng/ml, achieved by a bolus of 10 μg/min followed by a maintenance infusion of 2 μg/min, were associated with haemodynamic stability (McQuay et al., 1979). In adults undergoing superficial operations, plasma fentanyl concentrations of 3—5 ng/ml, resulting from a bolus of 5 μg/kg and a constant infusion of 3 μg/kg per h maintained stable cardiovascular conditions (Andrews et al., 1982). During both studies, 67% nitrous oxide was administered. A plasma concentration of 8—10 ng/ml is associated with a reduction of about 50% of enflurane MAC, while 20 ng/ml causes unconsciousness and a 65% decrease in enflurane MAC (Murphy and Hug, 1982), without additional nitrous oxide. For cardiac surgery, plasma levels up to 20 ng/ml or more were needed to avoid hypertensive responses (Moldenhauer and Hug, 1982; Wynands et al., 1984) although with computer-assisted infusion techniques fentanyl requirements were less as the plasma fentanyl concentrations needed to maintain cardiovascular stability amounted to 10 ng/ml (Alvis et al., 1985). Clinically important respiratory depression is reported with plasma fentanyl concentrations in the range 1.5—3.0 ng/ml, the lower values observed in hyperventilated patients (Cartwright et al., 1983).

During fentanyl-oxygen anaesthesia, the filling pressures of the right and left heart remained constant when fentanyl was infused at different rates varying from 0.3 to 0.5 μg/kg per min following an initial bolus dose. However with the lower infusion rate, significant increases in cardiac output and heart rate and an initial fall of systemic vascular resistance, followed by a marked increase of this parameter upon surgical stimulation, occurred. At a higher infusion rate only heart rate changed with no change in cardiac output or afterload. This is in agreement with the clinical impression that higher doses of fentanyl will induce fewer haemodynamic changes (Sprigge et al., 1982; Hynynen et al., 1986). The degree of left ventricular (LV) function impairment produced by continuous fentanyl infusions will have an effect on the global haemodynamic profile during coronary artery surgery in spite of similar plasma levels of about 10 ng/ml (Wynands et al., 1983): in patients with impaired LV function heart rate increased after induction and remained elevated throughout surgery, raising cardiac index, whereas systemic vascular resistance fell significantly on induction and increased slightly thereafter without however reaching the preinduction values. Simultaneous infusions of fentanyl (100—200 μg/min) and droperidol (5 mg/min) have been compared with a similar infusion of fentanyl alone in cardiac patients (Milocco et al., 1985): only small differences appeared with cardiac output unchanged, mean arterial pressure decreasing and heart rate increasing in both groups, both effects being slightly more pronounced when droperidol was used.

*Alfentanil*

To provide adequate perioperative analgesia, alfentanil plasma levels of 200—250 ng/ml are needed for body surface (Shafer et al., 1983), general (Leysen et al., 1983) or lower abdominal surgery (Ausems and Hug, 1983) whereas higher levels of 300—400 ng/ml are required for upper abdominal surgery (Shafer et al., 1983), all these figures being subject to a wide margin of variation of at least 30% (Ausems et al., 1986). However, plasma alfentanil levels of at least 1.0 μg/ml must be reached to prevent haemodynamic, somatic and sympathetic responses during heart surgery (Bower and Hull, 1986) when alfentanil is the sole anesthetic agent; more recent investigations show, however, that neither 1.7 μg/ml (De Lange and De Bruijn, 1983) nor even 4.6 μg/ml (Hall et al., 1987) can ablate the circulatory responses in patients undergoing coronary artery surgery during maximal surgical stress. Anaesthetic conditions were, however, satisfactory when a large premedicant dose of lorazepam (0.08 mg/kg) was used in combination with alfentanil in the range 1.0—1.4 μg/kg (Hall et al., 1987). Total recommended cumulative alfentanil requirements for heart surgery span from at least 1 mg/kg (De Lange and De Bruijn, 1983) to 1.5 mg/kg (Sebel et al., 1982). Awakening and spontaneous respiration is unlikely to occur postoperatively until plasma levels have decayed to less than 200 ng/kg (Stanski and Hug, 1982; Fragen et al., 1983b; Norman, 1983). Maintenance infusion rates of alfentanil are usually between 0.5 and 3 μg/kg per min; but even at such a high rate of delivery additional boli of the drug are needed to treat sudden increases of blood pressure during surgical stimulation, while recovery is markedly delayed (Wyatt and Nestorowicz, 1984). The rationale of such an administration strategy has thus been questioned (Lavies, 1984). Alternatively, a variable-rate alfentanil infusion has been used successfully to adapt the alfentanil plasma concentrations required by variable surgical stimuli (Ausems and Hug, 1983). Haemodynamic instability could be somewhat reduced by giving a higher loading dose up to 125 μg/kg (Sebel et al., 1982) or even 150 μg/kg (Bovill et al.,

1984). Heart rate and cardiac output remained unchanged or decreased and the endogenous catecholamine output was reduced.

Such important induction boli are, however, not as safe and advisable as might appear from mean figures pooled from a patient population. Patients scheduled for coronary artery bypass grafting (CABG) have been reported to show impressive and potentially harmful haemodynamic changes after a 125 μg/kg alfentanil bolus given in 2 min. Acute hypotension or hypertension may occur despite increasing the bolus to 250 μg/kg (Sebel et al., 1982). Similar incidents are not reported during valve replacement surgery (Bovill et al., 1984). A progressive increase in systemic vascular resistance was also observed. When designing the optimal alfentanil dosing profile, inter-individual pharmacokinetic variability can be taken into consideration using computer algorithms proposing a dosing strategy, calculating a confidence interval for the time course of plasma concentrations, and adjusting the dosing scheme if the desired target concentration at a given time is not bracketed by the confidence interval (Maitre et al., 1987).

Data obtained in halothane-anaesthetized (1.5%) dogs (Kien et al., 1986) during alfentanil infusion (3 μg/kg per min, initial loading dose 45 μg/kg) suggest that a direct vasodilatory effect on the peripheral vasculature was responsible for a 20% decrease in systemic arterial pressure to which the sympathetic inhibition may have contributed, but left ventricular dynamics remained normal. Interestingly enough, myocardial and cerebral blood flows were well maintained, suggesting preservation of autoregulatory mechanisms. However, renal blood flow fell by 20% and hepatic arterial blood flow by 60%. The normal oxygen delivery to the liver thus could be jeopardized, which would be detrimental in patients with impaired liver function. The findings of this study are at odds with other investigations in canine models when no halothane was administered: alfentanil 200 μg/kg produces a significant increase in dP/d*t* in chronically instrumented dogs (De Bruijn et al., 1983), while 320 μg/kg induces an increase in ventricular afterload and in peripheral resistance (Schauble et al., 1983). Therefore, most of the untoward effects might be ascribed to a combination of halothane-mediated myocardial depression, direct vasodilatation and sympathetic inhibition.

For sedation and analgesia in intensive care, much lower infusion rates of alfentanil, such as 0.25—0.5 μg/kg per min, in ventilated patients (Yate et al., 1986) and 0.1—0.2 μg/kg per min in spontaneously breathing patients (Andrews et al., 1985), are required. They offer the advantage of stable haemodynamic conditions with satisfactory analgesia.

*Sufentanil*

Being highly lipophilic and distributing rapidly and extensively to all tissues, sufentanil differs from fentanyl on pharmacokinetic grounds by its smaller volume of distribution and shorter elimination half-life which explains its quicker onset of action and its shorter effect. Infusions up to 40 μg/kg per min have been shown to produce few cardiovascular changes in atropinized dogs, with or without nitrous oxide (Reddy et al., 1980). Sufentanil has been given by continuous infusion techniques at variable rates for outpatient anesthesia (De Lange et al., 1982) with infusion rates varying up to 7 μg/min. In this setting no significant haemodynamic changes were reported. In adult patients with beta-adrenergic blockade undergoing cardiac surgery, premedicated with lorazepam, cardiovascular dynamics were minimally altered throughout the operation with a continuous infusion of sufentanil (300 μg/min) in the absence of nitrous oxide (De Lange et al., 1982; De Lange et al., 1983). This beneficial effect can be explained by a blockade of some hormonal stress responses occurring during cardiopulmonary bypass, but cannot be achieved without continuous infusions: in similar patients given sufentanil 15 μg/min over 2 min with allowance for further additional boli only in case of persistent hypertension, episodes of hypotension on induction, tachycardia after tracheal intubation and hypertension following sternotomy have been mentioned (Sebel and Bovill, 1982). However, very little information is available on the relation between plasma concentration and effect for sufentanil. Plasma sufentanil levels associated with haemodynamic stability in the absence of nitrous oxide are 15—20 ng/ml (Rosow, 1984). Further research is needed to determine whether sufentanil is superior to other narcotics for use as an anaesthetic during heart surgery or non-cardiac surgery. Despite the theoretical advantage of sufentanil having fewer side effects than less potent drugs, a double-blind comparison of continuous infusions of fentanyl (up to 100 μg/kg) and sufentanil (as much as 30 μg/kg) showed that neither drug provided better 'haemodynamic stability' in patients undergoing CABG premedicated with morphine and scopolamine (Rosow et al., 1983).

In conclusion, when used for total intravenous anaesthesia, continuous infusions of hypnotics and narcotics induce only minimal changes in cardiac and haemodynamic parameters provided extremely high doses are avoided. They influence the cardiovascular system mainly by reducing preload and have a variable drug-specific and probably dose-dependent effect on myocardial contractility. In most instances, compensatory mechanisms maintain the cardiac output within normal limits. These include compensatory increases in heart rate through baroreceptor reflex pathways, splanchnic vasoconstriction and/or increased sympathetic outflow with preservation of myocardial contractility. Particular attention should be given to maintain a normal preload.

### Combination of opioids and hypnotics

The simultaneous use of continuous infusions of both an hypnotic and an opioid is an alternative advocated by some as an elegant and flexible strategy for general anaesthesia (Norman, 1983; Dundee, 1985), but the determination of target blood concentrations is further compounded by possible interactions of one drug on the pharmacokinetic constants of another. Even the evidence available on this account can be controversial as, e.g., fentanyl has been shown either to reduce propofol total body clearance, thereby increasing the level of propofol blood concentrations (Briggs et al., 1985), or conversely not to impair the clearance or distribution of propofol significantly. Such an interaction, if any, does not appear to increase either the hypnotic effect of propofol or the respiratory depressant action of fentanyl (Fragen et al., 1983c). The haemodynamic effects of simultaneous continuous infusion of fentanyl and hypnotics have at this date not yet been thoroughly investigated.

The analgesic effects of alfentanil are not potentiated by etomidate (Schüttler et al., 1983) but are slightly potentiated by propofol. This results from a propofol-induced decrease in apparent volume of distribution of alfentanil (Gepts et al., 1988). Conversely, alfentanil, having itself hypnotic properties, enhances the clinical effects but does not alter the disposition kinetics of propofol. The cardiovascular effects of continuous alfentanil infusions (1 μg/kg per min, loading bolus 10 μg/kg) administered simultaneously with either methohexitone (0.15 mg/kg per min, initial bolus 1.5 mg/kg) or propofol (200 μg/kg per min, initial bolus 2 mg/kg) have been recorded during major surgery and without premedication or concomitant administration of nitrous oxide (Kay, 1986). Methohexitone caused a significant rise in mean pulse rate and both systolic and diastolic pressures throughout anesthesia, those changes being maximal at intubation and 10 min thereafter. There was no change in pulse rate and a slight decline in systemic blood pressures during alfentanil-propofol infusions. Slightly different results were observed with alfentanil-propofol infusions during body surface surgery (Hilton et al., 1986). Although heart rate remained stable with the exception of a short gallamine-induced tachycardia, systolic and diastolic blood pressures constantly decreased and the magnitude of this fall increased with age. This was possibly related to a weaker surgical stimulation in the presence of lower rates of administration of alfentanil (0.25 μg/kg per min, loading bolus 5 μg/kg).

**Interactions with nitrous oxide**

As do all inhalation anaesthetics, nitrous oxide exerts a direct (albeit moderate) myocardial depressant effect (Eisele and Smith, 1972) but has a stimulating effect on the brain control of beta-adrenergic activity (Fukunaga and Epstein, 1973) thereby indirectly exciting the heart. Moreover, apart from increasing sympathetic tone, it also inhibits norepinephrine metabolism by the lung (Naito and Gillis, 1973) which explains a peak increase in plasma catecholamines after 15 min exposure to nitrous oxide (Eisele and Smith, 1972). It significantly depresses the baroreflex control of heart rate (Bristow et al., 1968) but bears little effect on hypoxia-induced pulmonary vasoconstriction (Price et al., 1969).

The net balance between those antagonistic factors depends not only on the inspired nitrous oxide concentration, but more on pre-existing sympathetic tone, concomitant drug administration and underlying pathological conditions.

Heart rate, blood pressure, cardiac output and stroke volume have been shown to increase and systemic vascular resistance to fall in volunteers breathing 60% nitrous oxide in oxygen for 2 h (Kawamura et al., 1980) while central venous pressure increased, due to a lower venous compliance.

Nitrous oxide does not produce any significant changes in pulmonary artery pressure, PCWP or pulmonary vascular resistance either in healthy patients (Price et al., 1969) or in case of coronary artery obstruction (Mc Cammon et al., 1980).

In contrast, perhaps because opioids block the sympathomimetic effects of nitrous oxide, adding nitrous oxide to a background of fentanyl 75 μg/kg in patients scheduled for heart surgery has been shown to result in a cardiovascular depression far exceeding the effects of either nitrous oxide or narcotics alone (Lunn et al., 1979): though heart rate and mean arterial pressure remained roughly unchanged, systemic vascular resistance increased markedly, leading to a significant fall in cardiac output and left ventricular stroke work.

The relationship between dose and response for this interaction between opioids and nitrous oxide is not well defined. Adequacy of depth of anaesthesia and extent of heart function impairment are likely to be related to these results: in cardiac patients given 50 μg/kg fentanyl (and 10 μ/kg flunitrazepam) the addition of 70% $N_2O$ in oxygen induced only moderate changes (Meretoja et al., 1985) in mean arterial pressure, a slight bradycardia and a moderate depression of cardiac index resulting in an unchanged systemic vascular resistance. Moreover, the myocardial depression was especially prominent in patients with hypokinetic areas of left ventricular wall, while the strongest decreases in cardiac output occurred in the patients with the lowest preoperative ejection fraction.

When administered to patients scheduled for CABG receiving a fentanyl infusion (10 μg/kg, loading dose 75 μg/kg), nitrous oxide caused heart rate, mean arterial pressure and cardiac index to drop significantly, while systemic vascular resistance remained virtually unchanged (Moffitt et al., 1984).

Those findings might cast a shadow of doubt on the safety of administering $N_2O$ to patients with ischaemic heart disease, the more $N_2O$ induces myocardial ischaemia in some animal models with jeopardized coronary perfusion, when superimposed on fentanyl (Philbin et al., 1975) or inhalation anesthesia (Nathan, 1988) — but not in all models (Cason et al., 1987).

However, $N_2O$ has been shown not to induce any myocardial ischaemia, as could be detected by ST-segment analysis and transoesophageal two-dimensional echocardiography, in patients with severe coronary narrowing under fentanyl anesthesia (15 μg/kg bolus, 0.2 μg/kg per min continuous infusion), in patients with either well-preserved (Calahan et al., 1987) or impaired (Mitchell et al., 1989) LV function. Transoesophageal echocardiography is, however, less sensitive by a factor of roughly 10 than the epicardially implanted microcrystals in the animal models. Although the use of $N_2O$ in patients with coronary artery disease has recently been claimed as safe (Nathan, 1989) provided stable haemodynamic conditions are maintained, it might induce myocardial wall dyskinesia too small to be detected by clinically applicable methods.

Limited information is available about the cardiovascular effects of intravenous infusions of alfentanil as a supplement to nitrous oxide anaesthesia. During lower abdominal gynecological operations (Ausems et al., 1983) mean blood pressure remained mostly unchanged while mild to moderate bradycardia occurred with

66% $N_2O$ in oxygen associated with an alfentanil bolus, 150 μg/kg, followed by an alfentanil infusion with a variable rate (25—150 μg/kg per h) according to the patient's response to stimulation. During general surgery (Ausems et al., 1986), the same anaesthetic regimen elicited hypotension (but never under 85 mmHg) on induction in 40% of the patients while blood pressure remained grossly stable throughout the procedures. Severe bradycardia occurred in 8% of the patients during induction, whereas heart rate later remained between 50 and 90 beats/min, with the exception of some episodes of moderate bradycardia. Finally, the fact that nitrous oxide augments the ventilatory depressant effects of narcotic analgesics should be kept in mind.

## CONCLUSION

Today, the clinical anaesthesiologist is able to control each component of the classical triad of anaesthesia — hypnosis, analgesia and muscle relaxation — specifically and independently from each other. On theoretical grounds, continuous infusion regimens allow an optimal drug titration against requirements and minimize the risk of overdosage, provided some simple pharmacokinetic principles are mastered. However elegant, this technique is not free of potential untoward cardiovascular effects for which thorough investigation is still lacking, especially in the field of interactions with other anaesthetic drugs or between multiple continuous infusions. Some further investigation is also needed to ascertain the effects of continuous infusions in patients with compromised myocardial function, with hypovolaemia or receiving treatments impairing the baroreceptor reflex. In such patients, the safety margin of continuous infusions of narcotics and hypnotics could be very narrow. Age-related changes in volume of distribution and elimination clearance of the drugs, cardiac output and renal function may also induce exaggerated responses of the elderly to standard doses of i.v. infused hypnotics. Therefore, adequate clinical observation and instrumental monitoring remain mandatory to optimize the infusion rate to the clinical end-points.

## REFERENCES

Adams, P., Gelman, S., Reves, J.G., Greenblatt, D.J., Alvis, J.M. and Bradley, E. (1985) Midazolam pharmacodynamics and pharmacokinetics during acute hypovolemia. *Anesthesiology* 63, 140—146.

Alvis, J.M., Reves, J.G., Covier, A.V., Menkhaus, P.G., Henling, C.E., Spain, J.A. and Bradley, E. (1985) Computer assisted continuous infusions of fentanyl during cardiac anesthesia: comparison with a manual method. *Anesthesiology* 63, 41—49.

Andrews, C.J., Sinclair, M., Dye, A., Dye, J., Harvey, J. and Prys-Roberts, C. (1982) The additive effects of nitrous oxide on respiratory depression in patients having fentanyl or alfentanil infusion. *Br. J. Anaesth.* 54, 1129.

Andrews, C.H.J., Robertson, J.A. and Chapman, J.M. (1985) Postoperative analgesia with intravenous infusion of alfentanil, *Lancet* 2, 671.

Arden, J.R., Holley, F.O. and Stanski, D.R. (1986) Increased sensitivity to etomidate in the elderly: initial distribution versus altered brain response. *Anesthesiology* 65, 19—27.

Ausems, M.E. and Hug, C.C., Jr (1983) Plasma concentration of alfentanil required to supplement nitrous oxide anaesthesia for lower abdominal surgery. *Br. J. Anaesth.* 55, (Suppl. 2), 191S—197S.

Ausems, M.E., Hug, C.C.. Jr and de Lange, S. (1983) Variable rate infusion of alfentanil as a supplement to nitrous oxide anesthesia for general surgery. *Anesth. Analg.* 62, 982—986.

Ausems, M.E., Hug, C.C., Jr, Stanski, D.R. and Burm, A.G.L. (1986) Plasma concentrations of alfentanil required to supplement nitrous oxide anesthesia for general surgery. *Anesthesiology* 65, 362—373.

Becker, K.E. (1978) Plasma levels of thiopental necessary for anesthesia. *Anesthesiology* 49, 192—196.

Becker, K.E. and Tonnesen, A.S. (1978) Cardiovascular effects of plasma levels of thiopental necessary for anesthesia. *Anesthesiology* 49, 197—200.

Blake, D.W., Donnan, G., Novella, J. and Hackman, C. (1988) Cardiovascular effects of sedative infusions of propofol and midazolam after spinal anesthesia. *Anesth. Intensive Care* 16, 292—298.

Bovill, J.G., Warren, P.J., Schuller, J.L., Van Wezel, H.B. and Hoeneveld, M.H. (1984) Comparison of fentanyl, sufentanil and alfentanil anesthesia in patients undergoing valvular heart surgery. *Anesth. Analg.* 63, 1081—1086.

Bower, S. and Hull, C.J. (1986) Comparative pharmacokinetics of fentanyl and alfentanil. *Br. J. Anaesth.* 54, 871—877.

Briggs, L.P., White, M., Cockshott, I.D. and Douglas, E.J. (1985) The pharmacokinetics of propofol ('Diprivan') in female patients. *Postgrad. Med. J.* 61 (Suppl. 3), 58—59.

Bristow, J.D., Prys-Roberts, C., Fisher, A., Pickering, T.G. and Sleight, P. (1968) Effects of anesthesia on baroreflex control of heart rate in man. *Anesthesiology* 31, 422—428.

Brown, C.R., Sarnquist, F.H., Canup, C.A. and Pedley, T.A. (1979) Clinical, electroencephalographic and pharmacokinetic studies of a water-soluble benzodiazepine, midazolam maleate. *Anesthesiology* 50, 467—470.

Bursztein, S. (1989) Sedation and reversal of sedation in intensive care. *Acta Anaesthesiol. Belg.* 40, 11—16.

Calahan, M.K., Prakash, O., Rulf, E.N., Calahan, M.T., Malaya, A.P., Lurz, F.C., Rosseel, P., Lachitjaran, E., Siphanto, K., Gussenhoven, E.J. and Roelandt, J.R. (1987) Addition of nitrous oxide to fentanyl anesthesia does not induce myocardial ischemia in patients with ischemic heart disease. *Anesthesiology* 67, 925—929.

Carbon, G.C., Kahn, R.C., Goldiner, P.L., Howland, W.S. and Turnbull, A. (1978) Long term infusion of sodium thiopental: hemodynamic and respiratory effects. *Crit. Care Med.* 6, 311—316.

Cartwright, P., Prys-Roberts, C., Gill, K., Dye, A., Stafford, M. and Gray, A. (1983) Ventilatory depression related to plasma fentanyl concentrations during and after anesthesia in humans. *Anesth. Analg.* 62, 966—974, 1983.

Cason, B.A., Mazer, C.D., Demas, K.A. and Hickey, R.F. (1987) Nitrous oxide does not worsen ischemic left ventricular dysfunction in the pig (Abstract). *Anesthesiology* 67, A46.

Christensen, J.H., Andreasen, F. and Jansen, J.A. (1980) Pharmacokinetics of thiopentone in a group of young women and a group of young men. *Br. J. Anaesth.* 52, 913—918.

Claeys, M.A., Gepts, E. and Camu, F. (1988) Haemodynamic changes during anaesthesia induced and maintained with propofol. *Br. J. Anaesth.* 60, 3—9.

Coates, D.P., Monk, C.R., Prys-Roberts, C. and Turtle, M.J. (1987) Hemodynamic effects of infusions of the emulsion formulation of propofol during nitrous oxide anesthesia in humans. *Anesth. Analg.* 66, 64—70.

Coetzee, A., Fourie, P., Coetzee, J., Badenhorst, E., Rebel, A., Bolliger, C., Uebel, R., Wium, C. and Lombard, C. (1989) Effect of various propofol plasma concentrations on regional myocardial contractility and left ventricular afterload. *Anesth. Analg.* 69, 473—483.

Crankshaw, D.P., Edwards, N.E., Blackman, G.L., Boyd, M.D., Chau, H.N.J. and Morgan, D.J. (1985) Evaluation of infusion regimens for thiopentone as a primary anaesthetic agent. *Eur. J. Clin. Pharmacol.* 28, 543—552.

Crankshaw, D.P., Boyd, M.D. and Bjorksten, A.R. (1987) Plasma drug efflux — a new approach to optimization of drug infusion for constant blood concentration of thiopental and methohexital. *Anesthesiology* 67, 32—41.

Dearden, N.M. and McDowall, D.G. (1985) Comparison of etomidate and althesin in the reduction of increased intracranial pressure after head injury. *Br. J. Anaesth.* 57, 361—368.

De Bruijn, N., Christian, C. and Fagraeus, L. (1983) The effects of alfentanil on global ventricular mechanics. *Anesthesiology* 59, A33.

De Grood, P.M.R.M., Ruys, A.H.C., Van Egmond, J., Booij, L.H.D.J. and Crul, J.F. (1985) Propofol emulsion for total intravenous anaesthesia. *Postgrad. Med. J.* 61 (Suppl 3), 65—69.

De Lange, S., Boscoe, M.J., Stanley, T.H., De Bruijn, N., Philbin, D.M. and Coggins, C.H. (1982) Antidiuretic and growth hormone response during coronary artery surgery with sufentanil-oxygen and alfentanil-oxygen anesthesia in man. *Anesth. Analg.* 61, 434—438.

De Lange, S. and De Bruijn, N.P. (1983) Alfentanil-oxygen anaesthesia: plasma concentrations and clinical effects during variable rate continuous infusion for coronary artery surgery. *Br. J. Anaesth.* 55 (Suppl. 2), 183S—190S.

De Lange, S., Stanley, T.H., Boscoe, M.J., De Bruijn, M., Berman, L., Green, O. and Robertson, D. (1983) Catecholamine and cortisol responses to sufentanil-$O_2$ and alfentanil-$O_2$ anaesthesia during coronary artery surgery. *Can. Anaesth. Soc. J.* 30, 248—254.

Doze, V.A., Westphal, L.M. and White, P. (1986) Comparison of propofol with methohexital for outpatient anaesthesia. *Anesth. Analg.* 65 1189—1195.

Dundee, J.W. (1985) Intravenous anaesthesia and the need for new agents. *Postgrad. Med. J.* 61 (Suppl. 3), 3—6.

Edbrooke, D.L., Newby, D.M., Mather, S.J., Dixon, A.M. and Hebron, B.S. (1982) Safer sedation for ventilated patients. *Anaesthesia* 37, 765—771.

Eisele, J.H. and Smith, N.T. (1972) Cardiovascular effects of 40 percent nitrous oxide in man. *Anesth. Analg.* 51, 956—963.

Ex, P. (1987) Use of midazolam infusion as sedative in a multi-disciplinary intensive care unit. *Acta Anaesthesiol. Belg.* 38, 5—8.

Fragen, R.J., Gahl, F. and Caldwell, N. (1978) A water soluble benzodiazepine, Ro 21-3981, for induction of anesthesia. *Anesthesiology* 49, 41—43.

Fragen, R.J., Arrain, M.J., Henthorn, T.K. and Caldwell, N.J. (1983a) A pharmacokinetically designed etomidate infusion regimen for hypnosis. *Anesth. Analg.* 62, 654—660.

Fragen, R.J., Booij, L.H., Braak, G.J., Vree, T.B., Heykants, J. and Crul, J.F. (1983b) Pharmacokinetics of the infusion of alfentanil in man. *Br. J. Anaesth.* 55, 1077—1081.

Fragen, R.J., Hanssen, E.H., Denissen, P.A., Booij, L.H. and Crul, J.F. (1983c) Disoprofol (ICI 35-868) for total intravenous anaesthesia. *Acta Anaesthesiol. Scand.* 27, 113—116.

Fukunaga, A.F. and Epstein, R.M. (1973) Sympathetic excitation during nitrous oxide-halothane anesthesia in the cat. *Anesthesiology* 39, 23—36.

Gautret, B. and Schmitt, H. (1985) Multiple sites for the cardiovascular actions of fentanyl in rats. *J. Cardiovasc. Pharmacol.* 7, 649—652.

Gepts, E., Camu, F., Cockshott, I.D. and Douglas, E.J. (1987) Disposition of propofol administered as constant rate intravenous infusions in humans. *Anesth. Analg.* 66, 1256—1263.

Gepts, E., Jonckheer, K., Maes, V., Sonck, W. and Camu, F. (1988) Disposition kinetics of propofol during alfentanil anaesthesia. *Anaesthesia* 43 (Suppl.), 8—13.

Hall, R.I., Angert, K.C., Reeder, D.A., Moldenhauer, C.C. and Hug, C.C., Jr (1987) Is alfentanil a complete anaesthetic in humans? *Can. J. Anaesth.* 34, S109—S110.

Hazeaux, C., Tisserant, D., Vespignani, H., Hummer-Siegel, M., Kwang Ning, V. and Laxenaire, M.C. (1987) Retentissement electroencephalographique de l'anesthésie au propofol. *Ann. Fr. Anesth. Reanim.* 6, 261—266.

Hebron, B.S., Edbrooke, D.L., Newby, D.M. and Mather, S.J. (1983) Pharmacokinetics of hypnomidate associated with prolonged IV infusions. *Br. J. Anaesth.* 55, 281—287.

Hermans, B., Gommeren, W., De Potter, W.P. and Leysen, J.E. (1983) Interaction of peptides and morphine-like narcotic analgesics with specifically labelled $\mu$ and $\delta$ opiate receptor binding sites. *Arch. Int. Pharmacodyn. Ther.* 263, 317—319.

Heykants, J.J.P., Meuldermans, W.E.G. and Michiels, L.J. (1975) Distribution, metabolism and excretion of hypnomidate, a short acting hypnotic drug, in the rat. *Arch. Int. Pharmacodyn. Ther.* 216, 113—129.

Hilton, P., Dev, V.J. and Major, E. (1986) Intravenous anaesthesia with propofol and alfentanil. The influence of age and weight. *Anaesthesia* 41, 640—643.

Holaday, J.W. (1983) Cardiovascular effects of endogeneous opiate systems. *Annu. Rev. Pharmacol. Toxicol.* 23, 541—594.

Hudson, R.J., Stanski, D.R. and Burch, P.G. (1983) Pharmacokinetics of methohexital and thiopental in surgical patients. *Anesthesiology* 59, 215—219.

Hynynen, M., Takkunen, O., Salmenperä, M., Haataja, H. and Heinonen, J. (1986) Continuous infusion of fentanyl or alfentanil for coronary artery surgery. Plasma opiate concentrations, haemodynamics and post-operative course. *Br. J. Anaesth.* 58, 1252—1259.

Jessop, E., Grounds, P.M., Morgan, M. and Lumley, J. (1985) Comparison of infusions of propofol and methohexitone to provide general anaesthesia during surgery with regional blockade. *Br. J. Anaesth.* 57, 1173—1177.

Kawamura, R., Stanley, T.H., English, J.B., Hill, G.E., Liu, W.S. and Webster, L.R. (1980) Cardiovascular responses to nitrous oxide exposure for two hours in man. *Anesth. Analg.* 59, 93—99.

Kay, B. (1986) Propofol and alfentanil infusion: a comparison with methohexitone and alfentanil for major surgery. *Anaesthesia* 41, 589—595.

Kien, N.D., Reitan, J.A., White, D.A., Wu, C.H. and Eisele, J.H. (1986) Hemodynamic responses to alfentanil in halothane-anesthetized dogs. *Anesth. Analg.* 65, 765—770.

Larsen, R., Rathberger, J., Bagdahn, A., Lange, H. and Riecke, H. (1988) Effects of propofol on cardiovascular dynamics and coronary blood flow in geriatric patients. A comparison with etomidate. *Anaesthesia* 43, (Suppl.), 25—31.

Lauven, P.M., Stoeckel, H. and Schwilden, H. (1982) Ein pharmakokinetisch begründetes Infusions-Modell für Midazolam. *Anaesthesist* 31, 15—20.

Lauven, P.M., Schwilden, H., Stoeckel, H. and Greenblatt, D.J. (1985) The effects of a benzodiazepine antagonist RO 15-1788 in the presence of stable concentrations of midazolam. *Anesthesiology* 63, 61—64.

Lauven, P.M., Schwilden, H. and Stoeckel, H. (1987) Threshold hypnotic concentration of methohexitone. *Eur. J. Clin. Pharmacol.* 33, 261—265.

Lavies, N.G. (1984) Accumulation of alfentanil. *Anaesthesia* 39, 1253.

Lebowitz, P.W., Cote, M.E., Daniels, A.L., Martyn, J.A., Teplick, R.S., Davison, J.R. and Sunder, N. (1983) Cardiovascular effects of midazolam and thiopentone for induction of anaesthesia in ill surgical patients. *Can. Anaesth. Soc. J.* 30, 19—23.

Leysen, J.E., Gommeren, W. and Niemegeers, C.J.E. (1983) $^3$H-sufentanil, a superior ligand for $\mu$-opiate receptors; binding properties and regional distribution in rat brain and spinal cord. *Eur. J. Pharmacol.* 7, 209—225.

List, W.F. and Ponhold, H. (1983) Vergleichende Untersuchungen der Wirkung von Midazolam und Hypnomidate auf die Herz- und Kreislauffunktion. *Anaesthesist* 32, 395—398.

Lunn, J.K., Stanley, T.H., Eisele, J., Webster, L. and Woodward, A. (1979) High dose fentanyl anesthesia for coronary artery surgery: plasma fentanyl concentrations and influence of nitrous oxide on cardiovascular response. *Anesth. Analg.* 58, 390—395.

Maitre, P.O., Vozeh, S., Heykants, J., Thomson, D.A. and Stanski, D.R. (1987) Population pharmacokinetics of alfentanil: the average dose-plasma concentration relationship and interindividual variability in patients. *Anesthesiology* 66, 3—12.

McCammon, R.L., Hilgenberg, J.C. and Stoelting, R.K. (1980) Hemodynamic effects of diazepam and diazepam-nitrous oxide in patients with coronary artery disease. *Anesth. Analg.* 59, 438—441.

McQuay, H.J., Moore, R.A., Paterson, G.M.C. and Adams, A.P. (1979) Plasma fentanyl concentrations and clinical observations during and after operation. *Br. J. Anaesth.* 51, 543—549.

Meretoja, O.A., Takkunen, O., Heikkilä, H. and Wegelius, U. (1985) Haemodynamic response to nitrous oxide during high-dose fentanyl-pancuronium anaesthesia. *Acta Anaesthesiol. Scand.* 29, 137—141.

Milocco, I., Löf, B.A., William-Olsson, G. and Appelgren, L.K. (1985) Haemodynamic stability during anaesthesia induction and sternotomy in patients with ischaemic heart disease. *Acta Anaesthesiol. Scand.* 29, 465—473.

Mitchell, N.M., Prakash, O., Rulf, E.N., Van Daele, M.E., Calahan, M.K. and Roelandt, J.R. (1989) Nitrous oxide does not induce myocardial ischemia in patients with ischemic heart disease and poor ventricular function. *Anesthesiology* 71, 526—534.

Moffitt, E.A., Scovil, J.E., Barker, R.A., Imrie, D.D., Glenn, J.J., Cousins, C.L., Sullivan, J.A. and Kinley, C.E. (1984) The effects of nitrous oxide on myocardial metabolism and hemodynamics during fentanyl or enflurane anesthesia in patients with coronary disease. *Anesth. Analg.* 63, 1071—1075.

Moldenhauer, C.C. and Hug, C.C., Jr. (1982) Continuous infusion of fentanyl for cardiac surgery. *Anesth. Analg.* 61, S 206.

Monk, C.R., Coates, D.P., Prys-Roberts, C., Turtle, M.J. and Spelina, K. (1987) Haemodynamic effects of prolonged infusion of propofol as a supplement to nitrous oxide anaesthesia. Studies in association with peripheral arterial surgery. *Br. J. Anaesth.* 59, 954—960.

Morgan, D.J., Blackman, G.L., Paul, J.D. and Wolf, L.J. (1981) Pharmacokinetics and plasma binding of thiopental. I. Studies in surgical patients. *Anesthesiology* 54, 468—473.

Murday, H.K., Hack, G., Hepmanus, E. and Rudolph, A. (1985) Hämodynamische Effekte einer Kombination von Etomidat, Flunitrazepam oder Midazolam zur Anästhesie-Einleitung bei Patienten mit Herzklappenvitien. *Anästh. Intensivther. Notfallmed.* 20, 175—178.

Murphy, M.R. and Hug, C.C., Jr. (1982) The anesthetic potency in terms of its reduction of enflurane MAC. *Anesthesiology* 57, 485—488.

Naito, H. and Gillis, C.N. (1973) Effects of halothane and nitrous oxide on removal of norepinephrine from the pulmonary circulation. *Anesthesiology* 39, 575—580.

Nathan, H.J. (1989) Control of hemodynamics prevents worsening of myocardial ischemia when nitrous oxide is administered to isoflurane-anesthetized dogs. *Anesthesiology* 71, 686—694.

Nathan, R.J. (1988) Nitrous oxide worsens myocardial ischemia in isoflurane-anesthetized dogs. *Anesthesiology* 68, 407—415.

Newman, L.H., McDonald, J.C., Wallace, P.G.M. and Ledingham, I. McA. (1987) Propofol infusion for sedation in intensive care. *Anaesthesia* 42, 929—937.

Nilsson, A., Tamsen, A. and Perrson, M.P. (1986) Midazolam-fentanyl anesthesia for major surgery. Plasma levels of midazolam during prolonged total intravenous anesthesia. *Acta Anaesthesiol. Scand.* 30, 66—69.

Nilsson, A., Persson, M.P., Hartvig, P. and Wide, L. (1988) Effect of total intravenous anesthesia with midazolam/alfentanil on the adreno-cortical and hyperglycemic response to abdominal surgery. *Acta Anaesthesiol. Scand.* 32, 379—382.

Norman, J. (1983) The IV administration of drugs (Editorial) *Br. J. Anaesth.* 55, 1049—1052.

Oldenhof, H., Dejong, M., Steenhoek, A. and Janknegt, R. (1988) Clinical pharmacokinetics of midazolam in intensive care patients, a wide interpatient variability? *Clin. Pharmacol. Ther.* 43, 263—269.

Pathak, K.S., Brown, R.H., Nash, C.L., Jr. and Cascorbi, H.F. (1983) Continuous opioid infusion for scoliosis surgery. *Anesth. Analg.* 62, 841—845.

Philbin, D.M., Foex, P., Drummond, G., Lowenstein, E., Ryder, W.A. and Jones, L.A. (1975) Postsystolic shortening of canine left ventricle supplied by a stenotic coronary artery when nitrous oxide is added in the presence of narcotics. *Anesthesiology* 62, 166—174.

Price, H.L., Cooperman, L.H., Warden, J.C., Morris, J.J. and Smith, T.C. (1969) Pulmonary hemodynamics during general anesthesia in man. *Anesthesiology* 30, 629—636.

Prys-Roberts, C., Sear, J.W., Low, J.M., Phillips, W.C. and Dagnino, J. (1983) Hemodynamic and hepatic effects of methohexital infusion during nitrous oxide anesthesia in humans. *Anesth. Analg.* 62, 317—323.

Reddy, P., Liu, W., Port, D., Gilmor, S. and Stanley, T.H. (1980) Comparison of haemodynamic effects of anaesthetic doses of alphaprodine and sufentanil in the dog. *Can. Anaesth. Soc. J.* 27, 345—350.

Reitan, J.A., Stengert, K.B., Wymore, M.L. and Martucci, R.W. (1978) Central vagal control of fentanyl-induced bradycardia during halothane anesthesia. *Anesth. Analg.* 57, 31—36.

Reiz, S., Balfors, E., Friedman, A., Hoggmark, S. and Peter, T. (1981) Effects of thiopentone on cardiac performance, coronary hemodynamics and myocardial oxygen consumption in chronic ischaemic heart disease. *Acta Anaesthesiol. Scand.* 25, 103—110.

Reves, J.G., Samuelson, P.N. and Lewis, S. (1979) Midazolam maleate induction in patients with ischemic heart disease: hemodynamic observations. *Can. Anaesth. Soc. J.* 26, 402—409.

Reves, J.G., Fragen, R.J., Vinik, H.R. and Greenblatt, D.J. (1985) Midazolam: pharmacology and uses. *Anesthesiology* 62, 310—324.

Rolly, G., Versichelen, L., Huyghe, L. and Mungroop, H. (1985) Effect of speed of injection on induction of anaesthesia with propofol. *Br. J. Anaesth.* 57, 743—746.

Rosow, C.E. (1984) Sufentanil citrate: a new opioid analgesic for use in anesthesia. *Pharmacotherapy* 4, 11—19.

Rosow, C.E., Philbin, D.M., Moss, J., Keegan, C.R. and Schneider, R.C. (1983) Sufentanil vs fentanyl. Suppression of hemodynamic responses. *Anesthesiology* 59, A323.

Samuelson, P.N., Reves, J.G., Smith, L.R. and Kouchoukos, N.T. (1981) Midazolam versus diazepam: different effects on systemic vascular resistance. *Arzneim.-Forsch. Drug Res.* 2268—2269.

Schauble, J.F., Chen, B.B. and Murray, P.A. (1983) Marked hemodynamic effects of bolus administration of alfentanil in conscious dogs. *Anesthesiology* 59, A85.

Schulte-Sasse, U. and Tarnow, J. (1984) Anästhesieeinleitung mit Midazolam/Fentanyl bei Patienten mit Koronarer Herzkrankheit und bei Patienten mit Herzklappenerkrankungen, In: *Midazolam in der Anästhesiologie*, Editor: J. Steffens, Editiones Roche, Basle, pp. 103—112.

Schüttler, J., Schwilden, H. and Stoeckel, H. (1983) Pharmacokinetics as applied to total intravenous anaesthesia. Practical implications. *Anaesthesia* 38, (Suppl.), 53—56.

Schüttler, J., Schwilden, H. and Stoeckel, H. (1985a) Infusion strategies to investigate the pharmacokinetics and pharmacodynamics of hypnotic drugs: etomidate as an example. *Eur. J. Anaesthesiol.* 2, 133—142.

Schüttler, J., Stoeckel, H. and Schwilden, H. (1985b) Pharmacokinetic and pharmacodynamic modelling of propofol ("Diprivan") in volunteers and surgical patients. *Postgrad. Med. J.* 61 (Suppl. 3), 53—54.

Scott, J.C., Ponganis, K.V. and Stanski, D.R. (1985) EEG quantitation of narcotic effect the comparative pharmacodynamics of fentanyl and alfentanil. *Anesthesiology* 62, 234—241.

Sear, J.W., Phillips, K.C., Andrews, C.J.H. and Prys-Roberts, C. (1983b) Dose response relationships for infusions of althesin or methohexitone. *Anaesthesia* 38, 931—936.

Sebel, P.S. and Bovill, J.G. (1982) Cardiovascular effects of sufentanil anesthesia. *Anesth. Analg.* 61, 115—119.

Sebel, P.S., Bovill, J.G. and Van Der Haven, A. (1982) Cardiovascular effects of alfentanil anaesthesia. *Br. J. Anaesth.* 54, 1185—1190.

Shafer, A., Coe, V. and White, P.F. (1983) Continuous intravenous infusion of alfentanil: defining the therapeutic concentration range. *Anesthesiology* 59, A348.

Sprigge, J.S., Wynands, J.E., Whalley, D.G., Bevan, D.R., Townsend, G.E., Nathan, H., Patel, Y.C. and Srikant, C.B. (1982) Fentanyl infusion anesthesia for aortocoronary bypass surgery: plasma levels and hemodynamic response. *Anesth. Analg.* 61, 972—978.

Stanski, D.R. and Hug, C.C., Jr. (1982) Alfentanil — a kinetically predictable narcotic analgesic. *Anesthesiology* 57, 435—438.

Stephan, H., Sonntag, H., Schenk, H.D., Kettler, D. and Khambatta, H.J. (1986) Effects of propofol on cardiovascular dynamics, myocardial blood flow and myocardial metabolism in patients with coronary artery disease. *Br. J. Anaesth.* 54, 871—877.

Todd, M.M., Drummond, J.C., Ostrup, R. and Stanski, D.R. (1982) Hemodynamic effects of high dose thiopental anesthesia in humans. *Anesthesiology* 57, A 39.

Todd, M.M., Drummond, J.C. and U, H.S. (1984) The hemodynamic consequences of high dose methohexital anesthesia in humans. *Anesthesiology* 61, 495—501.

Turcant, A., Delhumeau, A., Premel-Cabic, A., Granry, J.C., Cottineau, C., Six, P. and Allain, P. (1985) Thiopental pharmacokinetics under condition of long-term infusion. *Anesthesiology* 63, 50—54.

Van Aken, H., Meinshausen, E., Prien, T., Brüssel, T., Heinecke, A. and Lawin, P. (1988) The influence of fentanyl and tracheal intubation on the hemodynamic effects of anesthesia induction with propofol/$N_2O$ in humans. *Anesthesiology* 68, 157—163.

Van Hamme, M.J., Ghoneim, M.M. and Ambre, J.J. (1978) Pharmacokinetics of hypnomidate, a new anesthetic. *Anesthesiology* 49, 274—277.

Van Lambalgen, A.A., Bronsveld, W., Van Den Bos, G.C., Thys, L.G. and Teule, G.J.J. (1982) Cardiovascular and biochemical changes in dogs during etomidate-nitrous oxide anesthesia. *Cardiovasc. Res.* 16, 599—606.

White, P.F. (1983) Use of continuous infusion versus intermittent bolus elimination of fentanyl or ketamine during outpatient anesthesia. *Anesthesiology* 59, 294—300.

Wyatt, R. and Nestorowicz, A. (1984) Accumulation of alfentanil. *Anaesthesia* 39, 189—190.

Wynands, J.E., Wong, P., Whalley, D.G., Sprigge, J.S., Townsend, G.E. and Patel, Y.C. (1983) Oxygen-fentanyl anesthesia in patients with poor left ventricular function: hemodynamics and plasma fentanyl concentrations. *Anesth. Analg.* 62, 476—482.

Wynands, J.E., Wong, P., Townsend, G.E., Sprigge, J.S. and Whalley, D.G. (1984) Narcotic requirements for intravenous anesthesia. *Anesth. Analg.* 63, 101—105.

Yate, P.M., Thomas, D., Short, S.M., Sebel, P.S. and Morton, J. (1986) Comparison of infusions of alfentanil or pethidine for sedation of ventilated patients on the ITU. *Br. J. Anaesth.* 58, 1091—1099.

# 9

# *Recovery from total intravenous anaesthesia*

Griselda Cooper

## INTRODUCTION

The desire to reduce atmospheric pollution by inhaled anaesthetic agents coincided with the introduction of more suitable intravenous drugs, an enhanced knowledge of pharmacokinetics and more sophisticated and accurate delivery systems such that total intravenous anaesthesia has become a popular proposition for the anaesthetist of the 1990s. Despite the importance of the speed and quality of recovery from any anaesthetic technique early reviews of total intravenous anaesthesia (TIVA) concentrated on the problems of ensuring adequate anaesthesia and on the haemodynamic and ventilatory effects. Scant attention was paid to the problem of recovery. Even now our knowledge of the clinical recovery from TIVA is far from complete.

There are many reasons to desire a rapid and complete recovery. One of the early indications for TIVA was (and still is) anaesthesia for bronchoscopy where the traditional route for maintenance of anaesthesia is denied by the presence of the bronchoscope. Anyone who is involved in these procedures under general anaesthesia appreciates the need for rapid return of reflexes and conscious cooperation as well as rapid awakening. This rapidity of early recovery also has implications for the safety of all patients and for the staffing of recovery areas. Until consciousness is regained a patient requires the undivided attention of a trained person (nurse or doctor). If one anaesthetic technique results in an average wakening time of 5 min and another 20 min, the implications on the staff needed with a throughput of 3000 patients annually is an additional 750 h spent maintaining or ensuring an airway. Such differences in awakening times were found by Sear et al. (1980) when comparing minaxolone with Althesin supplemented by nitrous oxide for short procedures. Rapid recovery, provided that adequate analgesia is ensured, is also more pleasant for the patient. This particularly applies for minor operative procedures. The importance of the quality and speed of late recovery have been highlighted by the increased popularity of day case surgery where patients expect to return to normality in minimum time.

Assessing early recovery is not difficult. It soon becomes apparent if one technique is resulting in long wakening times or excessively somnolent or confused patients. Even so not all comparisons are valid as they may be made under different conditions or on different types of patients. The more subtle after effects of general anaesthesia are more difficult to quantify but are extremely important for the day case patient who may, contrary to instructions, be tempted to return home alone, or worse, drive a car. These difficulties in assessing recovery of course apply to patients recovering from inhalational anaesthesia. However, the problem is often knowing whether one is making fair comparisons. It is not enough to say that recovery is quicker from TIVA without knowing whether the depth of anaesthesia is comparable. Nobody is surprised if the patient who breathes 5% halothane for 15 min takes longer to wake than the patient who is only given increments of an induction agent when indicated because the patient moves. Yet the comparison between the inhalational and TIVA is an important one to make because it is this choice which is of clinical relevance. It is irrelevant to know whether one TIVA technique gives quicker recovery if we are unable to relate it to our current clinical practice.

Difficulties in comparisons of different agents are compounded by other factors affecting the speed or quality of recovery: these include the use of other sedative drugs, analgesics and considerations such as the age and general fitness of the patient. In reviewing published work on recovery from TIVA I shall try to indicate to the reader where these factors may play an important part.

## PHARMACOKINETICS

Pharmacokinetic properties which predict a rapid recovery from TIVA are a short distribution phase, high clearance and a short elimination half-life. These pharmacokinetic indices for various induction agents are illustrated in Table 9.1. The low clearance and long elimination half-life of thiopentone indicate that it is not suitable for TIVA. Personal experience of administering doses of 1—1.5 g thiopentone over periods of 30—40 min for electroencephalographic recordings showed very long wakening times, in some cases several hours.

In comparison with thiopentone, the clearance of methohexitone is four times greater and the elimination half-life is more than three times shorter. Before the advent of newer agents methohexitone was popular for TIVA, although it was mainly administered as intermittent boluses rather than as a continuous infusion. Further reference to the use of methohexitone will be made later.

Other agents as listed in Table 9.1 have acceptably short elimination half-lives. Althesin was popular for TIVA until it was withdrawn from the market because of an unacceptably high incidence of anaphylactoid reactions. The pharmacokinetic profile of etomidate suggests it to be a suitable agent for TIVA. Although its use

TABLE 9.1

Pharmacokinetic indices of induction agents

| Drug | Distribution half-life (min) | Clearance (ml/kg per min) | Elimination half-life (min) | Source |
|---|---|---|---|---|
| Methohexitone | 6.2 | 12.1 | 9.7 | Wood (1982) |
| Thiopentone | 2.8 and 48.7 | 3.3 | 342.0 | Wood (1982) |
| Propofol | 2.5 | 58.0 | 55.0 | Adam et al. (1983) |
| Althesin | 2.8 | 17.0 | 91.0 | Sear and Prys-Roberts (1982) |
| Etomidate | 2.7 | 11.7 | 68.0 | Schuttler et al. (1983) |
| Midazolam | — | — | 120.0 | Brown et al. (1979) |
| Ketamine | 11.0 | 17.0 | 150.0 | Wood (1982) |

for long term sedation in Intensive Care has been curtailed because of adrenocortical suppression (Ledingham and Watt, 1983) it remains used for anaesthesia for surgical procedures.

Undoubtedly the most popular agent in current use for TIVA is propofol. As seen in Table 9.1 it has not only a rapid elimination half-life but also a much higher clearance than the other agents.

## EARLY RECOVERY: INDIVIDUAL DRUGS

Before making comparisons between drugs it will be useful to those unfamiliar with the dosage regimens to look at the amounts of drug used and relate these, the duration of anaesthesia and the use of supplementary drugs to the time it takes patients to awaken and to become orientated. For ease of comparison all infusion schemes are quoted as mg/kg per h although, in some cases, the original work uses μg/kg per min. With TIVA, as with an inhalational technique, it is obvious that the end of surgery can be anticipated and the dosage can be adjusted appropriately such that quicker awakening times can be achieved in routine clinical practice.

### Propofol

In a study to determine the Minimum Infusion Rate for the emulsion formulation of propofol, Spelina et al. (1986) infused either 2.4, 3.0, 3.6, 4.2 or 4.8 mg/kg per h after induction with 2 mg/kg propofol in patients premedicated with morphine sulphate. Patients breathed 67% nitrous oxide in oxygen and the propofol infusion was continued for at least 30 min before surgery commenced. The main purpose of the study was to determine the proportion of patients who moved on surgical incision but it is particularly interesting to note that there was no correlation between the total dose of propofol infused and the length of time patients took to waken and to become orientated. Total doses of between 403 and 555 mg of propofol were received and the maintenance period lasted between 77 and 96 min. On average patients awoke 4—5 min after stopping the infusion and became orientated 1—3 min later. Surprisingly, the longest individual recovery times were in the patients who received maintenance with only 2.4 mg/kg per h.

Although none of the patients were aware, it is important to note that the infusion schemes above are of lower dosage than those in clinical practice because one is concerned that no patients should move or be aware. The $ED_{95}$ for propofol determined by Spelina et al. (1986) is 6.7 mg/kg per h under the conditions quoted above. However it is also important to appreciate that the confidence limits of this figure are wide (5.1—18.4 mg/kg per h) and hence explain the higher dosages which are now used in clinical practice.

Some of the infusion schemes in use for propofol are outlined in Table 9.2 and are placed in order of increasing duration of infusion. These schemes illustrate the problems in comparing different author's work as none of these regimens are identical. Firstly, it should be noted that the schedules of Zuurmond (1987) and Herregods et al. (1988) are not strictly total intravenous techniques as nitrous oxide has also been administered.

Secondly, in order to establish the adequacy of anaesthesia in the patients studied, it is important to note that there was only one occurrence of a patient being aware. This was reported by Mackenzie and Grant (1985) where anaesthesia was maintained by intermittent boluses of propofol given when indicated on clinical grounds. This is a danger when a drug with such rapid recovery is used but in this instance the patient was not distressed because analgesia was complete as regional blockade was being used. The mean infusion rate of propofol given by Mackenzie and Grant (1985) is equivalent to 8 mg/kg per h. Although this is at the lower end of doses used it is pertinent to notice that no other sedative drugs were given (in contradistinction to Spelina et al. (1986) where morphine sulphate and nitrous oxide were used).

With regard to the doses of propofol used the induction dose is between 2 and 2.6 mg/kg but the maintenance infusion rate differs quite markedly being anything from 4.8 mg/kg per h to 12 mg/kg per h. Despite these variations the average time to wakening is not greatly different, being from 5 to 12 min after cessation of infusion confirming the earlier observations of Spelina et al. (1986). It should also be noted that, in most cases, the patients become well orientated within a very few minutes of wakening. The two exceptions are those of Steegers and Foster (1988) and Ledderose et al. (1988) where the mean time to orientation was 8 min after wakening. One contributory factor may be the longer duration of propofol infusion but it should also be noted that the patients in the studies of Ledderose et al. (1988) received promethazine, pethidine, droperidol and fentanyl in addition to propofol and these drugs are likely to have a significant effect on the speed of recovery. Many of these papers comment on the clear-headed nature of recovery after propofol, even after relatively long durations of infusion.

TABLE 9.2

Propofol for TIVA

| Drug | *n* | Induction dose (mg/kg) | Maintenance dose (mg/kg per h, time) | Duration (min) | Other agents | Awake (min) | Orientated (min) | Comments | Source |
|---|---|---|---|---|---|---|---|---|---|
| Propofol | 15 | 2.0 | 12.0, 15 min<br>9.0, 10 min<br>6.0, thereafter | 17 | Alfentanil | 7 | 7 | Some elderly patients | De Grood et al. (1987a) |
| Propofol | 48 | 2.1 | 12.8, initially<br>11.5, thereafter | 18 | Fentanyl | 5 | 7 | Infusion rates adjusted clin. | Price et al. (1988) |
| Propofol | 40 | 2.0 | 12.0 | 20 | Temazepam<br>Alfentanil | 7 | 12 | | Bailie et al. (1989) |
| Propofol | 16 | 2.5 | 12.0, 15 min<br>9.0, 25 min<br>6.0, thereafter | 35 | Fentanyl | 8 | 9 | Extra boluses propofol given | De Grood et al. (1987b) |
| Propofol | 20 | 2—2.5 | 9.0, 30 min<br>6.0, thereafter | 39 | Fentanyl | 8 | 10 | | Harries et al. (1988) |
| Propofol | 20 | 2.0 | 10.0 | 51 | Nitrous oxide | 9 | 12 | | Zuurmond et al. (1987) |
| Propofol | 20 | 2.0 | 12.0, 30 min<br>9.0, thereafter | 51 | Nitrous oxide<br>Alfentanil | — | 7 | | Herregods et al. (1988) |
| Propofol | 20 | 2.5 | 8.0 | 52 | Regional block | 9 | 9 | Maintenance as boluses not constant infusion. 1 patient aware | Mackenzie and Grant (1985) |
| Propofol | 14 | 2.6 | 7.2, 10 min<br>4.8, thereafter | 54 | Diazepam<br>Alfentanil infusion | 11 | 13 | | Mayné et al. (1988) |
| Propofol | 20 | 2.0 | 12.0, 30 min<br>9.0, thereafter | 56 | Nitrous oxide | — | 8 | | Herregods et al. (1988) |
| Propofol | 25 | 2—2.5 | 7.2 | 64 | Alfentanil<br>Midazolam | 12 | 20 | Infusion rate adjusted for depth of anaesthesia | Steegers and Foster (1988) |
| Propofol | 25 | 2.2 | 12.0, 10 min<br>6.0, thereafter | 110 | Promethazine<br>Pethidine<br>Droperidol<br>Fentanyl | 10 | 18 | | Ledderose et al. (1988) |

## Methohexitone

Similar data to those of propofol for infusion schemes of methohexitone are set out in Table 9.3. Anaesthesia is induced with 1.5 mg/kg of methohexitone and anaesthesia is maintained with 5—10 mg/kg per h methohexitone. These figures compare with an $ED_{95}$ of 4.6 mg/kg per h as estimated by Sear et al. (1983) in patients premedicated with morphine sulphate. It is noteworthy that there are three reports of awareness in the two studies using the lowest maintenance doses. These are above the $ED_{95}$ but in the absence of morphine premedication.

Apart from the study of Ogg et al. (1983) where anaesthesia lasted only an average of 8 min, the wakening times are somewhat longer than after propofol maintenance. Of greater significance is the longer time it takes for patients to become orientated once they have woken, being of the order of 6—12 min later. The occurrence of awareness suggests that it is not a practical proposition to reduce the maintenance dose in order to speed awakening — that is until we are able to accurately assess depth of anaesthesia in each of our patients.

## Etomidate

The data related to two studies using TIVA with etomidate are also shown in Table 9.3. With infusions lasting 20—30 min patients become orientated some 5—6 min after awakening. A further study by Russell (1986) showed that patients awoke 9.5 min after etomidate infusion but did not become orientated until 10 min later. The range of values for awakening times were from 4 to 44 min compared with an average wakening time of 2 min after a 'balanced' technique using nitrous oxide and fentanyl. The difference in recovery times leads one to suppose that perhaps the depth of anaesthesia was not comparable and indeed this was the case. Using the isolated forearm technique 44% of those who received the 'balanced' technique were found to be wakeful and one patient was aware whereas no patient who received an etomidate infusion was aware and only 7% were wakeful.

## Thiopentone

An early study of TIVA by Jolly (1960) demonstrated the unsuitability of thiopentone for use in this way. Patients who received thiopentone awoke 26 min after removal of retained products of conception compared with 8 min if methohexitone was the agent used. The wakening times after thiopentone ranged from 4—102 min compared to 2—30 min after methohexitone. It is relevant to note that these patients were premedicated with papaveretum and hyoscine.

## Midazolam

Midazolam has been more popular as a sedative agent than for TIVA but a study by Raeder et al. (1988) showed wakening times of 21—28 min after 0.4 mg/kg

TABLE 9.3

Methohexitone and etomidate for total intravenous anaesthesia

| Drugs | *n* | Induction dose (mg/kg) | Maintenance dose (mg/kg per h, time) | Duration (min) | Other agents | Awake (min) | Orientated (min) | Comments | Source |
|---|---|---|---|---|---|---|---|---|---|
| Methohexitone | 20 | 1.5 | 9.7 | 8 | Fentanyl | 2 | | Increments, not infusion. | Ogg et al. (1983) |
| Methohexitone | 14 | 1.5 | 6—18 | 36 | Pethidine Nitrous oxide | 22 | 34 | Infusion rate adjusted for depth of anaesthesia. | Vinik et al. (1987) |
| Methohexitone | 20 | 1.5 | 4.8 | 40 | Fentanyl | 7 | 13 | One patient aware | Harries et al. (1988) |
| Methohexitone | 20 | 1.5 | 5.3 | 59 | Regional Block | 9 | 9 | Increments, not infusion 2 patients aware | Mackenzie and Grant (1985) |
| Methohexitone | 25 | 1.5—2.0 | 7 | 74 | Midazolam Alfentanil | 13 | 25 | Extra boluses given. | Steegers and Foster (1988) |
| Etomidate | 15 | 0.3 | 1.8, 10 min<br>1.5, 10 min<br>1.0, thereafter | 21 | Alfentanil | 6 | 12 | Some elderly patients | De Grood et al. (1987a) |
| Etomidate | 15 | 0.3 | 1.8, 15 min<br>1.0, thereafter | 30 | Fentanyl | 14 | 19 | Extra boluses given | De Grood et al. (1987b) |

midazolam and 0.03 mg/kg alfentanil for gynaecological dilatation and curettage. Patients who received the benzodiazepine antagonist, flumazenil, were awake and orientated within 1 min. Less sedation, better orientation and cooperation were also demonstrated by Klausen et al. (1988) when midazolam anaesthesia was reversed by flumazenil. In a technique combining midazolam with ketamine for laparoscopy Bailie et al. (1989) found that the patients awoke after 3 min and became orientated at 12 min after anaesthesia.

In summary, the pharmacokinetic predictions of early recovery appear to be borne out in clinical practice. The reliability of reasonably quick awakening and orientation times after propofol anaesthesia justifiably place it as the favoured agent in current practice. The place of reversal of benzodiazepine-induced anaesthesia in this respect deserves further investigation.

## LATER RECOVERY

There are much less data on the quality of later recovery and it seems appropriate to look at individual comparisons in order to put the results into perspective.

### Propofol and thiopentone, halothane

In a study of children undergoing outpatient dental anaesthetics Puttick and Rosen (1988) compared propofol induction and maintenance with thiopentone induction and halothane maintenance. Both techniques included nitrous oxide. Recovery as assessed by the time to open eyes, stand unaided and to be ready for discharge was 3—7 min shorter in those who received propofol. The authors themselves comment that this may have been influenced by differing depths of anaesthesia with the two techniques because propofol increments were only given in response to movement. Nevertheless these differences in recovery are clinically important because the caseload can be high in dental outpatients. My own experience in this field has been that propofol is particularly suitable because of the quick orientation resulting in less tearfulness and restlessness. More formal attempts at the psychomotor assessment of recovery in children have not been employed much and nor were they in this study. The relevance of these could be directed towards when children are safe to play on climbing frames (if they ever are!).

### Propofol and thiopentone, isoflurane

In patients undergoing laparoscopy, De Grood et al. (1987b) found that patients who received TIVA with propofol awoke more quickly than those who received thiopentone induction and isoflurane maintenance. This was despite the anaesthetic time being on average 10 min longer in those who received TIVA. Recovery was further assessed at 1 and 3 h by the *p* deletion test of Dixon and Thornton (1973). No differences were detected between the techniques although it is stated that some patients were unable to complete the test because of severe side effects or psychomotor dysfunction but not how many were from each group. Both groups performed at about 80% of their preoperative values at 3 h postoperatively.

In gynaecological patients, Vinik et al. (1987) found enhanced recovery in those who received propofol TIVA compared to those who received thiopentone induction and isoflurane maintenance. This was assessed by the Trieger test as described by Newman et al. (1969). In comparing the results the impairment is quoted as the time and accuracy ratio compared to baseline and is 0.71 for those who received propofol and 0.5 for those who received thiopentone and isoflurane. This is despite an anaesthetic time of 80 min in the propofol group and 51 min in the other group.

**Propofol and propofol, isoflurane**

This comparison eliminates the effect of a different induction agent and looks at the differences between maintenance with propofol and with isoflurane.

No differences in recovery were found by Zuurmond et al. (1987) who studied patients undergoing arthroscopy. Recovery was assessed by the measurement of ocular imbalance using a Maddox Wing and by a modified form of the *p* deletion test. The subjective view of the patients, questioned 1 month later, was that they felt back to normal 1 day after their anaesthetic and there were no differences between the groups. Herregods et al. (1988) using the *p* deletion test and the Trieger test were also unable to demonstrate a difference in recovery between patients maintained with propofol and those with isoflurane, albeit in the presence of nitrous oxide. Milligan et al. (1987) found initial recovery more rapid with propofol TIVA but not by 1 h after anaesthesia using the *p* deletion test and a four choice reaction timer. Likewise De Grood et al. (1987b) were unable to demonstrate differences using the *p* deletion test. These findings are all in contrast to those of Nightingale and Lewis (1990) who find quicker recovery from propofol (and alfentanil) than from isoflurane using a six choice reaction timer and critical flicker fusion threshold. In summary it seems that differences in recovery from propofol or isoflurane maintenance are small and not easily detected.

**Propofol and methohexitone**

In a comparison of single doses of propofol (3 mg/kg) or methohexitone (2 mg/kg) for patients undergoing dental extraction Logan et al. (1987) were able to find few differences in recovery using choice reaction timing and critical flicker fusion threshold. The same tests of recovery were used by Mackenzie and Grant (1985) who infused propofol or methohexitone to maintain anaesthesia in patients undergoing surgery under spinal analgesia. No differences in recovery from these agents were seen in these patients who were tested for 4 h. However the comment was made by an independent assessor that the quality of recovery was superior from propofol with fewer side effects.

It is this quality of recovery which is commented on by many anaesthetists but has been difficult to prove objectively. A non-blind assessment of the quality of recovery after TIVA for extracorporeal shock-wave lithotripsy judged 6 out of 20 patients to have a poor quality recovery after methohexitone compared to none out of 20 who received propofol. Steegers and Foster (1988) found that 96% of patients were clear-headed 20 min after propofol whereas only 46% of patients were clear-headed at this time after methohexitone.

However these are subjective assessments. The study by Vinik et al. (1987) in gynaecological patients was able to show an impressive difference between propofol and methohexitone by the Trieger test. The impairment (reflecting speed and accuracy) one hour after wakening was 0.71 after propofol and only 0.16 after methohexitone. Although this is stated as impairment in this short abstract it appears that performance was 71% of baseline after propofol and 16% of baseline after methohexitone. It should be noted that this was an open study and it is not possible to exclude an element of bias.

### Propofol and etomidate

De Grood et al. (1987b) found in patients who had undergone laparoscopy that those who received etomidate took longer to awaken. However, there were no demonstrable differences in recovery as assessed by the *p* deletion test. Again it is stated that some patients were unable to complete the test because of severe side effects but it is not indicated which anaesthetic these patients had received. It is obvious that excluding patients with the worst recovery improves the results!

### Propofol and midazolam

After sedation provided for patients undergoing surgery with spinal analgesia. Wilson et al. (1988) found markedly less impairment after propofol than after midazolam for the first 2 h after surgery using critical flicker fusion threshold. Using choice reaction time there was little impairment after propofol but significantly impaired performance after midazolam for 3 h after surgery. No differences were demonstrable at 4 h after surgery.

### Propofol with nitrous oxide and propofol with alfentanil

Herregods et al. (1988) found the inclusion of nitrous oxide to propofol TIVA preferable to that of alfentanil because of a swifter return to full recovery with few side-effects and more predictable depth of anaesthesia. This was evidenced by the Trieger test and *p* deletion test showing greater impairment at 30 min after anaesthesia when alfentanil was used.

### Midazolam and midazolam with flumazenil

Raeder et al. (1988) have found better recovery in flumazenil reversed patients in the first 30 min after midazolam anaesthesia as assessed by the degree of cooperation. The use of flumazenil also appeared to shorten the duration of postoperative amnesia. However, there were no differences shown in the *p* deletion test or in choice reaction timing whether the patients had received flumazenil or not.

## SUMMARY

It seems unlikely that there are no differences in the speed and quality of recovery from different anaesthetic agents with regard to higher mental functioning in the first 24—48 h following anaesthesia. The tests currently available are not good at demonstrating differences and the above reviews of the current state of our knowledge only demonstrates how little is known. At present we seem to have little better to go on than the subjective view of the patients which indicates that the quality of recovery after TIVA is at least as good as after inhalational anaesthesia. See also Chapter 15.

## REFERENCES

Adam, H.K., Briggs, L.P., Bahar, M., Douglas, E.J. and Dundee, J.W. (1983) Pharmacokinetic evaluation of ICI 35868 in man. Single induction doses with different rates of injection. *Br. J. Anaesth.* 55, 97—103.

Bailie, R., Craig, G. and Restall, J. (1989) Total intravenous anaesthesia for laparoscopy. *Anaesthesia* 44, 60—63.

Brown, C.R., Sarnquist, F.H., Canup, C.A. and Pedley, T.A. (1979) Clinical, electroencephalographic, and pharmacokinetic studies of a water-soluble benzodiazepine, midazolam maleate. *Anesthesiology* 50, 467—470.

De Grood, P.M.R.M., Mitsukuri, S., Van Egmond, J., Rutten, J.M.J. and Crul, J.F. (1987a) Comparison of etomidate and propofol for anaesthesia in microlaryngeal surgery. *Anaesthesia* 42, 366—372.

De Grood, P.M., Harbers, J.B., Van Egmond, J. and Crul, J.F. (1987b) Anaesthesia for laparoscopy. A comparison of five techniques including propofol, etomidate, thiopentone and isoflurane. *Anaesthesia* 42, 815—823.

Dixon, R.A. and Thornton, J.A. (1973) Tests of recovery from anaesthesia and sedation: intravenous diazepam in dentistry. *Br. J. Anaesth.* 45, 207—215.

Harries, A., Bagley, G. and Lim, M. (1988) Anaesthesia for shock-wave lithotripsy. A comparison of propofol and methohexitone infusions during high frequency jet ventilation. *Anaesthesia* 43, 100—105S.

Herregods, L., Capiau, P., Rolly, G., De Somner, M. and Donadoni, R. (1988) Propofol for arthroscopy in outpatients. *Br. J. Anaesth.* 60, 565—569.

Jolly, C. (1960) Recovery time from methohexital anaesthesia. *Br. J. Anaesth.* 32, 576—579.

Klausen, N.O., Juhl, O., Sorensen, J., Ferguson, A.H. and Neumann, P.B. (1988) Flumazenil in total intravenous anaesthesia using midazolam and fentanyl. *Acta Anaesthesiol. Scand.* 32, 409—412.

Ledderose, H., Rester, P., Carlsson, P. and Peter, K. (1988) Recovery times and side effects after propofol infusion and after isoflurane during ear surgery with additional infiltration anaesthesia. *Anaesthesia* 43, 89—91S.

Ledingham, I. McA. and Watt, I. (1983) Influence on mortality in critically ill multiple trauma patients. *Lancet* i, 1270.

Logan, M.R., Duggan, J.E., Levack, I.D. and Spence, A.A. (1987) Single-shot IV anaesthesia for outpatient dental surgery. Comparison of 2,6 Di-isopropyl Phenol and methohexitone. *Br. J. Anaesth.* 59, 179—183.

Mackenzie, N. and Grant, I.S. (1985) Comparison of propofol with methohexitone in the provision of anaesthesia for surgery under regional blockade. *Br. J. Anaesth.* 57, 1167—1172.

Mayne, M., Joucken, K., Collard, E. and Randour, P. (1988) Intravenous infusion of propofol for induction and maintenance of anaesthesia during endoscopic carbon dioxide laser ENT procedures with high frequency jet ventilation. *Anaesthesia* 43, 97—100S.

Milligan, K.R., O'Toole, D.P., Howe, J.P., Cooper, J.C. and Dundee, J.W. (1987) Recovery from outpatient anaesthesia: A comparison of incremental propofol and propofol-isoflurane. *Br. J. Anaesth.* 59, 1111—1114.

Newman, M.G., Trieger, N. and Miller, J.C. (1969) Measuring recovery from anesthesia — a simple test. *Anesth. Analg., Curr. Res.* 48, 136—140.

Nightingale, J.J. and Lewis, I.H. (1990) Recovery from anaesthesia: A comparison of total intravenous anaesthesia with an inhalational technique. *Br. J. Anaesth.* 65, 287—288P.

Ogg, T.W., Jennings, R.A. and Morrison, C.G. (1983) Day-case anaesthesia for termination of pregnancy. Evaluation of a total intravenous anaesthetic technique. *Anaesthesia* 38, 1042—1046.

Price, M.L., Walmsley, A., Swaine, C. and Ponte, J. (1988) Comparison of a total intravenous technique using a propofol infusion, with an inhalational technique using enflurane for day case surgery. *Anaesthesia* 43, 84—87S.

Puttick, N. and Rosen, M. (1988) Propofol induction and maintenance with nitrous oxide in paediatric outpatient dental anaesthesia. A comparison with thiopentone-nitrous oxide-halothane. *Anaesthesia* 43, 646—649.

Raeder, J.C., Nilsen, O.G., Hole, A., Arnulf, V. and Grynne, B.H. (1988) The use of flumazenil after total IV anaesthesia with midazolam in outpatients. *Eur. J. Anaesth.* Suppl. 2, 257—264.

Russell, I.F. (1986) Comparison of wakefulness with anaesthetic regimens. Total IV v. balanced anaesthesia. *Br. J. Anaesth.* 58, 965—968.

Schuttler, J., Schwilden, H. and Stoeckel, H. (1983) Pharmacokinetics as applied to total intravenous anaesthesia. Practical implications. *Anaesthesia* 38, 53—56S.

Sear, J.W., Cooper, G.M., Williams, N.B., Simpson, P.J. and Prys-Roberts, C. (1980) Minaxolone or Althesin supplemented by nitrous oxide. A study in anaesthesia for short operative procedures. *Anaesthesia* 34, 169—173.

Sear, J.W. and Prys-Roberts, C. (1982) Effect of antihypertensive therapy on the pharmacokinetics of Althesin by infusion to man. *Br. J. Anaesth.* 54, 1130—1131.

Sear, J.W., Phillips, K.C., Andrews, C.J.H. and Prys-Roberts, C. (1983) Dose response relationships for infusions of Althesin or methohexitone. *Anaesthesia* 38, 931—936.

Spelina, K.R., Coates, D.P., Monk, C.R., Prys-Roberts, C., Norley, I. and Turtle, M.J. (1986) Dose requirements of propofol by infusion during nitrous oxide anaesthesia in man. I. Patients premedicated with morphine sulphate. *Br. J. Anaesth.* 58, 1080—1084.

Steegers, P.A. and Foster, P.A. (1988) Propofol in total intravenous anaesthesia without nitrous oxide. *Anaesthesia* 43, 94—97S.

Wood, M. (1982) Intravenous anaesthetic agents. In: *Drugs and Anaesthesia.* 1st edition. Chapter 8. Editors: M. Wood and A.J.J. Wood, Williams and Wilkins, Baltimore, pp. 199—237.

Vinik, H.R., Shaw, B., Mackrell, T. and Hughes, G. (1987) A comparitive evaluation of propofol for the induction and maintenance of anaesthesia. *Anesth. Analg.* 66, 184S.

Wilson, E., Mackenzie, N. and Grant, I.S. (1988) A comparison of propofol and midazolam by infusion to provide sedation in patients who receive spinal anaesthesia. *Anaesthesia* 43, 91—94S.

Zuurmond, W.W.A., Van Leeuwen, L. and Helmers, J.H.J.H. (1987) Recovery from propofol infusion as the main agent for outpatient arthroscopy. A comparison with isoflurane. *Anaesthesia* 42, 356—359.

# 10

# *Intra-operative monitoring of awareness*

Harvey L. Edmonds, Jr. and Markku P.J. Paloheimo

## INTRODUCTION

The term intra-operative awareness and its usual synonym, consciousness, are difficult to define precisely and unambiguously. Casual definitions often focus on the cognitive and perceptual aspects of these phenomena (Papper, 1987). However, such emphasis may exlude certain individuals, e.g., infants, who are clearly aware of their surroundings (Russell, 1989). A distinction between the two states was drawn by Jones and Konieczko (1986), who identified several levels of intra-operative awareness. We have altered their scheme somewhat for the sake of clarity.

| Level | Characteristics |
|---|---|
| 1 | Conscious awareness with normal storage and conscious recall |
| 2 | Conscious awareness with normal storage but imperfect conscious recall |
| 3 | Unconscious awareness with imperfect storage and no conscious recall, with persistance of subconscious recall |
| 4 | Imperfect awareness with imperfect storage and no conscious recall |
| 5 | Absent awareness with no storage or conscious recall |

This continuum parallels the concept of the depth of anaesthesia and suggests a wide range of altered states of consciousness between level 1 and level 5. Note that since the definition includes elements of postoperative recall, it would be impossible to detect the level of awareness from intra-operative monitoring alone. Thus, although such definitions may be of interest to psychologists, they are of little use to anaesthesiologists and others concerned about identifying periods of unintended awareness during surgery or painful diagnostic procedures.

In contrast, Vickers (1987) chose a binary approach to define unconsciousness. He viewed it as a state equivalent to level 5 in the scheme above — the absence of intra-operative awareness and storage as well as a lack of postoperative conscious and subconscious recall. By this definition, any state other than unconsciousness is non-unconsciousness, regardless of its level. This approach seems well-suited to the needs of anaesthesiologists since only by the total abolition of awareness, both conscious and unconscious, can we be certain to prevent all aspects of recall.

Like Vickers, our pragmatic definition of awareness is a binary construct, based on stimulus-response coupling. Therefore, detection of such coupling in the surgical patient becomes prima facie evidence of inadequate anaesthesia. To our knowledge, there are no prospective reports of conscious or subconscious recall of intra-operative events in carefully monitored patients who have demonstrated complete unresponsiveness to a range of effective physiological stimuli. The monitoring of responsiveness as an objective indicator of inadequate anaesthesia (awareness) then becomes a matter of choosing the most reliable physiological measurement system(s). Our purpose here is to compare the currently available approaches for monitoring patient responsiveness.

## AUTONOMIC SIGNS

For many years, anaesthesiologists have relied primarily on skeletal movement and autonomic signs to monitor anaesthetic adequacy. This approach persists despite numerous reports of its ineffectiveness, especially when used with modern anaesthetic techniques that rely on complex polypharmacy (Artusio, 1955; Parkhouse, 1960; Robson, 1969; Saunders, 1981; Breckenridge and Aitkenhead, 1983; Prys-Roberts, 1987). The widely used movement-based concept of minimal alveolar concentration (MAC) becomes meaningless when large boluses of neuromuscular blockers are administered. Similarly, the coadministration of a wide range of anaesthetic adjuvants may diminish or abolish autonomic signs of inadequate anaesthesia. Ausems et al. (1983) even point to the unreliability of autonomic indicators in the absence of such adjuvants.

Evans et al. (1983) sought to minimize the subjectivity of autonomic monitoring by establishing a scoring system based on changes in blood pressure, pulse rate, sweating and tear formation (PRST). However, Russell (1989) assessed the reliability of the PRST scoring system using the isolated forearm technique (described below). Reflex movements or appropriate arm/hand responses to verbal commands occurred at nearly all PRST scores, suggesting the system was a poor indicator of awareness. Russell summarized these findings and concluded: 'Neither changes in blood pressure, heart rate, sweating nor tear production, taken individually or in aggregate, can reliably predict when a patient may be awake during certain general anaesthetic techniques.' We can add little to his well-substantiated opinion.

## SKELETAL MUSCLE MOVEMENT (ISOLATED FOREARM TECHNIQUE)

The isolated forearm technqiue (IFT) was first used by Tunstall (1979). By use of a padded tourniquet on the arm, movement in the hand distal to the cuff remained possible during neuromuscular blockade. With this technique we have noted signs of conscious awareness (intentional volitional signalling), unconscious awareness (response to voice command without postoperative conscious recall) and imperfect unconsciousness awareness (reflex movements without appropriate response to voice command) in patients lacking autonomic signs of inadequate anaesthesia (Edmonds, Couture and Stolzy, unpublished observations). Our experience is completely consistent with results from the recent report by Russell (1989) described above.

Despite the technique's seeming appeal and simplicity, it has not been widely used. Authors of the few negative reports on IFT reliability have had methodological inconsistencies or seem to have not understood the purpose of the measurement. For example, Breckenridge and Aitken-Mead (1981) concluded that the IFT was of little clinical utility because of vigorous arm movement during the operative procedure.

Another negative perception has been that the IFT is limited to very brief surgical procedures. However, Russell (1989) shows that by using repeated bolus dosing of short-acting neuromuscular blockers the cuff can be deflated and reinflated at regular intervals during a long surgery to prevent compressive nerve injury or forearm ischaemia.

## SMOOTH MUSCLE MOVEMENT (OESOPHAGEAL CONTRACTILITY)

The lower oesophagus is composed of smooth muscle that is controlled centrally by the brainstem vagal motor nucleus and nearby reticular activating system. Thus, both the levels of vigilance and autonomic tone have powerful influences on oesophageal motility. Therefore, it is not surprising that emotional or psychological stress may enhance the non-propulsive or spontaneous lower oesophageal contractility (SLOC) (Faulkner, 1940; Nagler and Spiro, 1961; Rubin et al., 1961).

Evans et al. (1984) were the first to measure SLOC and provoked lower oesophageal contractility (PLOC) in anaesthetized patients using a water-filled manometry balloon attached to the tip of a disposable probe. SLOC during anaesthesia resembles non-peristaltic contractions that occur in awake subjects exposed to mild stress (Stacher et al., 1979). PLOC, provoked with a second cephalad balloon, disappear during anaesthesia adequate for endotracheal intubation. Because the amplitude of SLOC is so highly variable, contractile activity has generally been quantified by the frequency of contractions. Maccioli et al. (1987) transformed these two variablies into a single value, the oesophageal contractility index (OCI), which is calcuated as 70 × (SLOC rate) + PLOC amplitude.

The clinical utility of SLOC, PLOC or OCI for the objective assessment of intra-operative awareness remains to be established. This is particularly true for the anaesthetic techniques that rely solely on intravenous agents or employ extensive use of adjuvants. Even though the oesophageal smooth muscle is relatively insensitive to neuromuscular blocking drugs, it is depressed by smooth muscle relaxants like sodium nitroprusside (Evans and White, 1987) and anticholinergic drugs (Kantrowitz et al., 1970). Isaac (1989) recently reviewed the published reports on the usefulness of SLOC. His thoughtful and balanced conclusion stated, 'When interpreted alone, the interpatient variability of the presence and magnitude of contractions makes lower oesophageal contractility unreliable in predicting light anaesthesia or conscious awareness.'

## FACIAL MUSCLE MOVEMENT

Of the commercially available methods for objectively monitoring intra-operative awareness, that of facial electromyography (FEMG) is undoubtedly the least familiar to most readers. Because of this general unfamiliarity and our long-standing research interest in this topic, we have devoted a large part of this chapter to a detailed description of the clinical experience with FEMG as well as the underlying physiology. For an even more extensive description, we refer the interested reader to our recent monographs (Edmonds et al., 1988; Paloheimo, 1990).

The muscles of facial expression have their evolutionary origin in the gill arches, the breathing apparatus of vertebrate fish. Both because of this embryologic origin and the extensive autonomic connections between these muscles and the facial nerve, many anatomists classify them as viscera (Noback and Demarest, 1975; Crelin, 1981). The facial nerve innervates at least 24 separate muscles, somatotopically represented in the facial nucleus (Ferguson, 1978). Facial mimic muscles are composed of relatively thin striate muscle fibres which never have both origin and attachment to bone (Hjortsjo, 1969). Since contraction of these muscles causes movement of facial landmarks, they receive the most prominent emotional motor output.

Based on innervation, the muscles of the face can be separated into two distinct groups: pure mimic muscles innervated by the facial nerve (cranial nerve VII) and masticatory muscles innervated by the trigeminal nerve (cranial nerve V) (Wilson-Pauwels et al., 1988). Alternatively, Ekman and Friesen (1978) divided the face into three regions: *upper face* including the forehead and the brows; *midface* including the eyes, lids and upper nose; and *lower face* including the cheeks, mouth, lower nose and chin. This division was based on the observations of regional motor independence. Behaviorally, these regions make independent contributions to facial messages (Rinn, 1984).

The *temporofacial* division contains a temporal branch (to the upper face) and a zygomatic branch (to the midface). The *cervicofacial* division contains buccal and mandibular branches (to the lower face) and a cervical branch (to the platysma). The temporofacial division differs from the cervicofacial division in that the latter carries impulses only from the contralateral hemisphere of the brain, while the temporofacial division, especially the temporal branch, carries impulses originating from both hemispheres (Wilson-Pauwels et al., 1988).

Duchenne used electrical stimulation for contraction of facial muscles to make them 'speak the language of passions and sentiment' (Duchenne, 1959). He placed the active stimulation electrode 'exactly to the points of entry of nerve filaments to the muscle' in order to obtain the contraction of all the fibres. Based on his experimental studies of partial contraction, he classified these muscles into four functional groups, of which the first one, completely expressive muscles, is most useful for the detection of intra-operative awareness. Expressions produced by these muscles can be understood even if the lower part of the face is covered.

There are four major mimic muscle groups of the upper face. The frontalis muscles signify attention and, in concert with other muscles, surprise, admiration and fright. Muscles of the orbicularis oculi group indicate pensive reflection, while the procerus muscle (pyramidalis nasi) expresses aggression and hostility. Functionally, the procerus is an antagonist of the frontalis and they never contract simultaneously in the absence of psychopathology. Pain is signified by the corrugator supercilii which are located under the orbicularis oculi.

These mimic muscles are composed of mixed Type I ('slow') and II ('fast') motor units, which are distinguished by histochemical methods. Type I fibres in the m. frontalis comprise 43—87% of the total, but in the orbicularis oculi the range is 0.5—23% (Johnson et al., 1973). These markedly different ratios are consistent with function, since the frontalis acts by sustained contraction while the orbicularis is involved in blinking and other transient movements. Furthermore, electrophysiological evidence shows the frontalis and corrugator to be very resistant to fatigue (van Boxtel et al., 1983).

An unusual aspect of mimic muscle physiology is that their force output is a linear function of the firing rate. In contrast to the limb muscles and those of mastication that regulate their contraction force by recruitment, control of the facial mimic muscles depends heavily on firing rate modulation. When large force outputs are in use, the frequency spectrum shows a decrease in amplitude of the low frequency peak. This leftward shift in peak frequency reflects diminished firing synchronization with increasing recruitment. Power spectral density functions of recordings during static contractions indicate that frequencies to 300 Hz can be detected in the frontalis and corrugator supercilii muscles (van Boxtel and Schomaker, 1984). Another unique feature of the mimic muscles is their apparent lack of muscle spindles. This absence reflects the fact that there are no unexpected changes in their lengths or in the loads imposed on them (Brown, 1984). These two unusual characteristics emphasize, in contradistinction to other striate muscles, that control of the mimic group is exclusively of central origin. Therefore, the EMG activity of these muscles provides an exquisitely sensitive continuous measure of CNS function.

Compared to the skeletal muscles, the mimic muscle motor endplate zone occupies a disproportionately large area (Buchtal, 1965; Schwarting et al., 1982). The oversized zone may reflect dual innervation, since Hertting et al. (1961) detected direct sympathetic innervation of mimic muscle motor endplates.

The terms 'tonic' and 'phasic' are not found in newer textbooks. These adjectives were formerly used when referring to two categories of motor units with different firing patterns and orders of recruitment. Small tonic motor neurons were described as having a low threshold of firing, a low discharge frequency and a high propensity for post-tetanic potentiation. Phasic motor neurons, on the other hand, have high firing thresholds, high discharge frequencies and a low potential for tetanic stimulation (Granit, 1970). Here, the terms tonic and phasic are used in relation to the muscle activity pattern. Tonic activity refers to the basic tension or spontaneous FEMG activity and phasic denotes transient increases from resting activity.

Dual control of the facial motor nucleus by higher motor centers stems from the voluntary cortical pyramidal pathway and the involuntary extrapyramidal system employed for emotional expression. Aside from the corticobulbar tracts, the facial motor nucleus receives supranuclear information from the extrapyramidal system with its wide multisynaptic interconnections (May, 1986). Bilateral indirect corticobulbar pathways are relayed from the brain stem reticular formation. In addition, there are innumerable connections between the facial, trigeminal, intermediate, vestibular, glossopharyngeal, vagus, spinal accessory, hypoglossal and upper cervical nerves as well as between the sympathetic and parasympathetic nerves. Facial motoneurons differ from spinal motoneurons in that they lack recurrent inhibitory (Renshaw) circuits (Brown, 1984).

Klein and Davis (1977) were the first to take advantage of the unique properties of mimic muscles for the monitoring of anaesthetic adequacy. They used the mean integrated amplitude of full-wave rectified FEMG activity as an indicator of patient relaxation during surgery. Later, Harmel, Klein and Davis (1978) used filtering techniques to separate 'contaminating' electromyographic activity from the EEG signal. They concluded that 'the FEMG can serve both as a reliable guide to patient muscular relaxation and an indicator of unacceptable muscle contamination of the EEG.'

The work of Klein and his colleagues was based on Fink's earlier reports on the use of abdominal EMG during anaesthesia (Fink, 1960; Fink, 1961). He suggested that 'the anaesthetist can regulate muscle activity centrally with general depressants or peripherally with myoneural depressants. Either method is susceptible to electromyographic control, but the EMG does not distinguish between them and is accordingly unsafe as a guide to anaesthetic depression when muscle relaxants are being used at the same time.' Hollmen et al. (1982) reported on their method of analyzing logarithmically compressed EMG energy values in the frequency domain (1—30 Hz). Their common finding was 'an instantaneous increase of EMG energy at intubation, at skin incision and during other sensory stimuli . . .The trend of increase in EMG activity served as a useful sign of lightening of the level of anaesthesia and warned of an impending reaction to surgical stimuli.'

Based on these early studies, development of the first commercial anaesthetic monitor incorporating FEMG analysis, the DATEX Anaesthesia and Brain Activity Monitor (ABM) was developed as the first commercial anaesthetic monitor incorporating FEMG analysis. Edmonds et al. (1983) published an initial clinical study utilizing FEMG capability of the ABM to detect changing levels of vigilance in anaesthetized and comatose patients. It was clear, even at this early stage, that in the absence of excessive chemical paralysis the FEMG was useful in detecting periods of inadequate anaesthesia.

Tammisto et al. (1983) simultaneously monitored spontaneous FEMG activity and electrically evoked hypothenar EMG responses in 18 anaesthetized patients using the ABM. They reported that thiopentone induction halved the pre-anaesthetized FEMG value of 80 ABM scale units (10 $\mu$V on log scale display). The anaesthetized FEMG signal was then nearly obliterated by the typical dose of succinylcholine used to facilitate endotracheal intubation. However, the powerful stimuli of laryngoscopy and intubation occasionally elevated FEMG amplitude, suggesting inadequate anaesthesia. Recovery from the initial neuromuscular blockade was always accompanied by increased FEMG amplitude. Half of the patients responded to skin incision with further elevations in FEMG amplitude, without other indication of inadequate anaesthesia. At the termination of the anaesthesia, FEMG amplitude reliably increased to pre-anaesthetized levels prior to visible patient reaction to the presence of the endotracheal tube. These authors concluded that FEMG amplitude was certainly influenced by neuromuscular blockade. However, even during near-complete (80—90%) neuromuscular block, powerful central activation in response to intense nociceptive stimulation could evoke transient (phasic) amplitude increases in the depressed FEMG tracing. Concurrent monitoring of the evoked hypothenar EMG and the FEMG response permitted reliable detection of inadequate anaesthesia, a necessary precondition for intra-operative awareness.

In another early clinical evaluation of the ABM, Kay (1984) relied on the FEMG to maintain adequate anaesthesia produced by repeat bolus dosing of etomidate. Periods of inadequate anaesthesia were readily detected by the FEMG. The author suggested that 'in clinical use the FEMG is of most use in indicating impending awareness during surgery on a paralyzed patient.' Rating and Kuypers (1984) used the ABM to monitor FEMG in 200 anaesthetized patients and found that mimic muscle activity during anaesthesia was influenced by the degree of psychosomatic stimulation. It thus reflected the depth of hypnosis, analgesic quality, supraspinal and spinal influences on muscle tone, and the nature of surgical stimulation. These workers described FEMG changes during induction with intravenous agents and inhalational anaesthetics and contrasted them with depressed muscle activity associated with administration of neuromuscular blocking agents.

Hynynen et al. (1985) compared the antinociceptive effects of fentanyl and three doses of alfentanil when administered before thiopentone induction. In close agreement with Edmonds et al. (1983) and Tammisto et al. (1983) they found pre-anaesthetized FEMG amplitude to be near 80 scale units. Although they found significant group differences in arterial pressure, heart rate, tolerance to endotracheal tube insertion and reactions to abdominal pinching, FEMG amplitude did not parallel these changes. However, increases in mimic muscle reliably predicted periods of impending inadequate anaesthesia characterized by patient intolerance to the endotracheal tube.

Watt et al. (1985) used two ABMs to compare FEMG activities from frontalis and trapezius or sternocleidomastoid muscles. FEMG changes at two sites exhibited a high degree of correlation. They concluded that spontaneous FEMG was a good predictor of impending arousal particularly in lightly anaesthetized patients. Nightingale et al. (1985) considered the change in FEMG pattern to be a useful indicator of emergence from propofol anaesthesia. Doze et al. (1986) compared the effects of propofol with methohexitone outpatient anaesthesia. Both induction and maintenance doses of propofol produced a significantly lower FEMG amplitude.

Edmonds et al. (1987) used the two ABMs to study FEMG activity during altered levels of vigilance. We concluded that although the FEMG alone was insufficient for sleep staging, it did discriminate between wakefulness and non-wakefulness in the non-drug state. We also observed a time-related increase in the coefficient of variation of the FEMG amplitude indicating increased variability associated with a rising state of vigilance over time in recovery room patients.

Our group also used both the EEG and FEMG signals from the ABM to examine the relation between purposeful movement intra-operatively (using the isolated forearm technique (IFT) previously discussed) and postoperative signs of subconscious recall (Stolzy et al., 1986, 1987). We detected evidence of subconscious recall for intra-operative events, even though patients experienced no conscious recall. There were high correlations between the presence of subconscious recall and intra-operative responsiveness as measured by either the FEMG or IFT. Thus, both these objective measures seem capable of detecting the anaesthetic conditions requisite for the development of postoperative recall, be it conscious or subconscious.

Herregods (1987), from the Department of Anaesthesia, State University of Ghent, based his doctoral thesis on a thorough evaluation of the ABM. Since this important work is not widely available, it is discussed here in some detail. Herregods final conclusion was that the ABM did not measure anaesthetic depth as described with other techniques (such as stages of general ether anaesthesia). Instead, it reliably detected the binary states of adequate or inadequate anaesthesia.

To reach his conclusion, Herregods carefully analyzed the cranial biopotentials obtained from the selectively filtered (70—300 Hz) and EEG (1—20 Hz) bandwidths. The dual aim of this craniobiopotential monitoring was to: (1) reveal excessive depression of cerebral activity by hypoperfusion, hypoxia or anaesthetic overdose, and (2) detect periods of inadequate anaesthesia in order to prevent the development of intra-operative awareness.

Herregods described characteristic EEG and FEMG patterns observed during the administration of different anaesthetic and pre-anaesthetic agents. Although scopolamine was without effect, diazepam (20 mg) significantly decreased FEMG amplitude within 25 min to a level of 30 scale units. FEMG reductions of similar magnitude were seen with intravenous administration of thalamonal 2 ml (dehydrobenzperidol 5 mg and fentanyl 100 $\mu$g). It thus appeared that clinically adequate sedation was signified by an FEMG amplitude of approximately 40 scale units, while hypnosis generally began when the value fell to 30 units. During adequate induction of anaesthesia with thiopentone (4 mg/kg), etomidate (300 $\mu$g/kg) or alfentanil (120 $\mu$g/kg) FEMG amplitude fell to 10—12 ABM scale units, about 5 units above the noise level of the system. Higher FEMG values were frequently associated with other signs of insufficient induction. Maintenance of presumably adequate anaesthesia with volatile agents, but without neuromuscular blockade, sustained the low FEMG amplitude achieved during induction. Recovery from inhalational anaesthesia was characterized by a sudden large FEMG increase to near pre-anaesthesia levels.

Herregods used two techniques for maintenance of total intravenous anaesthesia. The first consisted of loading doses of fentanyl (15 $\mu$g/kg) + dehydrobenzperidol (150 $\mu$g/kg) followed by intermittent bolus administration of fentanyl (5 $\mu$g/kg); alternatively, he used a bolus of fentanyl (120 $\mu$g/kg) for induction followed by its infusion at an initial rate of 300 $\mu$g/kg per h. Although the magnitude of FEMG depression during apparently adequate anaesthesia was similar to that achieved with the inhalational agents, the rate of increased mimic muscle activity during anaesthesia recovery was generally more gradual.

In the experimental part of his thesis, Herregods studied propofol as an agent for induction and maintenance of anaesthesia. Propofol (2 mg/kg) caused a sudden decrease in FEMG close to the 5 scale unit noise level. This remarkably low mimic muscle tone was achieved a few seconds before the loss of eyelash reflex in all patients. However, 10/20 patients reacted at incision with abrupt FEMG increase to more than 60 scale units if anaesthesia was maintained with nitrous oxide/oxygen (2:1) and a propofol infusion of 200 $\mu$g/kg per min in the absence of neuromuscular blockade.

Chang et al. (1988) evaluated the clinical utility of FEMG monitoring during short methohexitone anaesthesia. Continuous objective assessment of anaesthetic adequacy by the FEMG permitted reductions in infusion rate and resulted in a significantly shorter recovery time. During the induction and preparation period, low FEMG values were associated with no patient movements, i.e., adequate anaesthesia. The percentage change in the FEMG with surgical stimulation was significantly greater in patients who moved during surgery (175%) than in non-moving patients (72%). FEMG values at the end of the operation were consistently higher in patients who awoke quickly compared with those displaying prolonged emergence. Even though the authors noted that none of the patients with low FEMG amplitude moved during surgical stimulation, they concluded that FEMG monitoring did not significantly improve administration of methohexitone during brief outpatient procedures. However, this surprising conclusion seems at variance with their own results!

Recently, we used the ABM to compare heart rate, mean arterial pressure, EEG zero-crossing frequency and FEMG as predictors of responsiveness to verbal commands during wake-up tests in patients undergoing scoliosis surgery (Couture et al., 1991). Only the FEMG measure demonstrated significant state-dependent differences in responsiveness.

## SPONTANEOUS EEG

Since awareness is of cerebral origin, many investigators have sought to measure the phenomenon through electroencephalographic recordings of the brain's spontaneous activity (EEG) or by stimulus-evoked potentials (SEP). Conventional EEG is simply a graph of signal amplitude (voltage) expressed as a function of time. Cerebrobiopotentials obtained with surface electrodes reflect distance-weighted averages of electrical currents in the underlying cortical mantle. During undisturbed (level 1) awareness, this averaging results in a series of low amplitude waves primarily of variable high frequency. This desynchronized pattern is due to the differential activation of parallel cortical columns underlying the large surface electrode. The magnitude of desynchronization seems related directly to the extent of cognitive processing (awareness). Diminished information exchange by neighbouring cortical columns results in more synchronized activity. The summed surface potentials generated by columns discharging in synchrony will therefore be larger in amplitude and lower in frequency. This inverse relationship between EEG amplitude and frequency remains unless normal neuronal function is perturbed pharmacologically or pathologically. For example, simultaneous decreases in both amplitude and frequency may occur during hypoxia, ischaemia, hypothermia and with large doses of certain central nervous system depressants.

The use of visual analysis of conventional EEG recordings to monitor routinely intra-operative awareness is impractical as it requires a rare commodity, the highly trained clinical electroencephalographer. Therefore, numerous attempts have been made to compress and numerically analyze information contained in EEG signals and then display the results in a form suitable for interpretation by anaesthesia personnel (Edmonds and Wauquier, 1986).

The simplest computational methods of quantitative electroencephalography (QEEG) rely on time domain analysis, since it approximates the approach used in visual waveform interpretation. The amplitude and period (mean frequency) of waveform segments (epochs) are quantified and displayed as a function of time (the so-called period-amplitude analysis).

This approach was originally applied to intra-operative monitoring by Klein and Davis (1977) and later used extensively by our group (Edmonds and Paloheimo, 1985) and others (Herregods and Rolly, 1987). This form of QEEG analysis is appropriate if one views the EEG as a non-stationary series of discrete events (Bergmann et al., 1987).

Alternatively, the EEG may be viewed as the algebraic summation of oscillator outputs, each with fixed frequency characteristics but variable amplitude. In this case, frequency domain analysis is appropriate because it expresses amplitude as a function of frequency rather than time. The dynamic range of most commercial displays is increased by measuring amplitude in units of power ($volts^2$ or picowatts (pW)), while frequency is shown on a linear scale. This is in marked contrast to classical frequency analysis which measures amplitude in decibels (20 log (instantaneous voltage/reference voltage)) and displays frequency on a log scale.

Another method of frequency domain analysis was developed by Demetrescu et al. (1981). This aperiodic analysis examines each wave in the EEG signal and determines its amplitude and period. This is done by detecting wave peaks, valleys, zero-crossings and the inter-valley duration. Thus, the period (or its reciprocal, frequency) is defined as the time between adjacent valleys. Low frequency (slow) waves are defined as those with an intervening zero-crossing between successive peaks or valleys. In contrast, high frequency waves do not require a zero-crossing. This information is displayed as a pattern of vertical lines whose length ($y$ axis) is proportional to amplitude and whose position ($x$ axis) indicates wave period. Time is displayed on the $z$ axis.

These various QEEG techniques have been employed with relative success for the detection of awareness during some forms of anaesthesia (Lopez da Silva et al., 1972; Edmonds and Wauquier, 1986; Prior, 1987; Schwilden, 1989). The ability of the EEG to detect inadequate anaesthesia seems due, in part, to the relatively homogeneous action of the volatile halogenated anaesthetics and depressant barbiturates throughout the brain. Both plasma levels of these drugs and QEEG indices correlate reasonably well with level of responsiveness (Hudson et al., 1983).

In contrast, consensus is lacking on the reliability of QEEG monitoring to detect responsiveness (deviations from level 5 unconsciousness) during administration of other classes of intravenous anaesthetics. Although some reports note good agreement between QEEG measures and the level of responsiveness (Scott et al., 1985; Dutton et al., 1987), others have failed to document such relationships (Wauquier et al., 1988). Aside from the inherent strengths and weaknesses of each of the QEEG analytical techniques and display formats, there are two obvious reasons for this lack of unanimity. First, it is well-established that the EEG mirrors cortical function almost exclusively. Since some conscious awareness and much unconscious awareness are mediated by subcortical processes, a close correlation between the level of awareness and QEEG indices should not be expected.

Second, general anaesthetics represent several distinct classes of compounds with widely disparate pharmacologic effects on both behavior and EEG. We have recently proposed four distinct classes of intravenous anaesthetic agents based on a wide range of physiologic parameters (Couture and Edmonds, 1989). In addition to the depressant barbiturates (Class I), we distinguished mu-agonist opioids

(Class II), benzodiazepines (Class III) and agents with some excitatory properties (Class IV, includes etomidate, propofol, methohexitone and ketamine). Our classification scheme is based partly on the observations of Herregods (1987) who used combined period-amplitude EEG analysis and the upper facial electromyogram to discriminate among different anaesthetics. Therefore, it seems highly unlikely that a small number of QEEG descriptors can reliably distinguish level 5 unconsciousness from all other altered states produced by the various anaesthetic classes.

## STIMULUS-EVOKED EEG RESPONSES

Stimulus-evoked EEG potentials (SEP) are generally accepted as useful in measuring the integrity of afferent pathways. However, reliable assessment of intra-operative awareness with SEP is difficult because they measure primarily the highly stereotyped cortical response capacity to simple afferent stimuli. SEP waveforms detected at the scalp do not necessarily reflect the more complex cognitive processes associated with various levels of awareness. Nevertheless, several workers have reported some success using this technology for monitoring anaesthetic adequacy.

### Auditory evoked potentials (AEP)

Acoustic stimuli can evoke potentials of extremely small amplitude over a wide area of the skull. Because of their tiny size, averaging techniques are necessary to extract them from the underlying spontaneous EEG waveform. The short latency (early) components of the AEP represent volume-conducted potentials arising, respectively, from the acoustic nerve, pons and midbrain (Starr et al., 1977). Most workers now agree that late potentials with latencies greater than 50 ms have frontal and association cortex as their source. The early AEP components are moderately resistant to the effects of modern intravenous anaesthetic agents (Bertoldi et al., 1983; Thornton et al., 1985; Savoia et al., 1988) with the possible exception of the barbiturates (Mendel and Hosick, 1975; Kriss et al., 1984). In contrast, the late AEP components appear to be more affected by the presence of these intravenous agents. Therefore, several workers have used anaesthetic-induced amplitude decrements or latency prolongation of these late AEP components to monitor anaesthetic adequacy (Velasco et al., 1983).

Thornton and Newton (1989) used AEP and the isolated forearm technique (IFT) described above to identify characteristic late AEP components suggestive of some level of awareness. Specifically, they felt that latencies of a large negative peak, termed $N_b$ of less than 44.5 ms indicated patient responsiveness to voice command. They concluded that 'the auditory evoked response has great potential as a means of measuring anaesthetic depth. Its two main drawbacks, averaging time and noise interference, are likely to be overcome using advances in microprocessor technology.'

### Somatosensory evoked potentials (SSEP)

Sebel et al. (1987) compared patient responsiveness as assessed by somatosensory evoked potentials (SSEP) and autonomic indices. They observed that with either halothane or fentanyl anaesthesia, surgical stimulation resulted in an average 30% increase in SSEP amplitude. Although autonomic indices were also suggestive of arousal, there was no temporal correlation between the two types of measures. Of course, this disagreement may have been due, in part, to the delays encountered in averaging a thousand or more individual evoked responses. More recently, Sebel (1989) found a statistically significant decrease in latency (0.5 ms) occurring during surgical stimulation. However, he concluded that 'evoked potentials *could* [our underlining] lead to a useful indicator of depth of anaesthesia. It is likely to be some years before commercially available devices will be in use to monitor anaesthetic effects on the CNS using evoked potential technology.'

## CONCLUSIONS

Our purpose was to describe the current methods available for the objective quantification of intra-operative responsiveness. We hope that it has become clear to the reader that each technique has unique advantages and limitations. Although the largest space was devoted to the EMG monitoring of upper facial muscles, this was done so that our readers could become acquainted with information which is unfortunately found mostly in obscure literature. It would seem in the patient's best interest that a judicious mix of these techniques should be used to monitor anaesthetic conditions compatible with responsiveness and possible recall, conscious or subconscious. The ultimate choices must, of course, be determined by the patient's condition, the nature of the surgical procedure, the availability of monitoring modalities and the familiarity of the anaesthesiologist with their prudent application and thoughtful interpretation.

## ACKNOWLEDGEMENTS

The authors thank Professors Benjamin M. Rigor, Sr., M.D. and Tapani Tammisto, M.D. for their continued guidance and support. Ms. Pat Bensinger's expert editorial assistance is gratefully acknowledged.

## REFERENCES

Artusio, J.F. (1955) Ether analgesia during major surgery. *J. Am. Med. Assoc.* 157, 33—36.

Ausems, M.E., Hug C.C. and de Lange, S. (1983) Variable rate infusion of alfentanil as a supplement to nitrous oxide anesthesia for general surgery. *Anesth. Analg.*, 62, 982—986.

Bergmann, B.M., Mistlberger, R.E. and Rechtschaffen, A. (1987) Period-amplitude analysis of rat electroencephalogram: stage and diurnal variations and effects of suprachiasmatic nuclei lesions. *Sleep* 10, 523—536.

Bertoldi, G., Manno, E., Bruera, G., Gilli, M. and Vighetti, S. (1983) The influence of etomidate, flunitrazepam and ketamine on the BAEP of surgical patients with no audiological or neurological alterations. *Minerva Anestesiol.* 49, 349—356.

Breckenridge, J.L. and Aitkenhead, A.R. (1981) Isolated forearm technique for detection of wakefulness during general anaesthesia. *Br. J. Anaesth.*. 53, 665P—666P.

Breckenridge, J.L. and Aitkenhead, A.R. (1983) Awareness during anaesthesia: a review. *Ann. R. Coll. Surg. Engl.* 65, 93—96.

Brown, W.F. (1984) Electromyography and the cranial nerves. In: *The Physiological and Technical Basis of Electromyography.* Butterworths, Stoneham, pp. 42—48.

Buchtal, F. (1965) Electromyography in paralysis of the facial nerve. *Arch. Otolaryngol.* 81, 463—469.

Chang, T., Dworsky, W.A. and White, P.F. (1988) Continuous electromyography for monitoring depth of anesthesia. *Anesth. Analg.* 67, 521—525.

Couture, L.J. and Edmonds, H.L., Jr. (1989) Monitoring responsiveness during anaesthesia. In: *Baillière's Clinical Anaesthesiology*, Vol. 3, No. 3. Editor: J.G. Jones, Baillière Tindall, London, pp. 547—558.

Couture, L.J., Greenwald, B. and Edmonds, H.L., Jr. (1991) Detection of responsiveness during intravenous anesthesia. In: *Memory and Awareness in Anaesthesia.* Editor: K. Bonke, Swets & Zeitlinger, Amsterdam, in press.

Crelin, E.S. (1981) Development of the musculoskeletal system. *CIBA Clinical Symposia* 33, 21—34.

Demetrescu, M., Kavan, E. and Smith, N.T. (1981) Monitoring the brain condition by advanced EEG. *Anesthesiology* 55, A130.

Doze, V.A., Westphal, L.M. and White, P.F. (1986) Comparison of propofol with methohexital for outpatient anesthesia. *Anesth. Analg.* 65, 1189—1195.

Duchenne, J.B. (1959) Motion of the face. In: *Physiology of Motion.* Editor: E.B. Kaplan, W.B. Saunders, Philadelphia, pp. 573—602.

Dutton, R.C., Smith, W.D. and Smith, N.T. (1987) In: *Consciousness, Awareness and Pain in General Anaesthesia.* Editors: M. Rosen and J.N. Lunn, Butterworths, London, pp. 72—82.

Edmonds, H.L., Jr. and Paloheimo, M. (1985) Computerized monitoring of the EMG and EEG during anesthesia: an evaluation of the Anesthesia and Brain Activity Monitor (ABM). *Int. J. Clin. Monit. Comput.* 1, 201—210.

Edmonds, H.L., Jr. and Wauquier, A. (1986) *Computerized EEG Monitoring in Anesthesia and Critical Care.* Instrumentarium Science Foundation, Helsinki.

Edmonds, H.L., Jr., Stolzy, S.L. and Couture, L.J. (1987) Surface electromyography during low vigilance states. In: *Consciousness, Awareness and Pain in General Anaesthesia.* Editors: M. Rosen and J.N. Lunn, Butterworths, London, pp. 89—98.

Edmonds, H.L. Jr., Paloheimo, M. and Wauquier, A. (1988) *Computerized EMG Monitoring in Anesthesia and Intensive Care.* Malherbe Publishing Company, Weert, The Netherlands.

Ekman, P. and Friesen, W.V. (1978) *Facial Action Coding System.* Consulting Psychologists Press, Palo Alto, CA.

Evans, J.M., Fraser, A. and Wise, C.C. (1983) Computer controlled anaesthesia. In: *Computing in Anesthesia and Intensive Care.* Editor: O. Prakash, Martinus Nijhoff, Boston, pp. 279—291.

Evans, J.M., Davies, W.L. and Wise, C.C. (1984) Lower oesophageal contractility: a new monitor of anaesthesia. *Lancet* i, 1151—1154.

Evans, J.M. and White, D.C. (1987) Lower oesophageal contractility and anaesthesia. In: *Conscious Awareness and Pain in General Anaesthesia.* Editors: M. Rosen and J.N. Lunn, Butterworths, London, pp. 112—128.

Faulkner, W.B. (1940) Objective esophageal changes due to psychic factors. *Am. J. Med. Sci.* 200, 796—803.

Ferguson, J.H. (1978) Hypothesis: hemifacial spasm and the facial nucleus. *Ann. Neurol.* 4, 97—103.

Fink, B.R. (1960) A method of monitoring muscular relaxation by the integrated abdominal electromyogram. *Anesthesiology* 20, 178—185.

Fink, B.R. (1961) Electromyography in general anaesthesia. *Br. J. Anaesth.* 33, 555—559.

Granit, R. (1970) *The Basis of Motor Control.* Academic Press, New York, pp. 1—44.

Harmel, M.H., Klein, F.F. and Davis, D.A. (1978) The EEMG — a practical index of cortical activity and muscular relaxation. *Acta Anaesthesiol. Scand.* 70, 97—102.

Herregods, L. (1987) *Quantitative Evaluation of Adequacy of Clinical Anesthesia.* Academic dissertation, Department of Anaesthesiology, State University of Ghent, Belgium.

Herregods, L. and Rolly, G. (1987) The EMG, the EEG zero crossing frequency and mean integrated voltage analysis during sleep and anaesthesia. In: *Conscious Awareness and Pain in General on Anaesthesia.* Editors: M. Rosen and J.N. Lunn, Butterworths, London, pp. 83—88.

Hertting, G., Axelrod, J., Kopin, I.J. and Whitby, L.G. (1961) Lack of uptake of catecholamines after chronic denervation of sympathetic nerves. *Nature* 189, 61—62.

Hjortsjo, C.H. (1969) The mimic muscles of the face. In: *Man's Face and Mimic Language.* Studentlitteratur, Lund, Sweden, pp. 43—98.

Hollmen, A.I., Sulg, I., Eskelinen, P. and Arranto, J. (1982) Monitoring of EEG and EMG during anaesthesia. *Br. J. Anaesth.* 54, 241P.

Hudson, R.J., Stanski, D.R., Saidman, L.J. and Meathe, E. (1983) A model for studying the depth of anesthesia and acute tolerance to thiopental. *Anesthesiology* 59, 301—308.

Hynynen, M., Korttila, K., Wirtavuori, K. and Lehtinen, A.-M. (1985) Comparison of alfentanil and fentanyl as supplements to induction of anaesthesia with thiopentone. *Acta Anaesthesiol. Scand.* 29, 168—174.

Isaac, P.A. (1989) Lower oesophageal contractility and depth of anaesthesia. In: *Baillière's Clinical Anaesthesiology,* Vol. 3, No. 3. Editor: J.G. Jones, Baillière Tindall, London, pp. 533—546.

Johnson, M.A., Polgar, J., Weightman, D. and Appleton, D. (1973) Data on the distribution of fibre types in thirty-six human muscles: An autopsy study. *J. Neurol. Sci.* 18, 111—129.

Jones, J.G. and Konieczko, K. (1986) Hearing and memory in anaesthetized patients. *Br. Med. J.* 292, 1291—1293.

Kantrowitz, P.A., Siegel, C.I., Strong, M.J. and Hendrix, T.R. (1970) Response of the human oesophagus to *d*-tubocurarine and atropine. *Gut* 11, 47—50.

Kay, B. (1984) The anaesthesia and brain activity monitor (ABM) — concept and performance. *Acta Anaesthesiol. Belg.* 35, 167—174.

Klein, F.F. and Davis, D.A. (1977) Spontaneous frontalis muscle activity as an indicator of surgical patient relaxation. *Proceedings of the 30th Annual Conference on Engineering in Medical Biology* 19, 340.

Kriss, A., Prasher, D.K. and Pratt, R.T.C. (1984) Brainstem evoked potentials following methohexitone anaesthesia and unilateral ECT. In: *Proceedings of 2nd International Evoked Potential Symposium,* Cleveland, Ohio. Editors: R.H. Nodar and C. Barber, Butterworths, Boston, pp. 582—588.

Lopes da Silva, F.H., Smith, N.T. and Zwart, A. (1972) Spectral analysis of the EEG during halothane anesthesia. Input-output relations. *Electroencephalogr. Clin. Neurophysiol.* 33, 311—319.

Maccioli, G.A., Calkins, J.M., Greff, R. and Kuni, D. (1987) The lower esophageal contractility index: a measure of anesthetic depth. *J. Clin. Monit.* 3, 302—303.

May, M. (1986) *The Facial Nerve.* Thieme, New York, pp. 21—62.

Mendel, M.I. and Hosick, E.C. (1975) Effects of secobarbital on the early components of the auditory evoked potentials. *Rev. Laryngol. Otol. Rhinol.* 96, 178—184.

Nagler, R. and Spiro, H.M. (1961) Serial esophageal motility studies in asymptomatic young subjects. *Gastroenterology* 41, 371—379.

Nightingale, P., Healy, T.E.J., Hargreaves, J., McGuinness, K. and Kay B. (1985) Propofol in emulsion form: Induction characteristics and venous sequelae. *Eur. J. Anaesth.* 2, 361—368.

Noback, C.R. and Demarest, R.J. (1975) *The Human Nervous System: Basic Principles in Neurobiology,* 2nd Edn. McGraw-Hill, New York.

Paloheimo, M. (1990) Quantitative surface electromyography applications in anaesthesiology and critical care. *Acta Anaesthesiol. Scand.*, 34 (Suppl. 93) 1—83.

Papper, E.M. (1987) The state of consciousness: some humanistic considerations. In: *Conscious Awareness and Pain in General Anaesthesia.* Editors: M. Rosen and J.N. Lunn, Butterworths, London, pp. 10—11.

Parkhouse, J. (1960) Awareness during surgery. *Postgrad. Med. J.* 36, 674—677.

Prior, P.F. (1987) The EEG and detection of responsiveness during anaesthesia and coma. In: *Conscious Awareness and Pain in General Anaesthesia.* Editors: M. Rosen and J.N. Lunn, Butterworths, London, pp. 34—45.

Prys-Roberts, C. (1987) Anaesthesia: a practical or impractical construct? *Br. J. Anaesth.* 59, 1341—1345.

Rating, W., and Kuypers, R. (1984) Frontal EMG and brain-activity during and after anaesthesia. *Acta Anesthesiol. Belg.* 35 (Suppl), 457—462.

Rinn, W.E. (1984) The neuropsychology of facial expression: A review of the neurological and psychological mechanisms for producing facial expressions. *Psychol. Bull.* 95, 52—77.

Robson, J.G. (1969) Measurement of depth of anaesthesia. *Br. J. Anaesth.* 41, 785—788.

Rubin, J., Nagler, R.I, Spiro, H.M. and Pilot, M.L. (1961) Measuring the effect of emotions on esophageal motility. *Psychosom. Med.* 24, 170—176.

Russell, I.F. (1989) Conscious awareness during general anaesthesia: relevance of autonomic signs and isolated arm movements as guides to depth of anaesthesia. In: *Baillière's Clinical Anaesthesiology,* Vol. 3, No. 3. Editor: J.G. Jones, Baillière Tindall, London, pp. 511—532.

Saunders, D. (1981) Anaesthesia, awareness and automation. *Br. J. Anaesth.* 53, 1—3.

Savoia, G., Esposito, C., Belfiore, F., Amantea, B. and Cuocolo, R. (1988) Propofol infusion and auditory evoked potentials. *Anaesthesia* 43 (Suppl.), 46—49.

Schwarting, S., Schroder, M., Stennert, E. and Goebel, H.H. (1982) Enzyme histochemical and histographic data on normal human facial muscles. *Otol. Rhinol. Laryngol.* 44, 51—59.

Schwilden, H. (1989) Use of the median EEG frequency and pharmacokinetcs in determining depth of anaesthesia. In: *Baillière's Clinical Anaesthesiology,* Vol. 3, No. 3. Editor: J.G. Jones, Baillière Tindall, London, pp. 603—621.

Scott, J.C., Ponganis, K.V. and Stanksi, D.R. (1985) EEG quantitation of narcotic effect: the comparative pharmacodynamics of fentanyl and alfentanil. *Anesthesiology* 62, 234—241.

Sebel, P.S. (1989) Somatosensory, visual and motor evoked potentials in anaesthetized patients. In: *Baillière's Clinical Anaesthesiology,* Vol. 3, No. 3. Editor: J.G. Jones, Baillière Tindall, London, pp. 603—621.

Sebel, P.S., Glass, P. and Neveille, W.K. (1987) Do evoked potentials measure depth of anaesthesia? *Int. J. Clin. Monit. Comput.* 5, 163—166.

Starr, A., Amlie, R.N., Martin, W.H. and Saunders, S. (1977) Development of auditory function in newborn infants revealed by auditory brainstem potentials. *Pediatrics* 60, 831—839.

Statcher, G., Schmierer, G. and Landgraf, M. (1979) Tertiary oesophageal contractions evoked by acoustic stimuli. *Gastroenterology* 77, 49—54.

Stolzy, S.L., Couture, L.J. and Edmonds, H.L., Jr. (1986) Evidence of partial recall during general anesthesia. *Anesth. Analg.* 65 (25), S154.

Stolzy, S.L., Couture, L.J. and Edmonds, H.L., Jr. (1987) A study of spontaneous and purposeful movement as a predictor of postoperative recall during fentanyl/nitrous oxide/diazepam anesthesia. *Anesthesiology* 67, 3A.

Tammisto, T., Wirtavuori, K. and Rantala, B. (1983) Estimation of anaesthetic depth by monitoring spontaneous scalp EMG and evoked hypothenar EMG. In: *Mortality in Anaesthesia,* Vol. 3. Editors: M.D. Vickers and J.N. Lunn, Springer-Verlag, Berlin, pp. 131—135.

Thornton, C. and Newton, D.E.F. (1989) The auditory evoked response: a measure of depth of anaesthesia. In: *Baillière's Clinical Anaesthesiology,* Vol. 3, No. 3. Editor: J.G. Jones, Baillière Tindall, London, pp. 559—585.

Thornton, C., Heneghan, C.P.H., Navaratnarajah, M., Bateman, P.E. and Jones, J.G. (1985) The effect of etomidate on the auditory evoked response. *Br. J. Anaesth.* 57: 554—561.

Tunstall, M.E. (1979) The reduction of amnesic wakefulness during caesarean section. *Anaesthesia* 34, 316—319.

van Boxtel, A., Goudswaard, P., van der Molen, G.M. and van den Bosch, W.E.J. (1983) Changes in electromyogram power spectra of facial and jaw-elevator muscles during fatigue. *J. App. Physiol.* 54, 51—58.

van Boxtel, A. and Schomaker, L.R.B. (1984) Influence of motor unit firing statistics on the median frequency of the power spectrum. *Eur. J. App. Physiol.* 52, 207—213.

Velasco, M., Velasco, F., Castaneda, R. and Sanchez, R. (1983) Effect of fentanyl and naloxone on somatic and auditory evoked potentials in man. *Proc. West. Pharmacol. Soc.* 26, 291—294.

Vickers, M.D. (1987) Detecting consciousness by clinical means. In: *Conscious Awareness and Pain in General Anaesthesia.* Editors: M. Rosen and J.N. Lunn, Butterworths, London, pp. 12—17.

Watt, R.C., Hameroff, S.R., Cork, R.C., Calcins, J.M., Keys, C.A. and Mylrea, K.C. (1985) Spontaneous EMG monitoring for anesthetic depth assessment. *Proc. Assoc. Adv. Med. Instrum.* 20, 92.

Wauquier, A., De Ryck, M., Van den Broeck, W., Van Loon J., Mellis, W. and Janssen, P.A.J. (1988) Relationships between quantitative EEG measures and pharmacodynamics of alfentanil in dogs. *Electroencephalogr. Clin. Neurophysiol.* 69, 550—560.

Wilson-Pauwels, L., Akesson, E.J. and Stewart, P.A. (1988) *Cranial Nerves.* Marcel Decker, Toronto.

# 11

# *Infusion equipment for total intravenous anaesthesia*

Brian Auty

## INTRODUCTION

There are five different types of equipment available for the control of intravenous (i.v.) infusions (Auty, 1989a). Of these, two are gravity controlled instruments and three are pumped systems.

(a) Gravity controlled — drip rate controllers and volumetric controllers.

(b) Pumped systems — syringe pumps, volumetric pumps and drip rate peristaltic pumps.

It is considered that two of these types of equipment (syringe pumps and volumetric pumps) would be suitable for total i.v. anaesthesia and the rest are either unsuitable or will pose difficulties in use. Syringe pumps are most likely to prove ideal, particularly if they have been designed specifically for this application.

In addition, there are battery powered ambulatory pumps but these are not designed for intravenous anaesthesia as will be seen later.

Because volumetric accuracy is a pre-requisite in this application, the use of equipment with a calibrated volumetric output is essential. It would also be preferable to have a pump which automatically converted from body weight and drug concentration to flow rate so that the anaesthetist would have few calculations to perform and the precise dose would be delivered. This, of course, would require the design of a special pump tailored specifically for i.v. anaesthesia.

These requirements rule out drip rate peristaltic pumps, which have other major disadvantages anyway (Department of Health, 1989) and drip rate gravity controllers because of the complications arising when attempting to convert drops to volumes.

The three volumetric instruments to be considered are syringe pumps, volumetric pumps and volumetric controllers.

## SYRINGE PUMPS

If small volumes only (up to 50 ml) of anaesthetic agent are required to be infused, then syringe pumps are by far the most practical type of pump to use in this application. Conventional mains/battery powered syringe pumps are very easy to operate, give a smooth and continuous output and infuse quite accurately over the full stroke of the syringe. Should the mains power supply fail or be accidently disconnected, these pumps are designed to continue to infuse without change of infusion rate or loss of memory of volume infused by automatically switching over to the internal battery supply. Flow rates available cover the range 0.1 to 99.9 ml/h in 0.1 ml/h increments and the decimal facility is very important in this application. This range of flow rates is rather restricted and syringe pumps designed specifically for intravenous anaesthesia have a wider range.

The choice of syringe pump is very important because some models only provide basic facilities and additional features are desirable — in particular, a display of volume infused and a calibrated bolus delivery mode. In addition, there can be a problem with mechanical backlash and variations in accuracy of delivered output can occur over short periods of time (minute to minute) depending on the particular design of the pump. These factors are particularly relevant to the control of intravenous anaesthesia and are not well understood by the majority of users.

Pocket-sized battery powered ambulatory pumps are to be avoided in this application because they are calibrated in length of travel of syringe plunger (mm) per unit time (minutes, hours or days). They deliver infusate in a quasi-continuous mode — small boli at infrequent intervals depending on the flow rate set. It might be difficult to control the effect of the anaesthetic in this mode and more difficult to calculate the precise dose required. Additionally, most of these pumps infuse at very low flow rates only and have very few alarms, if any. It is often not easy to determine whether they are actually running. It should be emphasised that these pumps were developed primarily for sub-cutaneous or intra-muscular infusion over periods of days rather than hours.

### Fundamental design problems

Most syringe pumps have inherent backlash in the drive mechanism which results in slow start up at low flow rates. This means that the set flow rate is not reached until the mechanical backlash has been taken up. It is possible to design a drive mechanism which has no backlash but this requires high-cost precision components which would result in a more expensive pump.

It is possible to take up the backlash prior to the infusion and manufacturers have a choice of methods of doing this. In particular, if the line is primed at a high rate before setting the flow rate required and connecting the cannula, most of the slack in the drive will be taken up and the pump will deliver within a few seconds of start-up. It is vital that the patient connection is not made until the rate has been adjusted down to the value required.

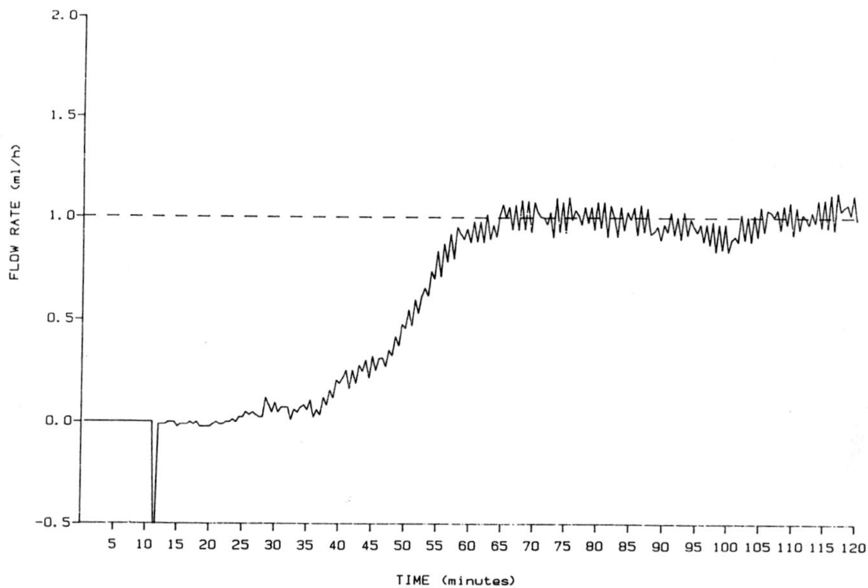


Fig. 11.1. Syringe pump start-up at 1 ml/h showing effect of backlash.

It is very important in this application that there is minimum delay in the anaesthetic reaching the patient. Another way of keeping the start up delay to a minimum is to dilute and then use a higher delivery rate. At rates of 10 ml/h and above, most syringe pumps will deliver an output almost immediately.

Figure 11.1 illustrates the output response of a syringe pump which has not been primed prior to start-up and in which there is no attempt in the design to take up backlash. The graph, which is in real time, displays the actual flow output against time. It can be seen that the set flow rate (in this case 1 ml/h) is not attained until about 60 min after the start of the infusion. The consequences of this in vivo could have been disastrous if it were not for the fact that the anaesthetist is monitoring the patient continuously and has other vital signs to indicate depth of anaesthesia. In other areas of a hospital, there might not be a competent clinician on the spot to notice or to make allowances for these problems.

Figure 11.2 displays the output of a syringe pump in which the line must be primed using the pump mechanism (as opposed to manual priming) before a rate can be set. It can be seen that the set rate is reached within a minute or so of start-up. Fortunately, when administering anaesthetic drugs, a loading dose is usually required at the start of the infusion (a large bolus delivered in a short time). This implies that the pump has to run at a high flow rate for a few seconds. The result is that all the mechanical backlash is taken up during the delivery of this bolus and when the pump is set to deliver at the basal rate (a relatively lower flow rate), the pump delivers its output immediately at the required rate assuming the two phases are consecutive.

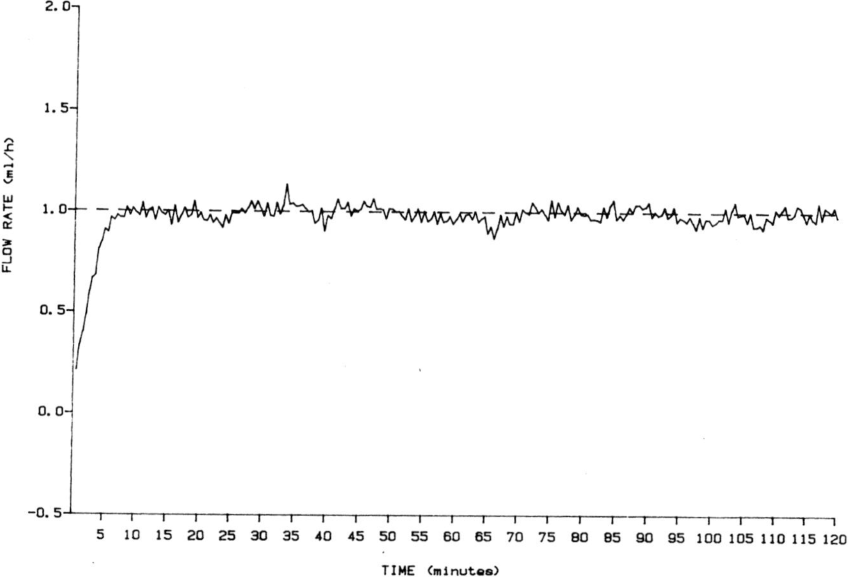


Fig. 11.2. Syringe pump start-up at 1 ml/h after pump priming at high rate.

In the induction phase, the speed of injection as well as the dose influences the intensity and duration of the effect of the anaesthetic. It is important that the pump starts up quickly and this can only be determined by observing the output as depicted in Figs. 11.1 and 11.2. These graphs are produced by gravimetric measurement of flow rate using a precision electronic balance interrogated by a computer system. In order to obtain sufficient accuracy of measurement, a balance reading to four decimal places of a gram is required to measure flow rates down to 1 ml/h.

A major problem with most syringe pumps is that the occlusion alarm setting is usually at a fairly high pressure level. This is because enough force must be available to drive a sticky syringe which implies a certain minimum value of motor current. The alarm threshold must be set at some level above this or else the motor will never run. This results in long alarm delays at low flow rates on total occlusion. If the occlusion is due to a blocked catheter, clotting, vein spasm or kinked tubing, a fairly large bolus may be injected on release of the occlusion. If the i.v. is out of position or extravasation has occurred, it is possible that the alarm will never activate.

There are some pumps in which this problem has been overcome by measuring pressure directly in the administration line using a pressure transducer. A dedicated line is required in which is moulded a small dome which locates in a pressure transducer housing on the pump. Using such a system, the occlusion alarm can be set to activate at any required level and this is totally independent of the drive system of the pump. The penalty for such an elegant system is the increased cost of the disposable item. More recent designs incorporate clever features which attempt to obtain a better occlusion response without the necessity of a dedicated line.

### Features and facilities

There are many different makes of syringe pump available and these fall broadly into two classes — basic pumps having very few features and facilities and high specification pumps. Only the latter can be considered suitable in this application. Key requirements to consider are:

1 basic accuracy measured over periods of 1 h
2 short-term accuracy measured over periods of minutes
3 occlusion response
4 alarm facilities
5 controls and displays
6 battery backup

### Basic accuracy

Most good syringe pumps can achieve a basic accuracy of ±5% measured over a 1-h period over the full range of flow rates (note that the measurement period can be less than 1 h depending on the syringe used). There is little point in choosing a pump which cannot match these standards. This accuracy can be achieved despite the manufacturing tolerances of disposable syringes. The better syringes are specified to be within ±2% of nominal dimensions. The fundamental drive accuracy of a good pump can be much better than ±1%.

### Short-term accuracy

When measured over periods of a few minutes, it may be a surprise to learn that the fluctuations in output from a syringe pump can be quite significant (Auty, 1988). These fluctuations are, however, of much less magnitude than those occurring in volumetric type pumps (see below). Figure 11.3 shows the short term flow rate errors of a typical syringe pump. This graph is called a trumpet curve. It should be noted that the $x$ axis is not plotted in real time but as a window of time (observation period). The data for the graph are determined by measuring the output over overlapping time intervals (of duration 1—31 min) during a 1-h infusion. The graph displays at a glance the maximum over and under infusion that can occur during any chosen time interval throughout the infusion. If the period of interest is 5 min, say, then the graph displays the greatest magnitude of error that can occur in the output, be it over or under infusion, during any 5-min period throughout the infusion. If high concentration, short half-life drugs were being infused, then these factors would assume significance.

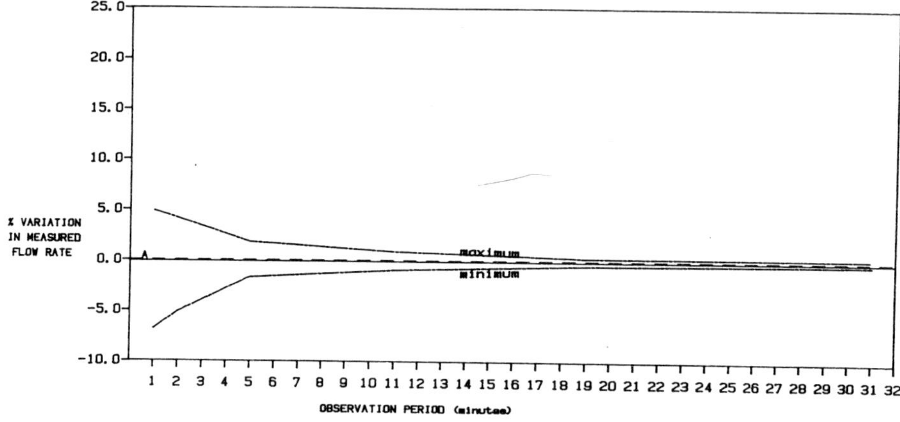


Fig. 11.3. Syringe pump — typical short-term flow rate errors (trumpet graph) at a set rate of 5 ml/h.

## Occlusion response

It is important to choose a pump with a good occlusion alarm response. Ideally, such a pump would have an alarm delay of less than 30 min on total occlusion at a flow rate of 1 ml/h and the bolus that might be released on release of the occlusion would be less than 0.5 ml. Regrettably, very few syringe pumps attain this level of performance. These data are not normally available in manufacturers' specifications but may be obtained, for instance, by consulting evaluation reports (Department of Health, 1986, 1987 and 1989). The new part II draft standard for infusion equipment (International Electrotechnical Commission, 1989) requires the manufacturer to disclose full information concerning the occlusion response of the pump.

Figure 11.4 shows the delay in alarm activation over the full range of flow rates for some typical syringe pumps having an occlusion alarm pressure setting of about 500 mmHg.

## Alarm facilities

The following alarms are considered essential:
occlusion
end of syringe
syringe removed
syringe not inserted correctly
incorrect size or brand of syringe inserted
drive disengaged
low battery
malfunction

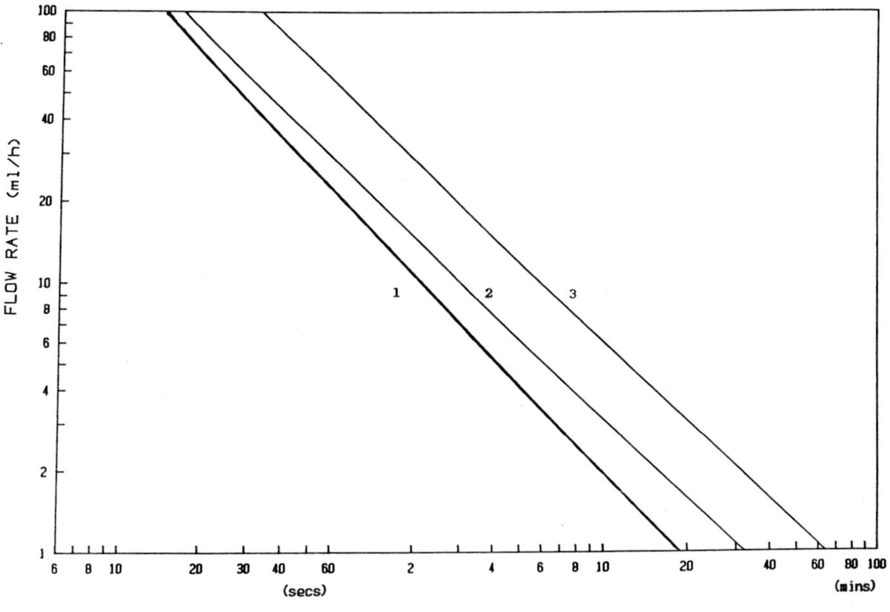


Fig. 11.4. Occlusion alarm delay times for typical syringe pumps.

In addition, there should be warnings for the following conditions:
mains supply failure/battery operation
nearly end of syringe
rate change attempted
bolus feature activated
preset volume infused

## Controls and displays

It is self-evident that the control layout of the pump should be neat and user-friendly. For normal i.v. applications, it is of utmost importance that all control functions except stop or hold are locked out during an infusion and it should not be possible to change flow rate and give an inadvertent over-infusion without using at least two key strokes. For intravenous anaesthesia, however, the anaesthetist requires to be able to give a bolus or change the infusion rate instantly. The two requirements are in conflict. Therefore, it is highly desirable that special syringe pumps be designed for this application, marked accordingly, and they should not be allowed to be used elsewhere in the hospital. There could be dangerous consequences if these rules are not followed.

Of particular importance in this application is a calibrated bolus function. This is the accurately controlled high flow rate used during the induction phase. It is essential that a volume infused display is coupled with this function and with the basal rate. The volume displayed may be reset to zero at the commencement of the infusion. A preset dose facility would also be valuable in the intended application. Combined with this should be a memory so that vital data are not lost due to a power failure (see battery backup below).

### Battery backup

In order to continue the infusion without interruption, it is essential that the pump contains a rechargeable battery and automatically switches over to battery power on failure of, or disconnection from, the mains supply without any change in the parameters set. In addition, a memory of volume infused and preset dose is important. These requirements must all be included to satisfy the new part II standard (International Electrotechnical Commission, 1989).

## VOLUMETRIC PUMPS

This type of pump is designed for infusing large volumes over long or short time periods. Flow rates from 1 ml/h up to 999 ml/h can be selected in increments of 1 ml/h and, in some designs, an additional range of 0.1 to 99.9 ml/h can be selected in 0.1 ml/h increments. The design of these pumps is usually of high quality and numerous features for safety in use and user convenience are included which are not always available in syringe pump designs. In particular, pressure sensing volumetric pumps can have a very low occlusion pressure setting with subsequent very fast response on occlusion. There is no reason why such pumps should not be used for intravenous anaesthesia provided a suitable small volume container is available. A burette administration set is probably the best choice.

### Types of volumetric pump

There are two main types of volumetric pump available; one having defined occlusion pressure settings and the other with variable pressure settings which the user can change as required. If used intelligently, the latter are capable of indicating an early rise in pressure which might be due to complications at the infusion site. These include extravasation, positional obstructions and vein spasm as well as total occlusion due to blocked catheter or kinked tubing. Some pumps can be programmed to run both a primary and a secondary infusion at different selected flow rates. Others can be programmed to run at a selected rate for a set period of time followed by another rate for a different time period.

Most volumetric pumps require the use of a dedicated administration set in order to achieve good accuracy of delivery. It is not possible to achieve this if the pump is designed to take any standard disposable set. In the main, most volumetric pumps can attain long-term accuracy equivalent to that from a good syringe pump. However, the output from such a pump is not nearly so smooth and the short-term accuracy is usually poorer.

## Pump mechanisms

There are several types of mechanism employed in the design of a volumetric pump (Auty, 1989b). The most common is the linear peristaltic and this can achieve quite a smooth output (see Fig. 11.5) if designed properly with compensation for the dead space. Other types of design include piston cassette, diaphragm cassette or rotary peristaltic mechanisms. Piston cassette mechanisms give an output as smooth as a syringe pump but the chamber only contains a few millilitres and has to be refilled automatically via a system of valves. Thus, there is a discontinuity in the output during the fill cycle whilst the chamber is being refilled (see Fig. 11.6). Diaphragm cassette mechanisms require a slightly more complex valve system and the timing has to be very precise. Even so, they tend to give a particularly spiky output (see Fig. 11.7). Rotary peristaltic mechanisms show large fluctuations unless there are a large number of rollers. Twin roller peristaltic mechanisms exhibit reverse infusion (suck back) for part of the cycle (see Fig. 11.8).

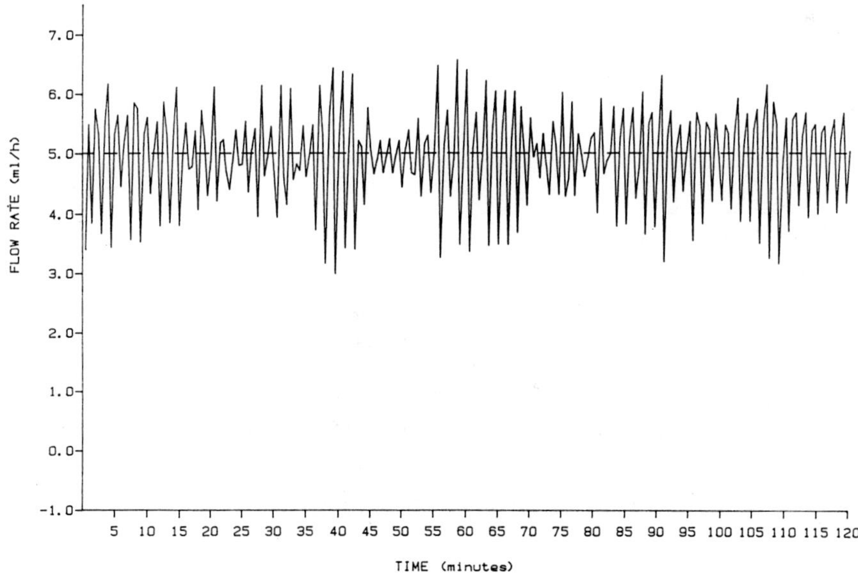


Fig. 11.5. Output from linear peristaltic volumetric pump at a set rate of 5 ml/h.

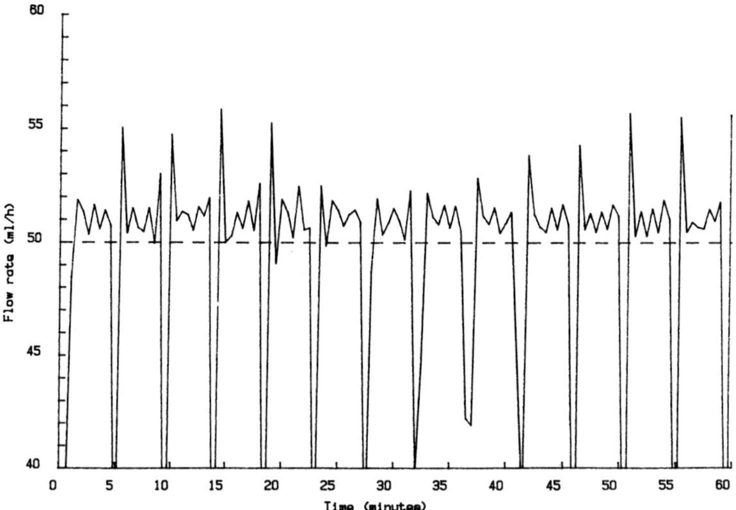


Fig. 11.6. Output from piston cassette type volumetric pump at a set rate of 50 ml/h.

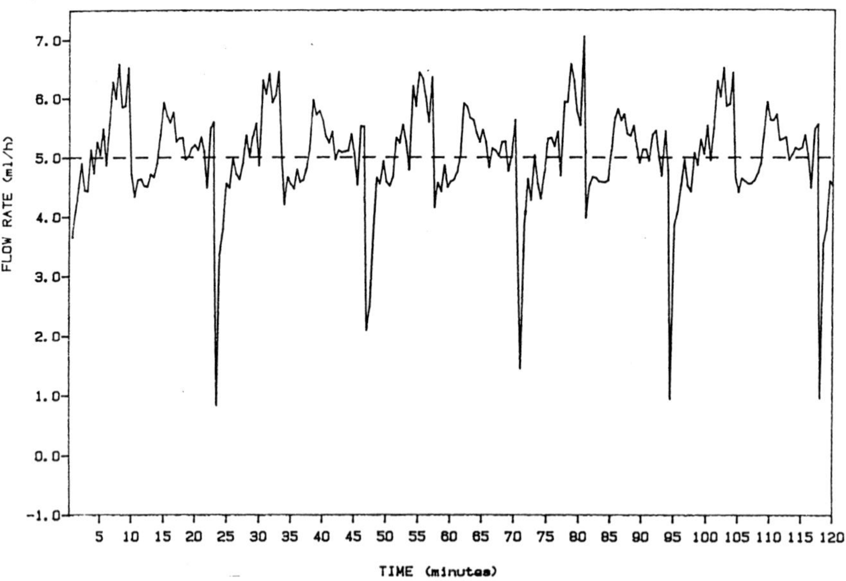


Fig. 11.7. Output from diaphragm cassette type volumetric pump at a set rate of 5 ml/h.

## Short-term accuracy

As already stated, the short-term performance of most volumetric pumps is not

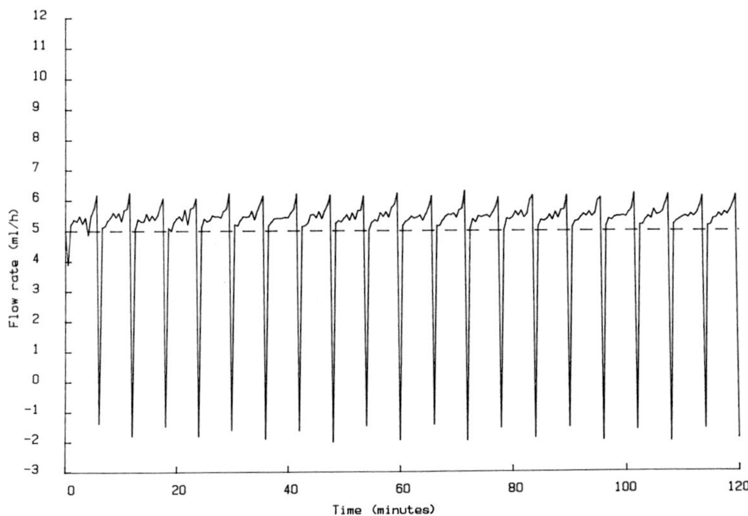


Fig. 11.8. Output from two roller rotary peristaltic volumetric pump at a set rate of 5 ml/h.

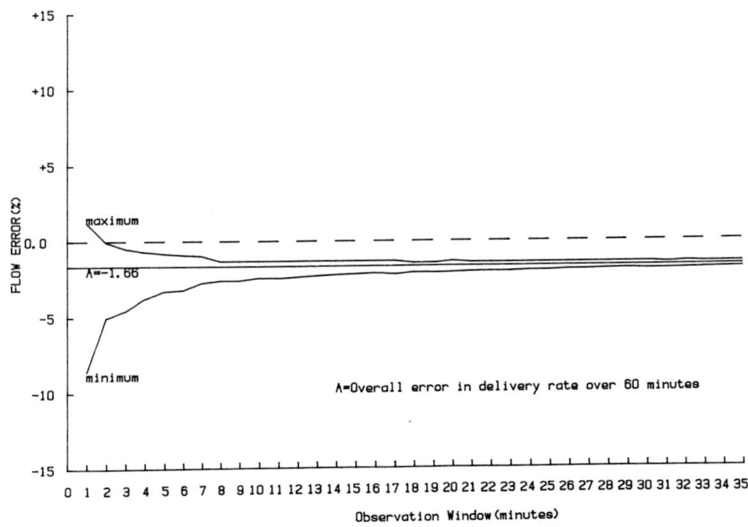


Fig. 11.9. Trumpet graph (linear peristaltic pump) showing typical short term flow rate errors at a set rate of 25 ml/h.

quite as good as that from a syringe pump. Figure 11.9 shows a trumpet graph for a typical linear peristaltic volumetric pump. In the main, linear peristaltic mechanisms tend to produce lower short-term fluctuations than other types of mechanism. Rotary peristaltic mechanisms tend to have the poorest performance. Start-up performance is, however, much improved over a syringe pump and even at the lowest rates, volumetric pumps deliver infusate practically instantaneously.

### Occlusion alarm response

Pressure sensing volumetric pumps in which the user can set the alarm level can give a very much better occlusion alarm response than most syringe pumps. This enables rapid activation of the alarm on total occlusion and a subsequent very small bolus on release of the occlusion. Some designs also display continuously the pressure in the infusion line and can aid the user in determining whether the i.v. is positionally obstructed or tissuing. If the latter occurs, the pressure in the line usually falls initially and then starts to rise to a level well above the original infusion pressure. If the alarm level can be set just a few millimeters of mercury above the working level, then it is quite feasible that the pump will alarm after the onset of extravasation with a short delay depending on the circumstances. This is important when infusing high concentration drugs at low flow rates if complications have arisen at the site. To mitigate against this, it is often preferable to dilute the drug and use a higher flow rate if at all possible.

### Controls and displays

It is interesting to note that the design of volumetric pumps has, in the past, attracted a higher level of engineering expertise than has been traditionally employed in the design of syringe pumps. This is now changing but the majority of volumetric pump designs have many more features and facilities and important internal safety systems. From the user's point of view, there are more displays of vital parameters such as volume preset, volume infused and, sometimes, pressure in the line. In addition, setting-up prompts and precise alarm conditions are often displayed.

Another useful facility often available is a secondary infusion capability thus allowing the user to infuse two different drugs or solutions. Separate programming of the primary and the secondary infusion rate is possible.

### Volumetric controllers

All types of controller depend on gravity for their operation and this means that the head height (the difference in height between the fluid level in the container and the infusion site) has to be sufficient to overcome resistance to flow due to venous pressure, pressure drop across the cannula and any resistance due to the tubing and the filter if one is used. In practice, this usually means that controllers are limited to peripheral infusions. Central lines can be used if the conditions are suitable. It is not possible to infuse arterially with controllers because of the difficulty of obtaining sufficient head height. For intravenous applications, a height of at least 90 cm is recommended.

Volumetric controllers are calibrated in volume per unit time (usually ml/h as are syringe pumps and volumetric pumps). They are intended to deliver an accurate volume of infusate in a given time. They do this by counting drops and calculating the volume of each drop (the assumption being that each drop will have the same size at a given drip rate). Unfortunately, drops are variable in size and many factors contribute to this (Hillman, 1989). Some of these factors are:

(i) drip rate
(ii) the size and nature of the drop-forming orifice
(iii) the properties of the fluid (surface tension, viscosity, density, etc.)
(iv) the nature of the fluid (whether a solution or suspension)
(v) temperature
(vi) pressure
(vii) the method of drip control

In order to compensate for all these factors, the designer of a gravity controller has to resort to compromise. Compensation for change in drop size due to drip rate is easily accommodated within the design of the controller. Careful design of the adminstration set which includes the drop forming orifice is essential and it is not, therefore, possible to use anything other than a dedicated unit. Compensation for the type of infusate being used is often accomplished by having several fluid codes from which the user may make a selection. This system attempts to group similar fluids together (for instance, simple electrolytes) and to compensate for their different properties by using an algorithm. Unfortunately, this process cannot be precise and accuracy is bound to suffer if an infusate is being used which does not have properties which place it amongst any of the available groupings. The effects of temperature are not usually compensated for but controllers attempt to maintain the drip rate set in spite of changes in back pressure.

**Flow status alarm system**

Most modern controllers incorporate a flow status alarm system which gives progressive warning of increased resistance to flow without activating the audible alarm. This system maintains the set rate in spite of variable resistance and has a long time constant so that the alarm is not activated when the increase in pressure is transient. This avoids nuisance alarms but alerts the user to conditions at the infusion site which may be deteriorating and require attention. Only when it becomes impossible to maintain the set rate (within a given tolerance) is the alarm activated and the set clamped off.

Such a system is very sensitive to changes in back pressure which could be due to positionally obstructed i.v. or to infiltration. Only pressure sensing pumps which have been set at a very low occlusion pressure will respond to such changes more quickly.

### Limitations in use

It is clear that the accuracy that can be obtained from conventional volumetric controllers is not expected to be much better than 10% measured over a period of 1 h.

The flow rate capability is usually limited to about 250 ml/h maximum and can be set in 1 ml/h increments only from a minimum of about 1 ml/h. The delivery of infusate will not be as accurate, nor can it be selected so precisely, as when using a syringe pump or a volumetric pump. Also, the maximum flow rate obtainable is probably not sufficient to give the loading dose.

For these reasons, the use of volumetric controllers to deliver anaesthetic drugs is probably not appropriate.

### Drip rate controllers

These instruments are identical in operation to volumetric controllers with the exception that they are calibrated in drops per minute (dpm) and are usually restricted to a range of 1 to 99 dpm selected in increments of 1 dpm. In the main, these instruments are low cost and are designed to use any standard solution set.

The problems of converting drops to volumes has already been discussed. This problem is exacerbated in a drop controller because the infusion set is not dedicated and the size and properties of the drop-forming orifice may not be known. It would be very difficult to calculate or predict reasonable levels of volumetric accuracy using these devices. Only by using empirical methods could accuracy be defined and this would most likely be considered unacceptable, thus ruling out this type of instrument.

### Drip rate pumps

These pumps are calibrated in drops per minute with a range usually from 1 to 99 dpm and are designed to take any standard tubing set. They exhibit the same problems as drip rate controllers in that no degree of volumetric accuracy can be expected and even if the same make of set is always used, there can be no expectations of consistency in volumetric performance despite the fact that the drip rate is highly accurate. Two main problems pertaining to this type of pump have been reported in the past (Department of Health, 1985). Most of them do not have an air detector and potentially they are capable of pumping air into the patient. The occlusion alarm pressure setting is usually extremely high making the use of these pumps potentially dangerous under certain conditions, particularly if the cannula has been misplaced or badly positioned. In addition, they can blow the infusion set apart should total occlusion occur.

The limited flow rate range and lack of any definable volumetric accuracy alone would rule out the use of this type of pump for anaesthetic applications. The additional complications are such that these pumps are not recommended by the Department of Health for use by the National Health Service in the U.K.

## AMBULATORY PUMPS

Ambulatory pumps are not designed for intravenous anaesthesia but are included here for completeness. These pumps are small and pocket sized, often powered by disposable batteries and intended to be worn on the person. Most of these pumps take small syringes in sizes from 1 ml up to 10 ml (sometimes a 20-ml syringe can be accommodated). Other designs are available working on the peristaltic pumping principle which have an integral fluid container in the form of a special cassette containing a collapsible bag. Such containers can be filled with up to 50 ml and sometimes 100 ml of infusate.

Most of these small pumps are designed for long-term delivery of drugs over periods of days and are intended for chemotherapy and pain relief and as such have very low flow rate capability. Only the cassette type can be set for rates up to about 90 ml/h. The small syringe pumps deliver their output in a quasi-continuous mode to conserve battery life.

## PUMPS DESIGNED SPECIFICALLY FOR INTRAVENOUS ANAESTHESIA

The only pumps identified on the market in the U.K. specifically for this application are syringe pump designs which accommodate 50-ml syringes. Such pumps are powered by disposable or rechargeable batteries. Some of these pumps look very much like conventional syringe pumps with additional features but the more sophisticated designs are obviously dedicated to intravenous anaesthetic applications only.

### Basic requirements

The pump should have the facility to deliver a basal rate plus a loading dose. In addition, it should be possible to preset the dose and display the volume and bolus infused. For the basal rate, a wide range of flow rates is required covering from 0.1 to 200 ml/h. The loading dose will require flow rates up to about 1000 ml/h and must be precisely calibrated. Accuracy of delivery should be within ±5% measured over an hour whilst short-term fluctuations in the output should be minimal and within ±5% measured over a 1-min period. The output should be reasonably continuous. All the other features and facilities of a good syringe pump are required together with a comprehensive alarm system.

### Advanced Medical Devices model PS6050

This model takes standard 50-ml syringes and can be calibrated for several different brands including BD and Monoject. Facilities provided: basal rate range, 1—200 ml/h (1 ml/h increments); bolus delivery, single rate of 600 ml/h; volume infused display, LCD; preset dose, not available; occlusion pressure, 600—900 mmHg; power supply, disposable batteries (separate mains power supply also available); alarms, comprehensive.

### Bard Infus O R

This revolutionary multi-drug system uses a series of smart labels which calibrate the pump automatically for a wide range of anaesthetic agents. Each smart label is clearly marked with drug dilution instructions and the required syringe size. They are colour coded by drug class according to the ASTM Drug Label Color Standard. The class and colour designations are as follows:

Narcotics — light blue
Muscle relaxants — fluorescent red
Vasopressors — violet
Hypotensive agents — violet/white stripes
Induction agents — yellow
Other agents — white

There are three types of smart label which provide for three different operating configurations of the front panel switches depending on the drug being delivered. These are bolus and basal rate delivery, basal rate without bolus, infusion delivery that is not based on body weight.

(i) Bolus and basal rate — for agents that are given as a loading or supplemental bolus and a continuous infusion, the upper panel switch selects infusion rate in $\mu$g/kg per min, the middle switch selects body weight in kg and the lower switch selects bolus settings (scaled by body weight) in $\mu$g/kg.

(ii) Infusion delivery without bolus — for agents that are given solely as a continuous infusion, the upper switch selects high infusion rate, the middle switch body weight and the lower switch low infusion rate, only one rate switch being active at any one time.

(iii) Infusion delivery not based on body weight — the upper and lower switches select high or low infusion rate, respectively, and the middle switch is not active.

The pump takes standard BD or Monoject 20 and 50 ml disposable syringes. The smart labels are magnetically coded and are magnetised to attach firmly to the front panel. Each coded label tells the microcomputer the delivery rate selections available when that specific label is used with the pump. The pump then calculates the correct volumetric delivery rate based on the infusion rate, the body weight of the patient and the drug concentration.

Typical selections available using propofol at a concentration of 10 mg/ml are:
Infusion rate: 0—300 μg/kg per min
Body weight: 30—100 kg
Bolus delivery: 0—3000 μg/kg

The front panel also contains a function switch having five positions — purge, off, stop, infuse and bolus start and a display showing total μg and (in bolus mode) μg/kg. The pump has a comprehensive alarm system with a maximum occlusion pressure of 570 mmHg using a 50-ml syringe. It is powered solely from disposable batteries.

**Ohmeda 9000**

This model takes standard 50-, 20- or 10-ml syringes and can be calibrated for Becton Dickinson, Monoject or Terumo syringes.
Facilities provided:
Basal rate range: 0.1—200 ml/h
Bolus infusion rates: 300, 600 or 1200 ml/h (50 ml syringes)
300, 350 or 450 ml/h (20 ml syringes)
180, 220 or 300 ml/h (10 ml syringes)
Display of total volume infused: 0.1—500 ml (0.1 ml increments up to 10 ml, 1 ml thereafter)
Two level occlusion alarm: low pressure for continuous infusion, high pressure for bolus infusion
Comprehensive alarm system
Optional RS232 computer interface
Powered by rechargeable batteries (power supply backbar available for pole mounting of one, two or three pumps which includes mains powered battery charger).

## CONCLUSIONS

The different types of instrumentation available for intravenous infusion have been explained giving advantages and limitations in use. It emerges that the most suitable pumps for intravenous anaesthesia are syringe pumps but that volumetric pumps chosen carefully could prove very capable in this application.

The features needed in a typical anaesthetic pump are, however, rather specialised and not always to be found in a pump designed for use in high care or special care areas. For this reason, several manufacturers have extended the basic syringe pump design to include the essential requirements. One pump of this new breed will even carry out all the calculations for the infusion automatically and is calibrated for most of the known agents. Such pumps are available now and will be of considerable assistance in promoting the use of this anaesthetic technique.

# APPENDIX

## Pumps and controllers available for intravenous infusion

| | |
|---|---|
| *Syringe pumps* | |
| Flo-gard 100 | Baxter Healthcare |
| Perfusor FT | B Braun Medical |
| Program 1 | Becton Dickinson |
| Program 2 | Becton Dickinson |
| SE200 series | Becton Dickinson |
| SE400 series | Becton Dickinson |
| SM90 | Critikon |
| Injectomat CP | Fresenius |
| MS 2000 | Graseby Medical |
| 710 | Ivac |
| P1000 | Welmed |
| P2000 | Welmed |
| P3000 | Welmed |
| *Volumetric pumps* | |
| Life Care 4 | Abbot Laboratories |
| Flo-gard 6100 | Baxter Healthcare |
| Flo-gard 6200 | Baxter Healthcare |
| Perfusa Secura | B Braun Medical |
| VIP II | Becton Dickinson |
| 920 | Imed |
| 960A series | Imed |
| 965A series | Imed |
| Gemini PC1 | Imed |
| Gemini PC2 | Imed |
| 560 series | Ivac |
| 565 series | Ivac |
| 590 | Ivac |
| 270 series | 3M Health Care |
| 275 series | 3M Health Care |
| *Volumetric controllers* | |
| Rateminder IV | Critikon |
| 281 | Ivac |
| Micromed II | Malem Medical |
| Micromed III | Malem Medical |
| *Drip rate controllers* | |
| Rateminder III | Critikon |
| 350 | Imed |
| Micromed I | Malem Medical |
| *Syringe pumps designed specifically for intravenous anaesthesia* | |
| PS6050 | Advanced Medical Devices |
| Infus O R | Bard |
| 9000 | Ohmeda |

# REFERENCES


Auty, B. (1988) Equipment for intravenous infusion — some aspects of performance. *Agressologie* 29, 824—828.

Auty, B. (1989a) Choice of instrumentation for controlled i.v. infusion. *ITCM Vol. 10, No. 4*, Medical Tribune Ltd., U.K., pp. 117—122.

Auty, B. (1989b) Controlled intravenous infusion — gravity feed or pumped systems? *Intensive Care World* 6, 149—153.

Department of Health (1985) *Infusion Pumps and Controllers — General Information Resulting from the Evaluation Programme HEI No. 135*, pp. 1—20.

Department of Health (1986) Evaluation of infusion pumps and controllers. *Sixth report HEI No. 157*, pp. 1—46.

Department of Health (1987) Evaluation of infusion pumps and controllers. *Seventh report HEI No. 175*, pp. 1—62.

Department of Health (1989) Evaluation of infusion pumps and controllers. *Eighth Report HEI No. 193*, pp. 37—38)

Hillman, M. (1989) The prediction of drop size from intravenous infusion controllers. *J. Med. Eng. Technol.* 13, 166—176.

International Electrotechnical Commission (1989) *Working group 8 of 62D — draft part II standard for infusion equipment.* British Standards Institution, Draft Document No. 90/51556.

B. Kay (ed.) Total Intravenous Anaesthesia



# 12

# *Total intravenous anaesthesia and postoperative sedation for cardiac surgery*

G.N. Russell

## INTRODUCTION

This chapter examines the specific considerations in the choice of anaesthetic technique in the context of cardiac surgery incorporating hypothermic cardiopulmonary bypass (CPB). As myocardial revascularisation is the most common form of cardiac surgery, this is examined in detail, although many of the considerations are equally applicable to other types of cardiac surgery.

The main considerations in the choice of intravenous anaesthetic technique for cardiac surgery are:

- prevention of perioperative myocardial ischaemia
- the balance between depth of anaesthesia and myocardial depression
- the requirement for postoperative respiratory support.

### Control of myocardial ischaemia

In 1985, Slogoff and Keats demonstrated the direct relation between the incidence of intraoperative myocardial ischaemia and subsequent postoperative myocardial infarction. This study prompted further investigation into the aetiology and incidence of perioperative myocardial ischaemia.

The imbalance between myocardial oxygen supply and demand that results in ischaemia may occur in a variety of circumstances (Fig. 12.1). Sternotomy and sternal spread are particularly potent stimuli that are unique to cardiac surgery, and inadequate suppression of tachycardia in response to these stimuli will result in haemodynamically related ischaemia.

Much controversy has surrounded the role of some anaesthetic agents in directly causing myocardial ischaemia. Isoflurane is a potent coronary arteriolar dilator and has the potential to cause a coronary steal effect (Reiz et al., 1983). Nitrous oxide may cause epicardial coronary artery constriction (Wilkowski et al., 1987),

**Detrimental Changes in the Myocardial Oxygen Balance**

| Decreased Myocardial Oxygen Supply | Increased Myocardial Oxygen Demand |
|---|---|
| 1. Decreased coronary blood flow | |
| a. Tachycardia | 1. Tachycardia |
| b. Diastolic Hypotension | 2. Increased wall tension |
| C. Increased preload | a. Increased preload |
| d. Hypocapnia | b. Increased afterload |
| e. Coronary spasm | 3. Increased contractility |
| 2. Decreased Oxygen Delivery | |
| a. Anemia | |
| b. Hypoxia | |
| c. Decreased 2.3 DPG | |

Fig. 12.1. Tachycardia is the most important single haemodynamic event to be associated with myocardial ischaemia.

although evidence of an association with an increased incidence of myocardial ischaemia in humans is lacking (Cahalan et al., 1986). None of the intravenous anaesthetics have been associated with coronary steal and further discussion of the subject is therefore beyond the scope of this chapter.

Between 50—90% of intra-operative ischaemic events are in fact entirely unrelated to adverse haemodynamic changes, and are due to fluctuations in coronary vascular tone. The incidence of this haemodynamically 'silent' ischaemia is identical to that experienced by the patient in the pre-operative period and is primarily a reflection of the severity of the patients' disease process (Knight et al., 1988) and thus beyond the immediate control of the anaesthetist.

Thus, the prime concern of the cardiac anaesthetist in the pre-bypass period is the prevention of additional haemodynamically related myocardial ischaemia. Control of tachycardia is of paramount importance in this respect.

## Depth of anaesthesia and myocardial depression

Anaesthesia for cardiac surgery incorporating cardiopulmonary bypass has traditionally been associated with a higher than normal incidence of awareness (Goldman et al., 1987). The likehood that any stimulus will lead to long term memory formation depends on the strength of the stimulus and the sensory threshold at the time the stimulus is experienced (Eisele et al., 1976). This problem of cardiac anaesthesia relates to the difficulty in achieving adequate depth of anaesthesia without the consequence of overt myocardial depression and there appear to be two high risk periods.

The first is during the intense surgical stimulus of sternotomy and sternal spread. Conditions conducive to memory formation will exist when light levels of anaesthesia are used to avoid hypotension, particularly in patients with poor ventricular function.

The second high risk period is during the rewarming phase of hypothermic cardiopulmonary bypass (CPB). Global myocardial ischaemia is an obligatory consequence of aortic crossclamping, even with modern techniques of cardioplegia. Any pre-operative ventricular dysfunction may be further compounded, making the restoration of the spontaneous circulation difficult. As virtually all true anaesthetic agents have some myocardial depressant effect, the concentration has traditionally been reduced or discontinued prior to attempts at weaning the patient from the bypass pump. The patient will then be normothermic and minimally anaesthetised, and although the degree of surgical stimulus at this time is not great, there is a very real risk of awareness.

The potential for recall, particularly during CPB, is compounded by the difficulty in assessing the depth of anaesthesia. Despite their well known limitations, sweating, hypertension and tachycardia are usually interpreted as signs of inadequate anaesthesia except in the context of cardiopulmonary bypass. Sweating during bypass, however, is often the consequence of a rapid rise in hypothalamic temperature and the haemodynamic signs are clearly of limited value. In view of the limitations of the traditional signs of inadequate anaesthesia, other techniques for monitoring depth of anaesthesia have been studied. The interpretation of the electroencephelogram (EEG), even in processed forms, is not without problems during hypothermic CPB. In addition, anaesthetic agents may produce differing characteristic EEG patterns (Kearse et al., 1989), further compounding analysis.

Recent interest has centered around the study of spontaneous and provoked patterns of lower oesophageal sphincter contraction as a guide to anaesthetic depth (Evans et al., 1987). Whilst initial studies of cardiac surgical patients have shown appropriate changes in contraction pattern with surgical stimulus (Thomas et al., 1989), the sensivity and specificity of this technique has yet to be determined.

Thus, the potential for awareness during cardiac surgery and CPB is high, and the ability to monitor anaesthetic depth is limited. The balance between anaesthetic depth and myocardial depression is one of the major considerations in the choice of anaesthetic technique for cardiac surgery.

### The requirement for postoperative respiratory support

There has in the past been much debate about the benefits of early extubation of patients following cardiac surgery. The term 'early' generally means within the first 8 h following surgery, a time period that allows adequate rewarming and assessment of cardio-respiratory function. There is no reason for a patient with good pre-operative ventricular function and uneventful cardiac surgery to remain attached to a ventilator beyond this initial assessment period and there is evidence that prolonged respiratory support in this group may actually be detrimental (Quasha et al., 1980). Whilst not the main consideration, the selection of an anaesthetic technique that permits the possibility of early extubation may have significant financial advantages to a busy cardiac surgical centre.

## PHARMACOLOGICAL CONSIDERATIONS SPECIFIC TO CARDIAC SURGERY

Fundamental to successful total intravenous anaesthesia is the knowledge of the pharmacokinetics of the agents used and the target concentration required for the procedure concerned. Cardiac surgery has the specific requirement of a high initial anaesthetic concentration to cover intubation and sternotomy and then a reduced level during periods of lesser stimulus such as accompanying mammary artery mobilisation.

The onset of hypothermic cardiopulmonary bypass will alter all major pharmacokinetic processes, making prediction of drug concentration difficult (Holley et al., 1982). Haemodilution and hypothermia are the two most important events in this respect.

### Haemodilution

The initiation of bypass is accompanied by the rapid infusion of the 3 l crystalloid pump prime. This will usually result in a reduction in the pre-bypass anaesthetic concentration, the magnitude of the fall being related both to the volume of distribution and the redistribution half-life of the drug. The initial fall may be further compounded by uptake, particularly of lipophylic drugs, onto the bypass apparatus.

By reducing the plasma protein binding sites available, acute haemodilution also increases the free drug concentration of many anaesthetic agents (Morgan et al., 1986). In addition, heparin administration causes a rise in plasma free fatty acids which may compete for protein binding sites to further increase the free drug fraction. Diazepam (99%), fentanyl (85%), sufentanil (93%) and propofol (95%) are all highly protein bound. Thus, even a 1% increase in the free diazepam concentration will effectively double the active drug and theoretically may increase the anaesthetic effect. However, the relationship between free drug and pharmacokinetic effect is extremely difficult to investigate and there have been few definitive studies relating these two factors. It would, therefore, be unwise to rely primarily on this effect to ensure adequate depth of anaesthesia (Wood et al., 1986).

### Hypothermia

Hypothermia has two potential pharmacokinetic effects. Firstly, it may cause intrahepatic shunting of blood and a reduction in effective hepatic blood flow (Larsen et al., 1971). Secondly, hepatic microenzyme activity will be reduced in direct relation to the fall in hepatic temperature. Both these effects will reduce the clearance of drugs dependent on hepatic metabolism.

The rapid and profound physiological changes associated with cardiopulmonary bypass preclude the achievement of steady states required to perform conventional pharmacokinetic analysis. Thus, the best guidelines available for ensuring the maintenance of anaesthesia are studies that simply define the trends in drug concentrations with the various phases of cardiopulmonary bypass.

## SPECIFIC ANAESTHETIC TECHNIQUES

### Opioid anaesthesia

In the mid 1960s, Lowenstein introduced the technique of high dose morphine anaesthesia for patients with impaired ventricular function requiring valve replacement. Since then, fentanyl, alfentanil and, most recently, sufentanil have been advocated as primary anaesthetic agents for cardiac surgery.

*Fentanyl*

High dose fentanyl as the sole anaesthetic was first introduced by Stanley in 1978, who reported excellent haemodynamic stability using a total dose of 74 μg/kg. The method has since been widely applied with total doses of up to 162 μg/kg (Wynands et al., 1983).

Fentanyl is frequently administered as a single bolus dose to induce and maintain anaesthesia for the entire duration of the operation. Although this produces a very high initial fentanyl concentration, loading doses of 60 μg/kg (Bovill et al., 1980) and 75 μg/kg (Hug et al., 1982) result in fentanyl concentrations of less than 10 ng/ml at the end of cardiopulmonary bypass. This is very close to the awakening concentration of 6.4 (2.1) ng/ml described by Hynynen et al. (1986). In order to overcome this problem, Lunn et al. (1979) suggested a loading dose of 50 μg/kg followed by a constant infusion of 0.5 μg/kg per min which achieved concentrations of 15—18 ng/ml throughout the procedure. A loading dose of 75 μg/kg and an infusion of 0.75 μg/kg per min results in plasma concentrations consistently above 20 ng/ml, the target concentration suggested by Wynands et al. (1983).

Even with these very high plasma concentrations the incidence of breakthrough hypertension and tachycardia during sternotomy and sternal spread is unacceptably high. (Edde et al., 1981). In fact, a concentration of 20 ng/ml appears to be a pharmacodynamic 'ceiling' as higher values are not associated with additional haemodynamic or hypnotic effect (Sprigge et al., 1982; Wynands et al., 1984).

It is not surprising that, when fentanyl is administered in these very high doses, there is an obligatory requirement for postoperative respiratory support, with extubation delayed for as long as 19 h (Wynands et al., 1983).

*Alfentanil*

Alfentanil is the shortest acting of the currently available opioids, with an elimination half-life of 90 min (Camu et al., 1982). It has been studied as the primary anaesthetic in the context of cardiac surgery with the hope of avoiding myocardial depression, whilst at the same time reducing the requirement for postoperative ventilation.

The haemodynamic profile of alfentanil anaesthesia seems generally less satisfactory than that of fentanyl. De Lange et al. (1983) reported good haemodynamic stability using a variable rate infusion and suggested a target concentration of 1000 ng/ml. However, using a priming infusion of 86 μg/kg per min for 10 min followed by a constant infusion of 7.8 μg/kg per min, Hug et al. (1983) found that even an alfentanil concentration as high as 2181 (62) ng/ml did not reliably suppress adverse haemodynamic responses in the majority of patients. The poor dose-response relationship of alfentanil was also noted by Robbins et al. (1990), who found poor haemodynamic control at both high and low plasma concentrations.

Unfortunately, the anticipated advantage of a short acting opioid in reducing the time to extubation does not seem to occur when alfentanil is used in these very high doses. The elimination half-life is increased following CPB, and prolonged respiratory depression is the inevitable consequence (Hynynen et al., 1986).

*Sufentanil*

Sufentanil is the opioid most recently introduced into the U.K. and is variously quoted as being five to ten times as potent as fentanyl. Given this wide range, comparative studies of other opiods in 'equipotent' concentrations are difficult to interpret. At 2.7 h, the half-life of sufentanil is somewhat shorter than that of fentanyl (Bovill et al., 1984) and thus it is kinetically even less suited to administration as a single bolus dose. An induction dose of 15 μg/kg results in very low plasma concentration with the onset of cardiopulmonary bypass and a further 10 μg/kg immediately pre-bypass is required to achieve the target concentration of 5 ng/ml (Fig. 12.2). An alternative approach is to use a pharmacokinetically driven, computer-assisted infusion based simply on pharmacokinetic data derived from general surgical patients (Flezzani et al., 1987). Plasma concentrations

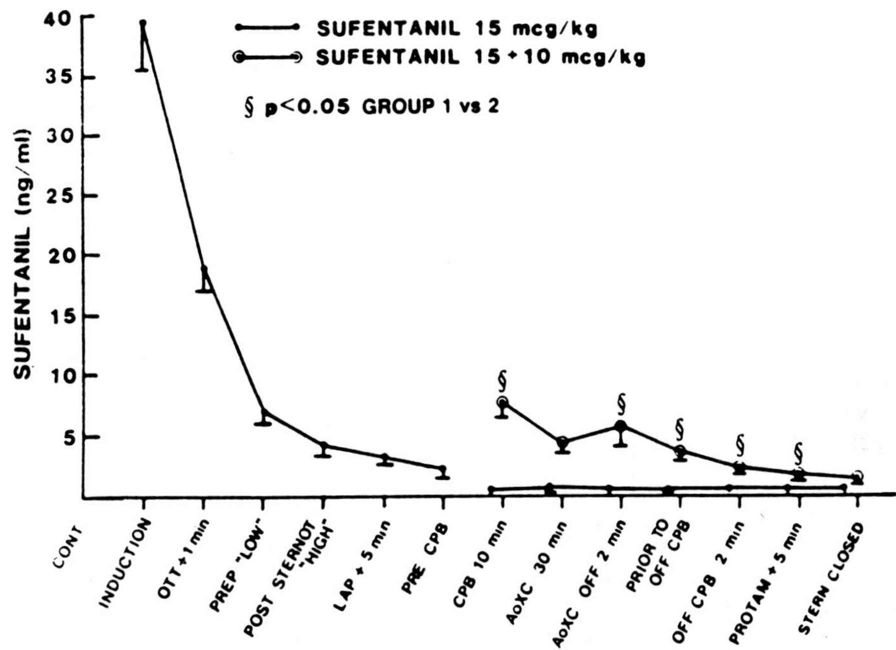


Fig. 12.2. Plasma levels of sufentanil following two administration techniques. The single bolus dose of 15 μg/kg is associated with very low concentrations at the end of CPB. The addition of a further 10 μg/kg immediatly pre-bypass significantly increases the plasma concentration during the high risk normothermic phase of bypass. Data from Samuelson et al. (1986). Reproduced with permission of authors and publisher.

within the target range can then reliably be achieved, although some accumulation will occur during the hypothermic phase of cardiopulmonary bypass as the clearance of sufentanil falls in direct proportion to hepatic temperature.

Despite the difficulty in ensuring equipotent doses, sufentanil does appear to be superior to fentanyl in the suppression of the haemodynamic responses to surgical stimuli (de Lange et al., 1982). This may be related to the fact that sufentanil has a more potent 'anaesthetic' effect as shown by the greater reduction in the MAC of inhaled agents (Hecker et al., 1983). Better protection from hypertension appears to be accompanied by a higher incidence of hypotension during induction, and the fall in blood pressure may be severe (Spiess et al., 1986).

A shorter elimination half-life does not confer a significant advantage for postoperative respiratory support (de Lange et al., 1982; Howie et al., 1985). Although Sanford et al. (1986) were able to extubate patients receiving sufentanil (10 μg/kg) earlier than those receiving fentanyl (95 μg/kg) the duration of ventilation was still over 10 h. A summary of the times to awakening and to endotracheal extubation with various opioid techniques is shown in Table 12.1.

TABLE 12.1

Times to awakening and endotracheal extubation following opioid anaesthetic techniques

| Opioid, total dose (μg/kg) Mean (S.E.M.) | Time to awakening following surgery (h) Mean (S.E.M.) | Time to extubation following surgery (h) Mean (S.E.M.) | Reference |
|---|---|---|---|
| Fentanyl 110 (10) | 3.3 (1.2) | 14.4 (3.2) | Hynynen et al. (1986) |
| Fentanyl 106 (2.4) | Not specified | 19.0 (1.0) | Moldenhauer et al. (1982) |
| Fentanyl 95.4 (9.9) | 1.03 (0.29) | 16.76 (1.3) | Sanford et al. (1986) |
| Fentanyl 100 | 8.11 (2.48)[a] | 19.96 (5.0)[a] | Thompson et al. (1987) |
| Fentanyl 100 | 6.5 (median value) | 17.0 (median value) | Howie et al. (1985) |
| Alfentanil 1089 (55.6) | 3.1 (0.6) | 9.7 (1.1) | Robbins et al. (1990) |
| Alfentanil 1379 (274) | 2.6 (1.3) | 11.8 (3.5) | Hynynen et al. (1986) |
| Sufentanil 18.9 (2.2) | 0.28 (0.15) | 8.8 (1.13) | Sanford et al. (1986) |
| Sufentanil 20 | 6.5 (median value) | 17.0 (median value) | Howie et al. (1985) |
| Sufentanil 15 | 7.48 (2.05)[a] | 17.31 (3.59) | Thompson et al. (1987) |

[a]Value relates to time following induction of anaesthesia.

TABLE 12.2

Propofol anaesthesia: induction by infusion (data from Roberts et al. (1988))

| Propofol dose (mg/kg per h) | Duration of infusion |
|---|---|
| 1 | 20 s |
| 10 | 10 min |
| 8 | 10 min |
| 6 | Continuously |

## Balanced intravenous anaesthesia

The application of balanced intravenous anaesthesia in the context of cardiac surgery has in the past been limited by the availabity of agents that are kinetically suited to continuous infusion. The advent of new short acting drugs means that the components of hypnosis, analgesia and reflex suppression can now be provided by separate infusions in a titratable fashion. Analgesia is provided by either a continuous infusion or intermittent injection of one of the previously described opioids but using much lower total doses. The adjuvant hypnotics are described below.

### *Propofol*

Propofol is the most recently introduced of the intravenous anaesthetic agents and, as such, data concerning its suitability for cardiac surgery are limited. Initial studies examined propofol as an induction agent in the presence of coronary artery disease. However, even with a bolus dose as low as 1.5 mg/kg Patrick et al. (1985) found a variable and sometimes severe reduction in arterial pressure. Using a similar dose preceded by 8 μg/kg fentanyl, Vermeyen et al. (1987) noted a mean reduction in systolic blood pressure of 28%, related primarily to a fall in SVR of 25%. Although no evidence of acute ischaemia was noted in this study, reductions in arterial pressure of this magnitude may be hazardous in the presence of coronary artery disease.The adverse haemodynamic effects of propofol when given by bolus dose relate to the overshoot in target blood concentration. Using a 1 mg/kg loading dose and a manual infusion regime (Table 12.2), Roberts et al. (1988) demonstrated that a target blood concentration of 3 μg/ml ($ED_{95}$ of propofol with $N_2O$) could rapidly be achieved without an overshoot in blood concentration and the consequent haemodynamic effects. Indeed, when preceded by 3 μg/kg of fentanyl this regime afforded excellent protection from the haemodynamic response to intubation (Fig. 12.3). These patients were not, however, receiving concurrent beta adrenergic or calcium channel blocker therapy and both of these may influence the haemodynamic effects of anaesthetic agents.

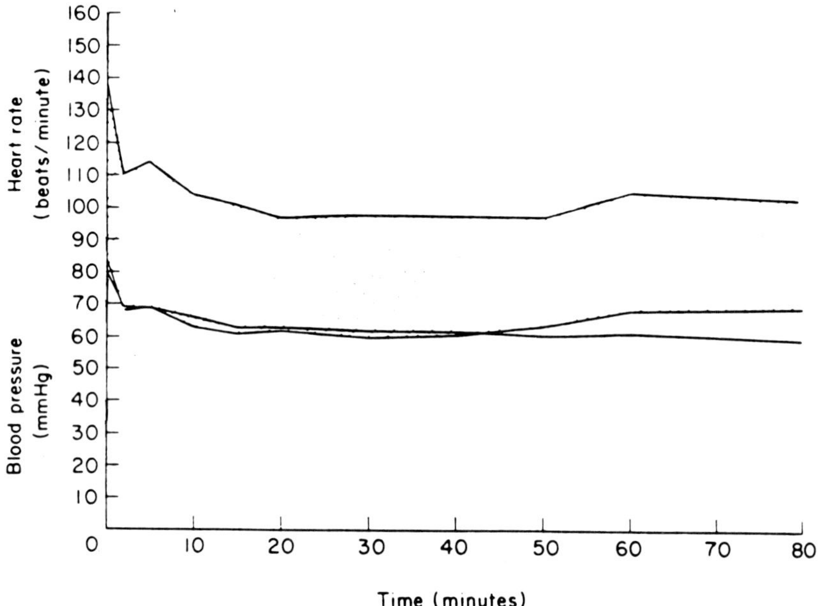


Fig. 12.3. Blood pressure and heart rate responses to induction of anaesthesia by infusion of propofol. Endotracheal intubation is accompanied by minimal haemodynamic change. Figure from Roberts et al., 1988. Reproduced with permission of authors and publisher.

An alternative approach has been to avoid the use of propofol for induction of anaesthesia (Russell et al., 1989). Moderate doses of fentanyl, when combined with a benzodiazepine, will produce transient blood levels that protect from the response to intubation, particularly if the patient is receiving beta blocker therapy. If a propofol infusion at 10 mg/kg per h is started following induction of anaesthesia in this way and continued to include sternotomy, excellent haemodynamic stability is achieved at this time. The infusion rate can then be decreased to 3—6 mg/kg per h with the reduction in surgical stimulus. Vermeyen et al. (1987) also noted good protection from the haemodynamic response to sternotomy using a combination of moderate dose fentanyl and propofol. The superior protection afforded by this combination compared to unsupplemented high dose fentanyl is probably related to two factors. Firstly, the addition of propofol may result in a mild negative inotropic effect. If the peak concentration is timed to occur at the period of maximal surgical stimulus then the reduction in myocardial oxygen consumption will be beneficial. Secondly, the addition of propofol will increase the depth of anaesthesia, an effect that cannot be achieved by simply increasing the dose of fentanyl due to the ceiling effect as described earlier.

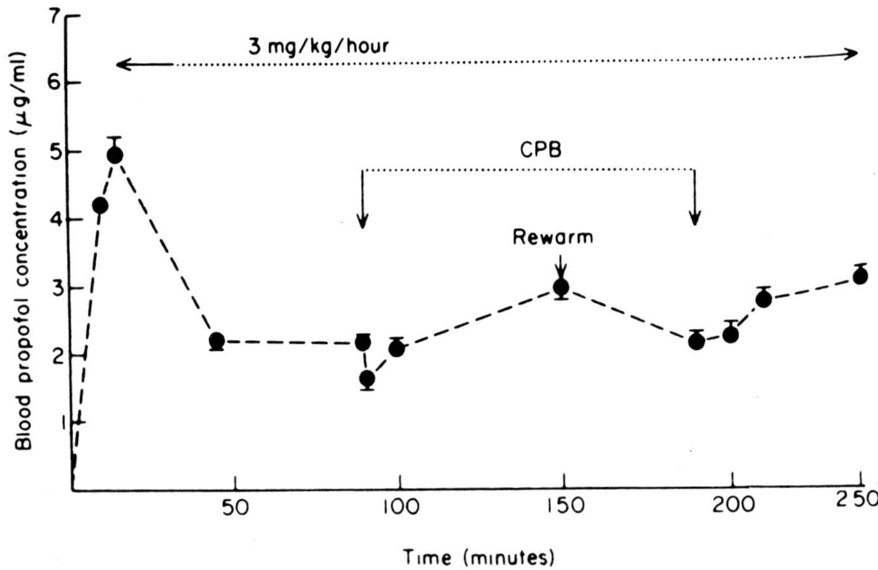


Fig. 12.4. Changes in blood concentration of propofol with a constant infusion during hypothermic cardiopulmonary bypass. Figure from Russell et al., 1989. Reproduced with permission of authors and publisher.

If a propofol infusion is continued throughout the procedure blood levels tend to follow a predictable pattern (Fig. 12.4). The onset of CPB is accompanied by a small decline in propofol concentration. The effect of haemodilution is offset in part by the large volume of distribution of the drug and the rapid redistribution half life of 2—4 min (Cockshott et al., 1987). The onset of the hypothermic phase of bypass is accompanied by a rise in propofol concentration to above the pre-bypass value. Rewarming results in a decline to the pre-bypass steady state value, indicating that the clearance of propofol during normothermic bypass is likely to be high. Weaning from bypass is accompanied by a small rise in propofol concentration, which may reflect a decrease in propofol clearance following the procedure (McMurray, 1989).

The use of a propofol infusion, combined with only moderate dose of fentanyl, for maintenance of anaesthesia during cardiac surgery is associated with good haemodynamic control. Weaning from bypass with this technique does not appear to be a problem — at least in patients with good ventricular function. There has been much debate as to the effects of propofol on ventricular function. In a definitive study using gated radionuclide ventriculography, Lepage et al. (1988) found that both propofol alone and the combination of propofol and fentanyl had little effect on end systolic volume or ventricular ejection fraction, which is in keeping with the clinical experience to date.

There is at present little data on the potential for early extubation using propofol and fentanyl for coronary artery surgery. The early experience of Mora et al. (1989) is encouraging in this respect. They found that the time to response and to extubation was significantly less in patients receiving propofol (total dose 9.4 mg/kg) and fentanyl (25 μg/kg) compared with fentanyl (122 μg/kg) alone.

Thus, it would appear that, if used appropriately, propofol may have significant advantages in cardiac anaesthesia. The combination of propofol and the newer opioids warrants further investigation as these combinations may permit even greater haemodynamic control and further reduction in the requirement for postoperative respiratory support.

*Midazolam*

Midazolam is a water soluble benzodiazepine with an elimination half-life of 185 min. When used as the sole agent for induction of anaesthesia, midazolam has few adverse haemodynamic effects (Marty et al., 1986). However, it has no analgesic effect and is therefore unsuitable as the primary anaesthetic agent for cardiac surgery. When administered in combination with high dose fentanyl, hypotension secondary to myocardial depression may result (Heikkila et al., 1984). This effect can be limited by slow administration and careful titration of the drug to the required endpoint (Raza et al., 1984) and this has become a popular induction technique in cardiac anaesthesia.

When midazolam is used as the hypnotic component of intravenous anaesthesia the target concentration is in the range 300—500 ng/ml (Persson et al., 1988). This can be acheived by an initial rapid infusion of 0.3 mg/kg over 10 min followed by a continuous infusion of 0.15 mg/kg per h. Few data are available concerning the effects of cardiopulmonary bypass on the kinetics of midazolam, although being primarily metabolised by the liver, accumulation during the hypothermic phase of bypass is likely.

With a constant background infusion of midazolam the most practical approach for cardiac surgery is the addition of a variable rate opioid infusion, titrated to the appropriate anaesthetic depth. Experience with fentanyl used in this way shows an effective plasma concentration of between 6 and 31 ng/ml and demonstrates the wide interpatient variability in dose requirements (Schweiger et al., 1989). The development of infusion pumps with the capability of high infusion rates and bolus drug delivery will greatly facilitate the closer titration of total intravenous anaesthesia.

Occasionally, a single bolus dose of midazolam is used to supplement high dose opioids during the high risk rewarming phase of CPB. The dose range is rather empirical but usually in the range 5—10 mg. The effect of this dose is uncertain.

There have been no formal studies of the requirement for postoperative ventilation with the combination of midazolam and opioid infusions. The awakening concentration of midazolam is around 100 ng/ml, approximately one third to one fifth of the therapeutic concentration. The elimination half-life of midazolam is 185 min and recovery might therefore be expected to be prolonged. In addition, there appears to be a group who metabolise midazolam very slowly and the elimination half-life in these patients may be as long as 16 h. Further studies are required to assess the potential benefits of midazolam and the newer opioids for cardiac anaesthesia.

*Thiopentone*

Although thiopentone has been used as an exponentially decreasing infusion to maintain anaesthesia during cardiopulmonary bypass (Morgan et al., 1986), it is clearly less suited than the newer agents previously described. There has, however, been a recent resurgence of interest in the use of thiopentone to reduce cerebral injury during open heart surgery.

The reported incidence of cerebral dysfunction following open cardiac chamber surgery ranges from 16 to 40% (Kollka et al., 1980; Slogoff et al., 1982). The probable cause is focal cerebral infarction secondary to both micro- and macro-emboli. Animal studies have demonstrated that this form of incomplete cerebral ischaemia may be responsive to the reduction in cerebral metabolic rate induced by pretreatment with barbiturates (Smith et al., 1974; Michenfelder et al., 1975). Based on this hypothesis, Nussmier and colleagues (1986) administered high dose thiopentone (mean dose 39.5 mg/kg) during CPB to patients having intracardiac surgery, and demonstrated a significant reduction in the incidence of cerebral dysfunction postoperatively. Hypothermia and arterial line filters were not used in their study and both these may have some influence on the incidence of embolic problems (Michenfelder et al., 1974). There was also an increased requirement for inotropic support in the study group and recovery was prolonged by the sedative effect of the drug. For these reasons, the administration of thiopentone during cardiopulmonary bypass is unlikely to be adopted as standard practice.

Neurological injury is one of the most catastrophic sequelae of bypass. In common with thiopentone, other intravenous hypnotic agents such as etomidate, propofol and midazolam reduce the cerebral requirement for oxygen. Further studies are required to assess the potential of these shorter acting drugs in the prevention of brain injury.

*Etomidate*

A very stable haemodynamic profile led to the recommendation of etomidate both for the induction and maintenance of anaesthesia in the cardiac surgical patient. If preceded by phenoperidine (0.04 mg/kg), an induction dose of 0.15 mg/kg and constant infusion of 20 $\mu$g/kg per min was associated with good haemodynamic stability and satisfactory anaesthesia (Oduro et al., 1983).

Etomidate, like propofol, is metabolised by the liver. Blood levels alter in a similar fashion with a rise in concentration during hypothermia and a decline to baseline levels during rewarming. Thus, there is no indication to alter the infusion rate during bypass.

Unfortunately, etomidate causes marked adrenal suppression and the finding of excessive mortality in trauma patients receiving continuous long term infusions of the drug (Ledingham et al., 1983) has led to a decline in its use. Transient adrenal suppression has also been demonstrated after even a single dose (Wagner et al., 1984). However, the clinical significance of this is unclear and etomidate still has a place for the induction of anaesthesia in the patient with poor left ventricular function.

### *Ketamine*

With a short distribution half-life and an elimination half-life of 150—240 min, ketamine is kinetically suited to the maintenance of anaesthesia by continuous infusion. Ketamine has two haemodynamic effects. The first is direct myocardial depression which can be demonstrated in isolated heart preparations (Valicenti et al., 1973). The second effect is a centrally mediated sympathetic response that tends to override the myocardial depression. The net effect is a significant increase in heart rate, cardiac index, systemic and pulmonary vascular resistances. Whilst this may be beneficial in situations of cardiac tamponade and constrictive pericarditis (Kingston et al., 1978), the increase in myocardial oxygen consumption may be detrimental in patients with coronary artery disease.

The sympathetic stimulation with ketamine is markedly attenuated by the addition of a benzodiazepine, and the combination of diazepam (0.3—0.5 mg/kg) and a ketamine infusion of 0.7 mg/kg per h provides excellent haemodynamic stability during induction, intubation and sternotomy (Hatano et al., 1976). Indeed, when compared to a diazepam/ketamine technique for coronary artery surgery, patients receiving high dose fentanyl had a significantly higher fluid and vasopressor requirement in the postoperative period (Tuman et al., 1988). In addition, the fentanyl group also had a longer stay in the intensive care unit.

There are few formal studies of the requirement for postoperative respiratory support using ketamine-based anaesthesia. The addition of diazepam to ketamine reduces the incidence of emergence delirium but significantly prolonges the recovery time. In fact extubation may be delayed to the same extent as occurs with high dose opioids (Tuman et al., 1988). Midazolam has a kinetic profile that is much closer to that of ketamine and may be a more appropriate combination.

## MUSCLE RELAXANTS FOR CARDIAC SURGERY

Rigidity of the chest and abdominal muscles is a frequent ocurrence with the use of high dose opiods (Jaffe et al., 1983) This may result in severe difficulties in maintaining ventilation prior to endotrachael intubation. Indeed, attempts at pulmonary inflation may result in high intrathoracic pressures causing a fall in venous return at the same time as the peak effect of the opioid. In an attempt to reduce time to intubation, higher than usual doses of muscle relaxant are often used, also ensuring profound muscular relaxation and a smooth intubation. The length of surgery and postoperative ventilation greatly exceeds the duration of any of the currently available muscle relaxants, even in these higher doses. Thus, the main criteria for selection of the relaxant relates primarily to the haemodynamic effects of the drugs.

Pancuronium, being virtually devoid of histamine releasing activity and having an indirect sympathomimetic effect, was the most popular of the older muscle relaxants for cardiac anaesthesia. The increasing awareness of the dangers of tachycardia in patients with coronary disease have probably led to a decline in its use and the closer examination of other relaxants. One approach is to combine pancuronium with metocurine or *d*-tubocurare which will not only minimise the heart rate changes associated with pancuronium alone but also potentiate the degree of neuromuscular blockade (Lebowitz et al., 1980).

Atracurium causes a dose-dependent release of histamine, which is responsible for the heart rate and blood pressure changes occasionally seen with the drug. In a study by Pokar et al. (1983), four out of nine patients receiving atracurium in a dose of 0.6—1.0 mg/kg had a fall in blood pressure of more than 10%. Indeed, even doses of 0.3 mg/kg have been associated with adverse haemodynamic changes when used for cardiac surgery (Philbin et al., 1983).

The margin between the neuromuscular blocking dose of vecuronium and the dose producing cardiovascular and autonomic effects is much wider than that of atracurium. It has little sympathomimetic activity and very large doses can be given without cardiovascular effect (Morris et al., 1983). The administration of 0.22 mg/kg (4 × $ED_{95}$) has an onset time as short as 1.3 min (Viby-Mogenson et al., 1980). Thus, vecuronium is the most cardiostable of currently available muscle relaxants with increasing application in coronary artery surgery. Ironically, the inherent cardiostability of vecuronium has led to reports of bradycardia when combined with vagotonic anaesthetic techniques such as very high dose opioids (Salmenpera et al., 1983). This is most likely to occur when the patients are also taking beta adrenergic antagonists and it is probably wise to substitute pancuronium for vecuronium if the presenting heart rate is less than 45 beats per min.

Pipecuronium, an analogue of pancuronium may soon be available for clinical use. It appears to be very similar to vecuronium in that it does not release histamine and is devoid of circulatory effects (Szenohradsky et al., 1982). It has, however, a longer duration of action than vecuronium, with an intubating dose of 0.08—0.1 mg/kg providing adequate surgical relaxation for 80—120 min. This may confer some additional advantage during cardiac surgery.

## OPIOID OR BALANCED ANAESTHESIA FOR CARDIAC SURGERY?

The choice of anaesthetic technique for cardiac surgery has formed the subject of much debate over many years. In the final analysis, the best technique is that which is associated with the best patient outcome in terms of cardiac morbidity and mortality. Two large studies by Tuman (1989) and Slogoff (1989) addressed this question directly. With data on over 2000 patients they could find no relationship between primary anaesthetic agent and the incidence of intra-operative ischaemia, postoperative myocardial infarction or death.

If outcome in terms of myocardial events is unchanged, then other aspects of anaesthetic technique assume increased importance. Awareness, even if pain is not experienced, is at best an unpleasant experience and may lead to protracted psychiatric morbidity in the form of a syndrome of traumatic neurosis (Blacher, 1975). Although there can be no doubt that most patients will be rendered unconscious by high dose opioids, there has been a disturbing number of reports of awareness (Mummaneni et al., 1980; Hilgenberg, 1981; Mark et al., 1983). Unlike true general anaesthetics, opioids have little or no direct effect on the cerebral cortex. Instead, they exert their pharmacological action on subcortical sites such as the limbic system, thalamus, mid-brain and spinal cord, acting so as to 'short circuit' ascending pathways (Snyder, 1977). Thus, used alone they cannot reliably be expected to produce unconsciousness and amnesia (Wong, 1983). It is likely that, were it not for the routine prescription of amnesic premedication as part of an opioid technique, the incidence of recall would be considerably higher. There is increasing evidence that balanced anaesthesia incorporating an hypnotic agent significantly increases the depth of anaesthesia and, hence, the risk of awareness (Silvay et al., 1989).

The single major advantage of opioid anaesthesia is the absence of a myocardial depressant effect in doses used clinically, and all cardiac anaesthesia techniques demonstrate the problem of the balance between ensuring adequate depth of anaesthesia and the avoidance of myocardial depression. Is the fear of the haemodynamic consequences of balanced anaesthesia justified? Outcome data would suggest not. One of the few studies that has directly addressed this question is that of Mora and colleagues (1989). They found similar inotrope requirements with techniques based on propofol, enflurane and high dose fentanyl. In addition, some indirect evidence is also available. As previously described, Nussmier (1986) administered large doses of thiopentone (39.5 mg/kg) during bypass to a group of patients having open heart surgery. Although there was an increased requirement for inotropic support, none of the patients failed to wean off the bypass pump. It should also be noted that the dose of thiopentone used was far in excess of that required simply to maintain anaesthesia. Thus, even if there were to be a small increase in inotrope requirement, this may not be unreasonable if adequate anaesthesia could be ensured.

The argument for pure opioid anaesthesia is strongest in the patient with severely impaired ventricular function. Indeed, this is the very group for whom it was originally designed and in whom the risk of awareness might be considered to be less important than the avoidance of myocardial depression. Since the prospect of early extubation generally does not apply to these patients, the requirement for prolonged respiratory support is of little consequence. The widespread application of this technique with all the inherent problems to patients with good ventricular function is both illogical and unnecessary.

Other potential benefits of balanced anaesthesia require further investigation. The possibility of reduced intensive care requirements both by a reduction in fluid and vasopressor requirements (Tuman et al., 1988) and early extubation may lead to financial savings. As neurological injury is one of the most catastrophic consequences of cardiac surgery, the possibility that the cerebral protective effects of hypnotic agents may positively influence patient outcome is a new and exciting development.

## SEDATION FOLLOWING CARDIAC SURGERY

There are three distinct groups of patients in a postoperative cardiac surgical intensive care unit, all with different requirements of a sedation technique.

The first group are those patients who have had uneventful cardiac surgery, and have little or no need for inotropic support. A short period of postoperative ventilation prior to extubation will allow assessment of cardiorespiratory status and permit rewarming following hypothermic bypass. In addition, the rate of mediastinal blood loss can be estimated. There is no evidence to suggest that light levels of sedation are beneficial during this period and indeed the incidence of postoperative hypertension may be reduced by deeper levels of sedation. The duration of respiratory support in this group depends on the philosophy of the unit and will vary from just a few hours to as long as 24 h. The argument for extubation early in this period has been presented earlier in this chapter. Thus, the sedative technique in this group must permit deep sedation that can be rapidly and reliably reversed to permit extubation. Both midazolam and propofol have been studied in this context, although the wide variety of dose regimens and preceding anaesthetic techniques makes comparison difficult. The results of studies by Grounds et al. (1987) and McMurray (1989) are, however, entirely in keeping with our own experience. Following awakening from an anaesthetic based on fentanyl (50 μg/kg) patients were sedated with either intermittent bolus doses of midazolam or by an infusion of propofol. Many workers prefer to administer midazolam in this way rather than by infusion because of the unpredictable elimination half-life even in normal patients. A comparison of times to extubation following discontinuation of sedation is shown in Table 12.3. The rapid and predictable recovery following even prolonged sedation with propofol is so impressive that it is likely to replace midazolam for the majority of patients having uneventful cardiac surgery.

TABLE 12.3

Recovery characteristics of propofol and midazolam following cardiac surgery

| Authors | Sedative and dose (μg/kg per min) Mean (S.E.M.) | | Time from stopping infusion to extubation (min) Mean (S.E.M.) | *P* value |
|---|---|---|---|---|
| McMurray (1989) | Propofol<br>Midazolam | 19.2 (1.2)<br>0.56 (0.03) | 7.46 (1.14)<br>125 (1.1) | <0.001 |
| Grounds et al. (1987) | Propofol<br>Midazolam | 13.13 (1.03)<br>0.27 (0.029) | 24.9 (2.97)<br>226.1 (22.8) | <0.001 |

The second group of patients to be considered are those with low cardiac output states following surgery. They may be receiving a number of inotropes, vasodilators and even intra-aortic balloon counterpulsation. The recovery period of these patients is likely to be prolonged and so the rapid reversibility is of less importance than the haemodynamic stability of the sedative technique. Muscle relaxants are frequently used in this group, both to reduce the work of breathing and to prevent shivering. The onset of shivering can cause a doubling of the whole body oxygen requirement (Guffin et al., 1987) which may have a catastrophic effect on the already compromised myocardium. The liberal use of relaxants therefore requires as deep a level of sedation as is compatable with haemodynamic stability. The best technique in this context is unclear, but will usually be based on an opioid infusion. Whilst Kenny et al. (1989) found a greater tendency to hypotension with propofol used as an adjuvant, Snellen et al. (1989) found that both midazolam and propofol had similar haemodynamic effects. The very low effective dose of propofol and the absence of the requirement to administer a bolus dose appears to attenuate any adverse haemodynamic effect of the drug (Morgan, 1989). Nonetheless, great care is required with the administration of any sedative agents to this group and insufficient data is available to strongly recommend any particular technique.

The third group are those patients with chronic respiratory failure. The initial acute haemodynamic problems have resolved and they generally have little requirement for inotropic support. Many weeks may be spent in weaning these patients from the ventilator. The aim is to maintain patients in a rouseable non-complaining condition with relief of pain, anxiety and the restoration of a natural sleep pattern. The administration of sedative agents should be minimised, although short acting agents such as propofol can be used to assist periods of sleep at appropriate times. The philosophy of sedation for the long stay intensive care patient has been recently reviewed more fully by Wallace (1989).

The introducton of short acting drugs such as propofol has significantly improved the quality of sedation following cardiac surgery. Further studies are currently underway to establish the safety of this drug when infused over longer periods of time.

# REFERENCES


Blacher, R.S. (1975) On awakening paralysed during surgery: a syndrome of traumatic neurosis. *J. Am. Med. Assoc.* 234, 67—68.

Bovill, J.G., Sebel, P.S. and Blackburn, C.L. (1984) The pharmacokinetics of sufentanil in surgical patients. *Anesthesiology* 61, 502—506.

Bovill, J.G. and Sebel, P.S. (1980) Pharmacokinetics of high dose fentanyl. A study of patients undergoing cardiac surgery. *Br. J. Anaesth.* 52, 795—801.

Cahalan, M.K., Prakash, O. and Rulf, E.N.R. (1986) Does nitrous oxide induce myocardial ischaemia in patients with ischaemic heart disease? *Anesthesiology* 65, A514.

Cockshott, I.D., Douglas, E.J., Prys-Roberts, C., Turtle, M. and Coates, D.P. (1987) Pharmacokinetics of propofol during and after i.v. infusion in man. *Br. J. Anaesth.* 59, 941P.

Camu, F., Gepps, E. and Rucquoi, M. (1982) The pharmacokinetics of alfentanil in man. *Anesth. Analg.* 61, 647—661.

De Lange, S. and de Bruijn, N.P. (1983) Alfentanil oxygen anesthesia. Plasma concentrations and clinical effects during variable rate continuous infusion for coronary artery surgery. *Br. J. Anaesth.* 55, 183—189(s).

De Lange, Boscoe, M.J., Stanley, T.H. and Pace, N. (1982) Comparison of sufentanil oxygen and fentanyl oxygen for coronary artery surgery. *Anesthesiology* 56, 112—118.

Edde, R. (1981) Hemodynamic changes prior to and after sternotomy in patients anesthetised with high dose fentanyl. *Anesthesiology* 55, 444—446.

Evans, J.M., Bithell, J. and Vlachonikolis, I. (1987) Relationship between lower oesophageal contractility, clinical signs and halothane concentration during general anaesthesia and surgery in man. *Br. J. Anaesth.* 59, 1346—1355.

Eisele, V., Weinreich, A. and Bartles, S. (1976) Perioperative awareness and recall. *Anesth. Analg.* 55, 513—518.

Flezzani, P., Alvis, M.J., Jacobs, J.R., Schilling, M.M., Bai, S. and Reeves, J.G. (1987) Sufentanil disposition during cardiopulmonary bypass. *Can. J. Anaesth.* 34 (6) 566—569.

Goldman, L., Shah, M.V. and Hebden, M.W. (1987) Memory of cardiac anaesthesia. *Anaesthesia* 42, 596—603.

Grounds, R.M., Lalor, J.M., Royston, D. and Morgan, M. (1987) Propofol infusion for sedation in the intensive care unit: preliminary report. *Br. Med. J.* 294, 397—400.

Guffin, A., Girard, D. and Kaplan, J.A. (1987) Shivering following cardiac surgery: haemodynamic changes and reversal. *J. Cardiothor. Anaesth.* 1 (1), 24—28.

Hatano, S., Keane, D.M. and Boggs, R.E. (1976) Diazepam ketamine anaesthesia for open heart surgery: a micro-mini drip administration technique. *Can. Anaesth. Soc. J.* 3, 648—656.

Heikkila, H., Jalonen, J., Arola, M., Kanto, J. and Laaksonen, V. (1984) Midazolam as an adjunct to high dose fentanyl anaesthesia for coronary artery bypass grafting operations. *Acta Anaesthesiol. Scand.* 28, 683—689.

Hecker, B.R., Lake, C.L., DiFazio, C.O., Mascicki, J.C. and Engles, J.S. (1983) Decrease in minimal alveolar concentration produced by sufentanil in rats. *Anesth. Analg.* 62, 987—990.

Hilgenberg, J.C. (1981) Intraoperative awareness during high dose fentanyl oxygen anesthesia. *Anesthesiology* 54, 341—344.

Holley, F.O., Stanski, D.R. and Ponganis, K.V. (1982) Effect of cardiopulmonary bypass on the pharmacokinetics of drugs. *Clin. Pharmacokinet.* 7, 234—251.

Howie, M.B., McSweeny, T.D. and Lingham, R.P. (1985) A comparison of fentanyl oxygen and sufentanil oxygen anesthesia for cardiac anesthesia. *Anesth. Analg.* 64, 877—887.

Hug, C.C. Jr, Hall, R.I., Angert, K.C., Reeder, D.A. and Moldenhauer, C.C. (1988) Alfentanil plasma concentration versus effect relationship in cardiac surgical patients. *Br. J. Anaesth.* 61 (4), 435—440.

Hug, C.C. and Moldenhauer, C. (1982) Pharmacokinetics and dynamics of fentanyl infusions in cardiac surgical patients. *Anesthesiology* 57, A45.

Hynynen, M., Takkunen, O., Salmenpera, M., Haataja, H. and Heinonen, J. (1986) Continuous infusions of fentanyl or alfentanil for coronary artery surgery. *Br. J. Anaesth.* 58, 1252—1259.

Jaffe, T.B. and Ramsey, F.M. (1983) Attenuation of fentanyl induced truncal rigidity. *Anesthesiology* 58, 562—564.

Kearse, L.A. and Fahmy, N.R. (1989) The electroencephalographic effects of propofol anaesthesia in humans: a comparison with thiopental/enflurane. *Anesthesiology* 71 (34), A121.

Kenny, G.N.C. and Chaudri, S. (1989) Investigation of propofol sedation following cardiac bypass surgery. *J. Drug Dev.* 2 (Suppl. 2), 125—126.

Kingston, H.G.G., Bretherton, K.W. and Holloway, A.M. (1978) Comparison between ketamine and diazepam as induction agents for pericardiectomy. *Anaesth. Intensive Care* 6, 66—70.

Knight, A.A., Hollenberg, M. and London, M.J. (1988) Perioperative myocardial ischaemia: importance of preoperative ischaemic pattern. *Anesthesiology* 68, 681—688.

Kolkka, R. and Hilberman, N. (1980) Neurologic dysfunction following cardiac operations with low flow, low pressure cardiopulmonary bypass. *J. Cardiothor. Surg.* 79, 432—437.

Larsen, J.A. (1971) The effect of cooling on liver function in cats. *Acta Physiol. Scand.* 81, 197—207.

Lebowitz, P.W., Ramsey, F.M. and Savarese, J.J. (1980) Potentiation of neuromuscular blockade in man produced by the combination of pancuronium and metocurine or pancuronium and *d*-tubocurarine. *Anesth. Analg.* 59, 604—609

Ledingham, I. and Watt, I. (1983) Influence of sedation on mortality of critically ill trauma patients. *Lancet* 1, 1270.

Lepage, J.-Y., Pinaud, M.L., Helias, J.H., Juge, C.M., Cozian, A.Y. and Farinotti, R. (1988) Left ventricular function during fentanyl and propofol anaesthesia in patients with coronary artery disease. Assessment with a radionuclide approach. *Anesth. Analg.* 67, 949—955.

Lowenstein, E., Hallowell, P. and Levine, F.H. (1969) Cardiovascular responses to large doses of intravenous morphine in man. *N. Engl. J. Med.* 281, 1389—1393.

Lunn, J., Stanley, T. and Eisele, J. (1979) High dose fentanyl anesthesia for coronary artery surgery. *Anesth. Analg.* 58, 390—395.

Mark, J.B. and Greenberg, L.M. (1983) Intraoperative awareness and hypertensive crisis during high dose fentanyl diazepam anesthesia. *Anesth. Analg.* 62, 689—700.

Marty, J., Nitenberg, A., Blanchet, F., Zouioueche, S. and Desmonts, J.M. (1986) Effects of midazolam on the coronary circulation in patients with coronary artery disease. *Anesthesiology* 64, 206—210

McMurray, T.J. (1989) Propofol sedation following open heart surgery — a clinical and pharmacokinetic study. *J. Drug Dev.* 2 (2) 131—132.

Michenfelder, J.D. (1974) The interdependence of cerebral function and metabolic effects following massive doses of thiopental in the dog. *Anesthesiology* 41, 231—236.

Michenfelder, J.D. and Milde, J.H. (1975) Influence of anaesthetics on metabolic, functional and pathological response to regional cerebral ischaemia. *Stroke* 6, 405—410.

Mora, C.T., Dudek, C., Epstein, R.H. and White, P.F. (1989) Cardiac anesthesia techniques. Fentanyl alone or in combination with enflurane or propofol. *Anesth. Analg.* 68, S202.

Morgan, D.J., Crankshaw, D.P., Prideaux, P.R., Chan, H.N.J. and Boyd, M.D. (1986) Thiopentone levels during cardiopulmonary bypass. *Anesthesia* 41, 4—10.

Morgan, M. (1989) Post cardiac surgery sedation. *J. Drug Dev.* 2 (Suppl. 2), 119—124.

Morris, R.B., Cahalan, M.K., Miller, R.D., Wilkinson, P.L., Quasha, A.L. and Robinson, S.L. (1983) The cardiovascular effects of vecuronium (ORG NC45) and pancuronium in patients undergoing coronary artery bypass grafting. *Anesthesiology* 58, 438—440.

Mummaneni, N., Rao, T.L.K. and Montoya, A. (1980) Awareness and recall with high dose fentanyl anesthesia. *Anesth. Analg.* 59, 948—949.

Nussmier, N.A., Arlund, C. and Slogoff, S. (1986) Neuropsychiatric complications following cardiopulmonary bypass. Cerebral protection by a barbiturate. *Anesthesiology* 64, 165—170.

Oduro, A., Tomlinson, A.A., Voice, A. and Davies, G.K. (1983) The use of etomidate infusions during anaesthesia for cardiopulmonary bypass. *Anaesthesia* 38, 66—69.

Patrick, M.R., Blair, I.J., Fenek, R.O. and Sebel, P.S. (1985) The comparison of the haemodynamic effects of propofol and thiopentone in patients with coronary artery disease. *Postgrad. Med. J.* 61, 23—27.

Perrson, P.M., Nilsson, A. and Hartvig, P. (1988) Relation of sedation and amnesia to plasma concentrations of midazolam in surgical patients. *Clin. Pharmacol. Ther.* 43 (3), 324—331.

Philbin, D.M., Machaj, V.R. and Tomichek, R.C. (1983) Hemodynamic effect of bolus injection of atracurium in patients with coronary artery disease. *Br. J. Anaesth.* 55, 131S.

Pokar, H. and Brandt, L. (1983) Haemodynamic effects of atracurium in patients after cardiac surgery. *Br. J. Anaesth.* 55 (Suppl. 1), 139S.

Quasha, A.L., Loeber, N., Feeley, T.W., Ulyot, D.J. and Roisen, M. (1980) Postoperative respiratory care: a controlled trial of early and late extubation following coronary artery bypass grafting. *Anesthesiology* 52, 135—141.

Raza, S.M.A., Masters, R.W., Vasireddy, A.R. and Zsigmond, E.K. (1988) Haemodynamic stability with midazolam-sufentanil analgesia in cardiac surgical patients. *Can. J. Anaesth.* 5, 518—525.

Reiz, S., Balfors, E., Sorensen, M.B., Ariala, S., Friedman, A. and Truedsson, H. (1983) Isoflurane — a powerful coronary vasodilator in patients with coronary artery disease. *Anesthesiology* 59, 91—97.

Robbins, R.G., Wynands, J.E., Whalley, D.G., Donnaty, F., Ramsay, J.G., Srikant, C.B. and Patel, Y.C. (1990) Pharmacokinetics of alfentanil and clinical responses during cardiac surgery. *Can. J. Anaesth.* 37 (1), 52—57.

Roberts, F.L., Dixon, J., Lewis, G.G.R., Tackley, R.M. and Prys-Roberts, C. (1988) Induction and maintenance of propofol anaesthesia. *Anaesthesia* 43(S), 14—17.

Russell, G.N., Wright, E.L., Fox, M.A., Douglas, E.J. and Cockshott, I.D. (1989) Propofol fentanyl anaesthesia for coronary artery surgery and cardiopulmonary bypass. *Anaesthesia* 44, 205—208.

Salmenpera, M., Peltola, K., Takkunen, O. and Heinonen, J. (1983) Cardiovascular effects of pancuronium and vecuronium during high dose fentanyl anesthesia. *Anesth. Analg.* 62, 1059—1064.

Samuelson, P.N., Reeves, J.G., Kirklin, J.K., Bradley, E., Wilson, K.D. and Adams, N. (1986) Comparison of sufentanil and enflurane $N_2O$ anesthesia for myocardial revascularisation. *Anesth. Analg.* 65, 217—226.

Sanford, T.J., Smith, N.T., Dec-Silver, H. and Harrison, W.K. (1986) A comparison of morphine, fentanyl and sufentanil anesthesia for cardiac surgery. *Anesth. Analg.* 65, 259—266.

Schweiger, I., Bailey, J. and Hug, C.C. (1989) Anesthetic interaction of computer controlled and constant infusions of fentanyl and midazolam for cardiac surgery. *Anesthesiology* 71(3A), A305.

Silvay, G., Salter, O., Grossbarth, D., Ostapkovich, N. and Kaplan, J.A. (1989) Depth of anaesthesia during hypothermic cardiopulmonary bypass. *Anesthesiology* 71(3A), A284.

Slogoff, S.T., Girgis, K.Z. and Keats, A.S. (1982) Etiologic factors in neuropsychiatric complications associated with cardiopulmonary bypass. *Anesth. Analg.* 61, 903—911.

Slogoff, S. and Keats, A.S. (1985) Does perioperative myocardlal ischaemia lead to postoperative myocardial infarction? *Anesthesiology* 62, 107—114.

Slogoff, S. and Keats, A.S. (1989) Randomised trial of primary anaesthetic agent on outcome of coronary bypass operations. *Anesthesiology* 70, 179—188.

Smith, A.L., Hoff, J.T., Nielsen, S.L. and Larson, C.P. (1974) Barbiturate protection in acute focal cerebral ischaemia. *Stroke* 5, 127—131.

Snellen, F.T.F., Demeyere, R., Mulier, J.P. and Lauwers, P. (1989) A comparison of propofol and midazolam for short term sedation after coronary artery bypass graft. *J. Drug Dev.* (Suppl. 2), 139—140.

Snyder, S.H. (1977) Opiate receptors and internal opiates. *Sci. Am.* 236, 44—56.

Speiss, B.D., Sathoff, R.H., el Ganzouri, A.R. and Ivankovich, A.D. (1986) High dose sufentanil: four cases of sudden hypotension on induction. *Anesth. Analg.* 65 (6), 703—705.

Sprigge, J.S., Wynands, J.E., Whalley, D.G., Bevan, D.R., Townsend, G.E., Nathan, H., Patel, Y.C. and Srikant, C.B. (1982) Fentanyl infusion anesthesia for aortocoronary bypass surgery. Plasma levels and hemodynamic response. *Anesth. Analg.* 61, 972—978.

Stanley, T.H. and Webster, L.R. (1978) Anesthetic requirements and cardiovascular effects of fentanyl oxygen and fentanyl diazepam anesthesia in man. *Anesth. Analg.* 57, 411—416.

Szenohradsky, J., Marosi, G. and Keresz, A. (1982) Clinical experience with pipecuronium bromide. *Sixth European Congress of Anaesthesiologists,* London.

Thomas, D. and Evans, J.M. (1989) Lower oesophageal contractility monitoring during anaesthesia for cardiac surgery: preliminary observations. *Ann. R. Coll. Surg. Engl.* 71, 311—315.

Tuman, K.J., McCarthy, R.J. and Spiess, B.D. (1989) Does choice of anaesthetic agent significantly affect outcome after coronary artery surgery? *Anesthesiology* 70, 189—198.

Tuman, K.J., Keane, D.M., Spiess, B.D., McCarthy, R.J., Silins, A.I. and Ivankovich, A.D. (1988) Effects of high dose fentanyl on fluid and vasopressor requirements after cardiac surgery. *J. Cardiothor. Anesth.* 2 (4), 419—429.

Valicenti, J.F., Newman, W.H. and Bagwell, E.E. (1973) Myocardial contractility during induction and maintenance of steady state ketamine anaesthesia. *Anesth. Analg.* 52, 190—194.

Vermeyen, K.M., Erpels, F.A., Janssen, L.A., Beechman, C.P. and Hanegreefs, G.H. (1987) Propofol fentanyl anaesthesia for coronary bypass surgery in patients with good left ventricular function. *Br. J. Anaesth.* 59, 1115—1120.

Viby-Mogensen, J., Jorgenson, B.C. and Engback, J. (1980) On Org NC45 and halothane anaesthesia. Preliminary results. *Br. J. Anaesth.*, 52 (Suppl. 1), 67S.

Wagner, R.L., White, P.F. and Kan, P.B. (1984) Inhibition of adrenal steriodogenesis by the anaesthetic etomidate. *N. Engl. J. Med.* 310, 1415—1421.

Wallace, P.G.M. (1989) Sedation in intensive care — current practice. *J. Drug Dev.* 2 (Suppl. 2), 9—14.

Wilkowski, D.A.W., Sill, J.C. and Bonta, W. (1987) Nitrous oxide constricts epicardial coronary arteries without effect on coronary arterioles. *Anesthesiology* 66, 659—665.

Wood, M. (1986) Plasma drug binding: implications for anesthesiologists. *Anesth. Analg.* 65, 786—804.

Wynands, J.E., Townsend, G.E., Wong, P., Whalley, D.G., Srikant, C.B. and Patel, Y.C. (1983). Blood pressure response and plasma fentanyl concentrations during high and very high dose fentanyl anesthesia for coronary artery surgery. *Anesth. Analg.* 62, 661—665.

Wynands, J.E., Wong, P., Townsends, G.E., Sprigge, J.S. and Whalley, D.G. (1984) Narcotic requirements for intravenous anesthesia. *Anesth. Analg.* 63, 101—105.

Wong, K.C. (1983) Narcotics are not expected to produce unconsciousness and amnesia. *Anesth. Analg.* 62, 625—626.

B. Kay (ed.) Total Intravenous Anaesthesia



# 13

# *Total intravenous anaesthesia and sedation for neurosurgery*

Edward Moss

## INTRODUCTION

The ideal anaesthetic agent for intracranial surgery would reduce brain bulk and intracranial pressure (ICP) and reduce cerebral metabolic rate giving some protection against ischaemic brain damage. Intravenous anaesthetics such as barbiturates, etomidate and propofol cause a reduction in cerebral metabolic rate, cerebral vasoconstriction and a reduction in brain bulk and ICP, whereas volatile agents cause cerebral vasodilation and an increase in ICP. Thus intravenous anaesthetics have theoretical advantages for induction and maintenance of anaesthesia for intracranial surgery, and for sedation and control of ICP on the intensive therapy unit. Hunter (1972a,b) first described the use of intravenous infusions of thiopentone and methohexitone for maintenance of anaesthesia during neurosurgery and since then neuroanaesthetists have searched for an agent which has similar effects on the cranial contents but is less cumulative than thiopentone and methohexitone.

Althesin was such an agent and proved useful until its withdrawal by the manufacturers. Etomidate was also used until its effect on adrenocortical function was recognised and now propofol is being used increasingly in this area.

This chapter will detail the theoretical background to the use of total intravenous anaesthesia in intracranial surgery, including discussion of the physiology and pathophysiology of the cranial contents, the anaesthetic requirements for intracranial surgery, the known effects of the available anaesthetic agents, both intravenous and inhaled, on the contents of the cranium, the advantages and disadvantages of total intravenous anaesthesia and the clinical and experimental experience of the use of intravenous anaesthetic techniques. The final section will discuss the use of intravenous sedation for neurosurgical patients.

## Physiology of the cranial contents

The adult cranium forms an almost rigid container which is in direct communication with the vertebral canal. It contains about 1400 g of brain, 130 ml of arterial and venous blood and 75 ml of cerebrospinal fluid (CSF). CSF is formed mainly in the choroid plexuses, which are present in all four ventricles, at a rate of about 0.4 ml/min. It is formed by active secretion with transependymal water following the pumping of sodium. CSF production is reduced by sympathetic stimulation and metabolic or respiratory alkalosis. CSF is mainly reabsorbed into the blood at the arachnoid villi; a process which is mechanical and depends on the pressure gradient between the CSF and the blood in the venous sinuses.

A change in volume of any one of the intracranial contents must lead to a change in ICP unless compensatory changes in the volumes of the other constituents occur. Under normal circumstances compensation occurs and returns ICP to normal. The compensatory mechanisms include a reduction in intracranial

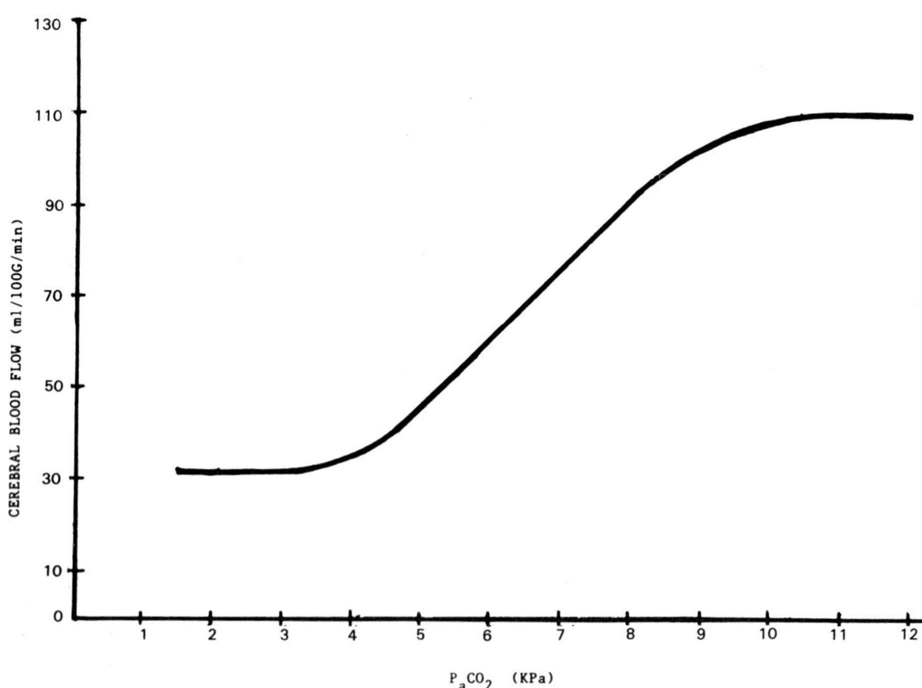


Fig. 13.1. The effects of changes in arterial carbon dioxide tension ($PaCO_2$) on cerebral blood flow.

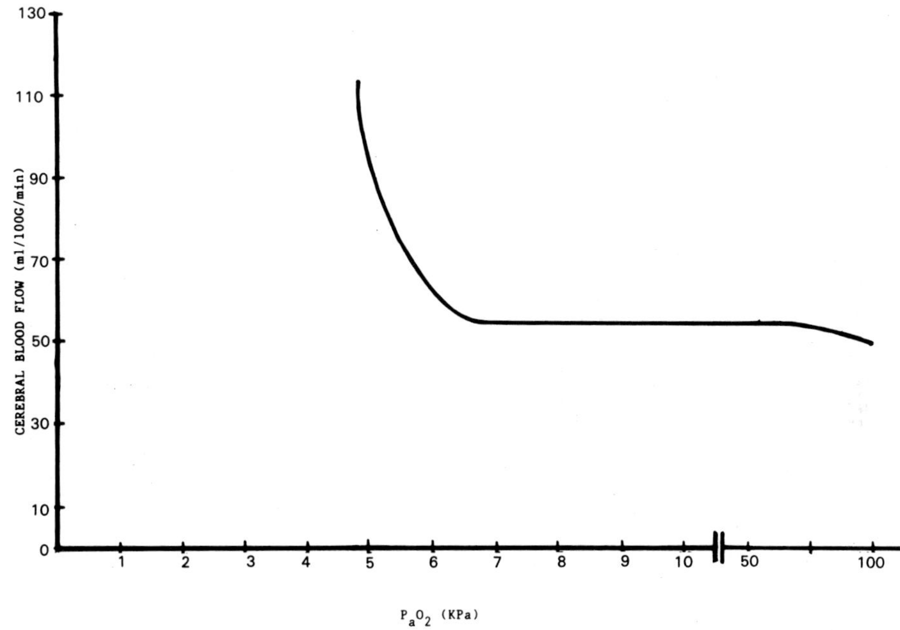


Fig. 13.2. The effect of changes in arterial oxygen tension ($PaO_2$) on cerebral blood flow.

blood volume due to the pressure exerted by the CSF on the thin-walled cerebral veins, displacement of CSF into the spinal subarachnoid space and increased reabsorption of CSF. There is a linear relationship between changes in cerebral blood flow (CBF) and cerebral blood volume (CBV) and an increase in CBV will lead to an increase in ICP because the volume of one of the contents of the non-expansile cranium has increased.

Changes in arterial blood gas tensions lead to alterations in CBF and ICP (Figs. 13.1 and 13.2). CBF is very sensitive to changes in $PaCO_2$ with hypocapnia causing a reduction and hypercapnia causing an increase in CBF. The relationship appears to be linear over the physiological range (3.3 to 7.3 kPa) with a levelling off at very low and very high $PaCO_2$ values (Thoresen and Walloe, 1980). No further increase in CBF occurs at a $PaCO_2$ of 10.6 kPa when CBF is increased to about 100% above normocapnic levels and very little further decrease occurs at $PaCO_2$ values below 2.6 kPa, at which values CBF is reduced to about 40% of normocapnic levels. The reduction in ICP associated with hypocapnia is a temporary effect lasting only 30 to 60 min because reduced reabsorption of CSF returns the volume of the cranial contents to normal. However, the longer lasting

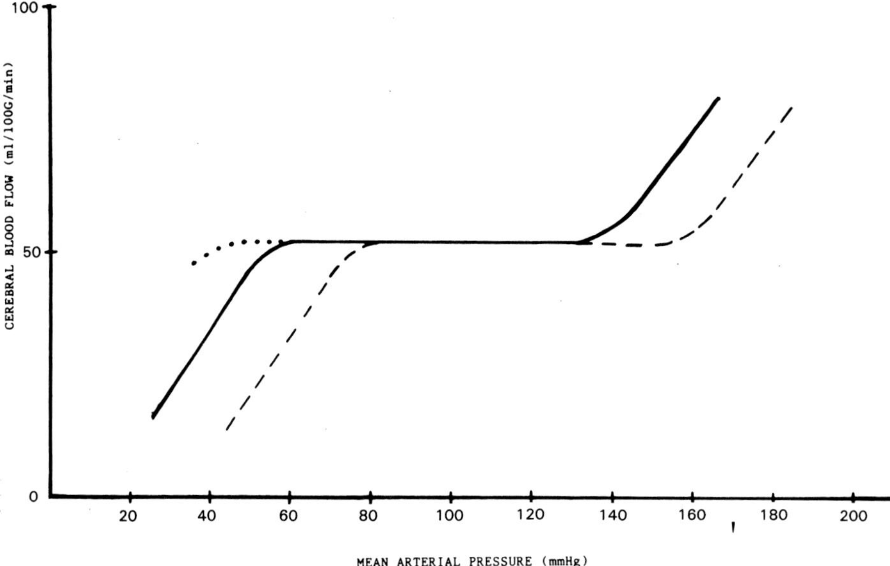


Fig. 13.3. Autoregulation of the cerebral circulation. ———, the autoregulation curve in normotensive man; - - - -, the autoregulation curve in hypertensive patients; · · · ·, demonstrates the effect of agents which dilate the cerebral vessels, such as halothane or sodium nitroprusside, on the lower limit of autoregulation. The reduction of cerebral blood flow is less when mean arterial pressure (MAP) is reduced below the lower limit of autoregulation by vasodilator drugs than when hypovolaemia reduces MAP.

reduction in CBV tends to produce good neurosurgical operating conditions. During prolonged hyperventilation the CSF, pH and CBF of normal brain return to normal over a period of from 6 h to 2 days. Damaged brain may react differently but Christensen et al.(1973) showed that during controlled hyperventilation in patients with stroke the CSF, pH and ICP had returned to normal after 30 h. Hypoxia causes an increase in CBF but not until the $PaO_2$ falls below 6.7 kPa (McDowall, 1966) (Fig. 13.1). At a $PaO_2$ of about 4.7 kPa CBF is nearly doubled (Cohen et al., 1968). Hyperoxia causes a reduction in CBF but this does not occur until the $FIO_2$ exceeds 0.8 (McDowall, 1966). It follows that the combination of hypoxia and hypercapnia is bad for the brain and should be avoided during intracranial surgery.

In normotensive man autoregulation maintains cerebral blood flow at 50 to 55 ml/100 g brain tissue per min, between mean arterial blood pressure (MAP) values of approximately 60 and 130 mmHg (Fig. 13.3). Above and below these limits

CBF becomes pressure passive. Hypertension shifts the curve to the right. CBF also autoregulates in response to increasing levels of ICP. Therefore, the cerebral circulation autoregulates to a change in cerebral perfusion pressure (CPP) which is defined as MAP − ICP because the pressure in the superficial cerebral veins must always be greater than ICP or they would collapse. If the jugular venous pressure (JVP) is higher than ICP (for example, when the patient is in the Trendelenberg position) JVP needs to be substituted for ICP in the above equation. However, situations where the JVP is raised are deliberately avoided during intracranial surgery. Autoregulation to a change in CPP is not immediate and a sudden increase in MAP may overcome autoregulation temporarily, while the same elevation occurring more slowly does not overcome autoregulation (Lassen and Agnoli, 1972). An increase in MAP above the autoregulation limit may cause distension of the cerebral arterioles and a large increase in CBF causing an increase in hydrostatic pressure in the capillaries and venules, focal disruption of the blood-brain barrier and oedema formation. If the blood pressure increase is abrupt it may cause dysfunction of the blood-brain barrier and cerebral oedema even when the change is within the limits of autoregulation. If autoregulation is impaired or abolished such damage could occur with less pronounced pressure changes. The upper limit of autoregulation may be lowered in the early stages of development of brain pathology, thus acute hypertension due to anaesthetic agents, laryngoscopy and intubation or surgical stimulation should be avoided during neurosurgical anaesthesia. Autoregulation is lost at a $PaCO_2$ value of 9 to 12 kPa and may be restored by hypocapnia. Autoregulation is impaired by hypoxia and is lost altogether with very severe hypoxia ($PaO_2 < 3.3$ kPa).

Stimulation of the sympathetic nerves supplying the cerebral vessels causes cerebral vasoconstriction and a reduction in CBV of no more than 10% (Harper et al., 1972). So anaesthetic agents with effects on the sympathetic nervous system may alter CBF.

Factors which alter nerve cell activity will alter CBF. Local changes in activity will produce local changes in CBF with no effect on global CBF, but factors which increase the overall metabolic activity in the brain will cause a global increase in CBF. Convulsions cause an increase in CBF and hypothermia decreases $CMRO_2$, CBF and ICP. Arousal and associated catecholamine release in the brain, due to pain and anxiety, induce marked increases in CBF and $CMRO_2$.

Changes in central venous pressure (CVP) or intrathoracic pressure can affect ICP by two mechanisms. Firstly, the increased pressure may be transmitted through the jugular and vertebral veins, thus increasing cerebral venous pressure, CBV and ICP. Secondly, the pressure may be transmitted to the epidural veins in the thoracic vertebral canal; the distension of these veins may elevate spinal CSF pressure and displace CSF from the spinal to the cranial compartment. The latter mechanism is probably the most important, particularly during rapid changes in intrathoracic pressure, for example, during coughing.

## The pathophysiology of the cranial contents

### *Effects of high ICP*

There is no evidence that increased hydrostatic pressure due to raised ICP has a direct effect on neuronal function or the structural integrity of the brain. A high ICP can have detrimental effects on the brain by two mechanisms. Firstly, it may cause a reduction in CPP which, in the absence of a compensatory increase in MAP, may cause cerebral ischaemia. Secondly, high ICP may cause brain shift through the foramen magnum, tentorium cerebelli or across the midline. Repeated insults to the brain in the form of elevations of ICP ultimately impair autoregulation, even if none of the individual increases in pressure has been suffi-

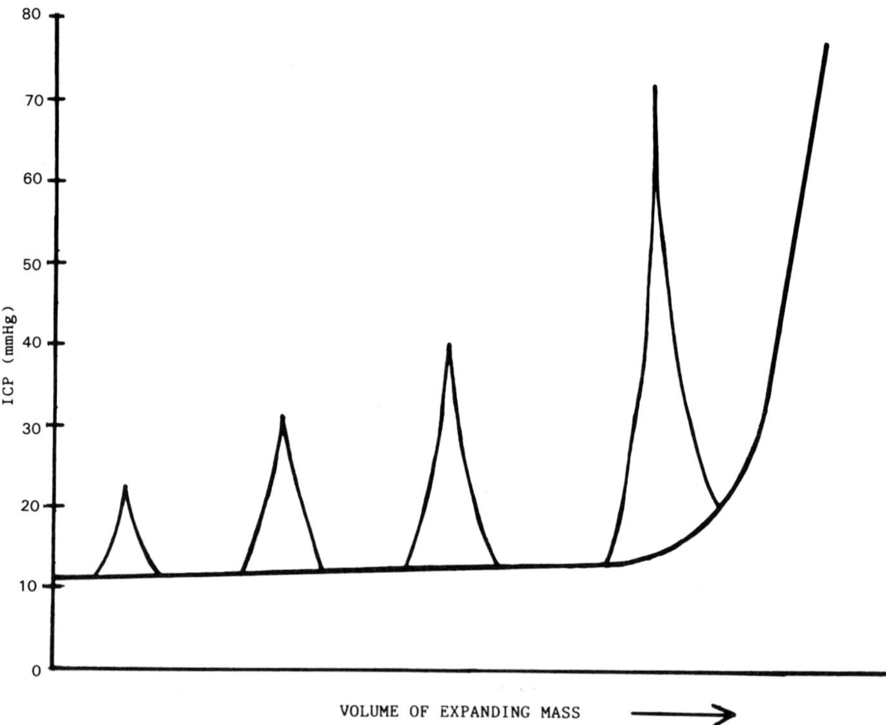


Fig. 13.4. The pressure volume curve of the cranial contents adapted from McDowall. As an intracranial mass expands ICP remains fairly constant until the compensatory mechanisms are exhausted when there is a steep increase in ICP. The isolated peaks of pressure increase represent the administration of an agent, such as halothane, which causes cerebral vasodilation. At the left hand end of the curve the resultant small increment in cerebral blood volume has a fairly small effect on ICP with a return to normal within a short time, but as the compensatory mechanisms are used up and the intracranial compliance is reduced the effect of the cerebral vasodilator on ICP increases.

cient to cause cerebral ischaemia (Miller et al., 1973) and if autoregulation is impaired an increase in ICP will cause a fall in CBF. Locally expanding mass lesions may affect local CBF by producing local tissue pressure differentials.

*The pressure volume curve*

The pressure volume curve of the cranial contents describes the ICP changes associated with increasing the volume of one of the cranial contents (Fig. 13.4) Due to compensation for the change in volume of the expanding mass the pressure remains fairly constant until the compensatory mechanisms are exhaused and there is a steep rise in pressure. An increase in CBV, for example, due to halothane administration will have little effect on ICP when the cranial contents are at the left hand end of the curve, but may cause a steep increase when the compliance is reduced at the right hand end of the curve. Most patients with intracranial pathology are on the flat compensated part of the pressure volume curve, though they are at various stages on the way to exhaustion of the compensatory reserve. It is only at a very late stage that patients reach the steep section of the curve and ICP rises rapidly. At this stage there is cerebral vasomotor paralysis with loss of both autoregulation and responsiveness to $PaCO_2$ changes and ICP follows the arterial pressure passively.

*Brain shift*

When a space-occupying lesion expands, the local tissue pressure around it is greater than the pressure in other areas of the brain. Such pressure gradients will tend to cause brain shifts. Actual shift of brain tissue may cause brain damage by direct effects on brain tissue, will cause distortion of the local blood supply and may cause obstruction of cerebral venous drainage by kinking the cortical veins as they enter the venous sinuses.

*Effects of disease on cerebrovascular control*

Impairment of autoregulation, which may be global or localised, is found in patients with head injuries, ischaemic brain lesions, subarachnoid haemorrhage, during seizure activity and in patients with cerebral tumours except for meningiomas in which autoregulation is usually well preserved. Carbon dioxide reactivity is also altered in patients with intracranial pathology including severe head injury, cerebral tumours and subarachnoid haemorrhage. Cerebrovascular carbon dioxide reactivity can also be significantly impaired in hypertensive patients and diabetics. Acute brain injury tends to affect autoregulation first and all vasomotor control later.

Focal loss of autoregulation and carbon dioxide reactivity in the region of a cerebral tumour, infarct or area of cerebral oedema may lead to intracerebral steal when there is cerebral vasodilation in normal brain tissue. This is a paradoxical decrease in flow through a damaged region when CBF through normal brain is increased, for example by an increase in $PaCO_2$ or halothane. Conversely, cerebral vasoconstriction due to hypocapnia will cause inverse intracerebral steal, increasing flow through the damaged region. However, hypocapnia does not always improve the blood supply to an area of focal cerebral ischaemia. If the lesion is receiving a collateral blood supply from vessels which are still sensitive to carbon dioxide, hypocapnia may reduce the blood flow to the ischaemic area.

### *Cerebral oedema*

Cerebral oedema is common after head injury and surgery on the brain. The commonest form is vasogenic cerebral oedema, which is caused by injury to the walls of the cerebral blood vessels damaging the blood brain barrier and leading to the escape of water and plasma constituents into the surrounding parenchyma. The driving force for the extravasation of fluid is the capillary transmural pressure gradient, so that an acute increase in the arterial pressure results in a dramatic increase in oedema formation. Hypoxic damage to brain cells causes cytotoxic cerebral oedema which directly affects the structural elements of the parenchyma, producing intracellular swelling, whilst vascular permeability remains relatively undisturbed. Osmotic diuretics will help in the treatment of cytotoxic cerebral oedema by reducing cellular oedema, but in vasogenic cerebral oedema avoidance of agents which cause cerebral vasodilation, control of hypertension, hyperventilation and possibly steroid therapy or the use of intravenous anaesthetic agents which cause cerebral vasoconstriction should prove to be more effective. Thus intravenous anaesthetic agents have properties which will help in the reduction of vasogenic cerebral oedema.

## ANAESTHETIC REQUIREMENTS FOR INTRACRANIAL SURGERY

During intracranial surgery the neuroanaesthetist uses this understanding of the physiology and pathophysiology of the cranial contents and aims to maintain a constant CPP by avoiding a marked reduction in MAP or an increase in ICP. Marked surges in arterial pressure may temporarily overcome normal cerebrovascular autoregulation and must be avoided because they initiate or increase cerebral oedema by increasing the pressure in the cerebral capillary bed. High ICP may have detrimental effects on the brain by reducing CPP or causing brain shift (see above) and avoidance of high ICP is essential when the cranium is still intact. When the dura mater is open, ICP decreases to zero so that CPP depends only on MAP, but herniation of the brain through the craniotomy defect will occur if ICP is high at the time of incision of the dura. Lesser degrees of increased brain bulk, and thus ICP lead to an increased pressure under the brain retractor which hinders the surgeon and increases brain trauma due to ischaemia.

Therefore, during intracranial surgery, the neuroanaesthetist keeps changes in brain bulk and ICP to a minimum by reducing $PaCO_2$, avoiding increases in CVP (by preventing the patient from coughing and straining, by careful positioning and by avoiding excessive inflation pressures or fluid overload), avoiding marked increases or decreases in arterial pressure and making appropriate choices of anaesthetic agents. The neurosurgeon may request a reduced arterial pressure at certain stages of the operation, to reduce bleeding from a vascular tumour or arteriovenous malformation or to reduce the tension in an aneurysm sac. A degree of cerebral protection against ischaemia is desirable during such periods of induced hypotension. Convulsions are detrimental because they cause an increase in $CMRO_2$ and eventually an imbalance between cerebral oxygen supply and demand resulting in cerebral ischaemia.

**Effects of anaesthetic agents on the contents of the cranium**

Anaesthesia can be induced and maintained with volatile anaesthetic agents, anaesthetic gases or intravenous anaesthetics, often supplemented by opioid analgesics. A reduction in $PaCO_2$ causes a reduction in CBF and brain bulk and this is normally achieved during intracranial surgery by using muscle relaxants and mechanical ventilation. Cerebrovascular autoregulation protects the brain from the detrimental effects of changes in arterial pressure. Therefore, it is desirable for anaesthetic agents to have little or no effect on cerebral autoregulation or on the carbon dioxide reactivity of the cerebral vessels. Anaesthetic agents influence ICP mainly through effects on vessel calibre, either directly or indirectly by depressing ventilation and increasing $PaCO_2$. Hatano and colleagues (1989) have shown that thiobarbiturates induce contraction in isolated cerebral arteries, having a greater effect on intracerebral arteries than on extracerebral arteries, probably by causing an influx of calcium into the cells. A change in vessel calibre causes a change in CBF and CBV which alters the volume of the cranial contents and thus ICP. Agents which reduce $CMRO_2$ reduce CBF and ICP and may provide some protection against cerebral ischaemia. Anaesthetic agents may also alter ICP by changing the rate of production or absorption of CSF. The effects of the individual agents are discussed below and summarised in Table 13.1.

**Volatile anaesthetic agents**

All volatile anaesthetic agents have been shown to increase CBF and ICP and reduce $CMRO_2$. This represents an uncoupling of the usual relationship between cerebral metabolism and CBF and indicates that the volatile agents have a direct vasodilating effect on the cerebral vessels. The changes in ICP are greater in those with increased ICP than in normal patients, due to the nature of the pressure volume curve of the cranial contents in that cerebral vasodilation adds a volume increment to the cranium and the associated increase in ICP is gradually

TABLE 13.1

Summary of the effects of anaesthetic agents on the cranial contents

| Agent | $CMRO_2$ | CBF | ICP | $CO_2$ reactivity | Cerebral autoregulation |
|---|---|---|---|---|---|
| **Intravenous anaesthetics** | | | | | |
| Thiopentone | ↓ | ↓ | ↓ | — | — |
| Methohexitone | ↓ | ↓ | ↓ | — | — |
| Althesin | ↓ | ↓ | ↓ | — | — |
| Etomidate | ↓ | ↓ | ↓ | — | — |
| Propofol | ↓ | ↓ | ↓ | — | — |
| **Volatile anaesthetics** | | | | | |
| Halothane | ↓ | ↑ | ↑ | ↑ | I |
| Enflurane | ↓ | ↑ | ↑ | ↑ | I |
| Isoflurane | ↓ | ↑ | ↑ | ↑ | I |
| Sevoflurane | ? | ↑ | ↑ | ? | ? |
| **Anaesthetic gases** | | | | | |
| Nitrous oxide | ↑ | ↑ | ↑ | — | — |
| Cyclopropane | ? | ↑ | ↑ | ↑ | ? |
| **Opioids** | | | | | |
| Morphine | ? | — | — | ? | — |
| Phenoperidine | — | ?↑ | ?↑ | ? | ? |
| Fentanyl | — | — | — | ↑ | — |
| Alfentanil | — | — | — | ? | ? |
| Sufentanil | — | ↑ | ↑ | ? | ? |
| **Muscle relaxants** | | | | | |
| Suxamethonium | — | — | ↑ | ? | ? |
| Non-depolarising | — | — | — | ? | ? |
| **Other agents** | | | | | |
| Diazepam | ↓ | ↓ | — | — | ? |
| Lorazepam | ↓ | ↓ | ? | ? | ? |
| Midazolam | ↓ | ↓ | — | ? | ? |
| Droperidol | — | ↓ | — | ? | ? |
| Lignocaine | ↓ | ↓[a] | ↓ | ? | ? |
| Ketamine | ↑ | ↑ | ↑ | — | — |

↑, increased; ↓, decreased; I, impaired; —, no effect; ?, unknown.
[a]Very large doses.

accentuated as the contents become more compressed (Fig. 13.4). CPP is reduced by the volatile agents because they decrease MAP and increase ICP. Halothane causes the greatest increase in CBF and ICP and isoflurane the least. The responsiveness of the cerebral circulation to carbon dioxide is increased during halothane, cyclopropane and isoflurane anaesthesia.

*Halothane*

Halothane causes an increase in CBF and ICP. A 1.6 minimum alveolar concentration (MAC) halothane trebles CBF (Eger, 1981). It reduces $CMRO_2$ but does not appear to offer any cerebral protection, in fact high concentrations can induce cerebral acidosis (Michenfelder and Theye, 1975). In patients with elevated ICP marked increases in ICP can be prevented by hyperventilation for at least 10 min before halothane is introduced, but even this may not be successful if ICP is increased considerably and halothane is best avoided until the dura is opened and the patient is hypocapnic. Autoregulation is disturbed by halothane in concentration of 1% or more and may not return to normal for 2 h after discontinuation of the halothane. Halothane does not cause abnormal EEG activity.

*Enflurane*

The majority of investigations show that enflurane has less effect on CBF and ICP than halothane and the largest reported increases in ICP with enflurane are significantly smaller than those reported with halothane. Concentrations of 1 MAC have little effect on CBF and ICP and one study showed that in patients with cerebral tumours 2% enflurane did not cause an increase in ICP, but MAP was significantly reduced and may have masked any cerebral vasodilation caused by the enflurane (Moss et al., 1983a). Like halothane, enflurane reduces $CMRO_2$. In concentrations of up to 1.5 MAC enflurane causes high voltage slow waves and hypersynchrony on the EEG but greater concentrations (>1.5 MAC) cause high amplitude spikes or spike and wave complexes, particularly during hypocapnia and auditory stimulation and this activity will increase $CMRO_2$ and CBF. However, enflurane is no more likely than isoflurane to cause convulsions after intracranial surgery (Christys et al., 1989). Enflurane increases the rate of production of CSF and decreases its absorption and these properties will contribute to the increase in ICP associated with its administration.

*Isoflurane*

Inspired concentrations of 0.6 to 1.1 MAC of isoflurane do not alter CBF in man, but 1.6 MAC isoflurane doubles CBF. ICP is similarly unaffected by isoflurane in concentrations of less than 1 MAC, but higher concentrations increase ICP (Gomez-Sainz et al., 1988). Isoflurane does not affect the rate of production or absorption of CSF. Isoflurane may enhance the carbon dioxide reactivity of the cerebral vessels which is maintained even when high concentrations are given (McPherson et al., 1989). Cerebral autoregulation is impaired significantly only by concentrations greater than 1 MAC (Van Aken et al., 1986). $CMRO_2$ is depressed to a greater extent with isoflurane than with halothane (Todd and Drummond, 1984) and progressive metabolic depression occurs with concentrations of isoflurane greater than 1 MAC until the EEG becomes isoelectric at approximately 2.5 MAC (Newberg et al., 1983). There is some evidence that isoflurane has a cerebral protective effect against ischaemia in man, but a study in primates showed that during profound hypotension isoflurane gave no more cerebral protection than halothane and sodium nitroprusside combined (Gelb et al., 1989). Isoflurane in concentrations up to 1.5 MAC has similar effects on the EEG to enflurane causing high voltage slow waves and hypersynchrony, but higher concentrations cause an isoelectric EEG. However, there are several case reports of convulsions occurring during or following isoflurane anaesthesia in patients who had not had fits previously.

### *Sevoflurane*

The limited amount of published work on sevoflurane in normocapnic animals indicates that, in concentrations of up to 1 MAC, it has a minimal effect on CBF and increases ICP very slightly (Scheller et al., 1988). It also has similar effects to isoflurane on the EEG.

## Anaesthetic gases

### *Nitrous oxide*

In dogs nitrous oxide increass $CMRO_2$ and CBF, but reports in man are conflicting. Nitrous oxide increases ICP during established anaesthesia with hypocapnia in patients with cerebral tumours (Misfeldt et al., 1974) and 50% nitrous oxide in oxygen increases ICP in hypocapnic patients with head injury (Moss and McDowall, 1979). These increases in ICP must be caused by cerebral vasodilation. Hyperventilation for 10 min before the administration of nitrous oxide effectively counteracts its effects on ICP so, in patients with raised ICP, nitrous oxide should not be introduced until after intubation and hyperventilation with 100% oxygen is established. Carbon dioxide reactivity is not affected by nitrous oxide. Nitrous oxide reverses the depression of $CMRO_2$ caused by 0.5 and 1 MAC isoflurane and therefore may attenuate any cerebral protection against ischaemia offered by isoflurane. In rats the addition of 0.5 MAC nitrous oxide to 0.5 MAC halothane anaesthesia produces similar increases in CBF to those produced by adding a further 0.5 MAC of halothane; also 0.5 MAC nitrous oxide added to 0.5 MAC isoflurane anaesthesia produces CBF values significantly greater than those measured with 1 MAC isoflurane alone (Hansen et al., 1989). However, it must be stressed that similar responses may not occur in man and the background anaesthetic may alter the response to nitrous oxide. The effect of nitrous oxide is less if an opioid is used (Drummond et al., 1987).

## Intravenous anaesthetic agents

Provided that respiratory depression does not occur, the intravenous anaesthetic agents reduce $CMRO_2$, CBF and ICP. The only exception is ketamine. Anaesthetic agents which reduce ICP cause a greater reduction in patients with higher initial ICP values (Ravussin et al., 1988). Studies of the effects of intravenous anaesthetic agents on CSF formation and reabsorption indicate that midazolam and thiopentone may increase the resistance to absorption whereas etomidate has no effect ( Artru, 1988). However, the response to different doses of these agents was variable so these results are unlikely to be clinically relevant.

*Thiopentone*

Thiopentone reduces $CMRO_2$ and CBF with a consequent reduction in ICP. It does not affect the carbon dioxide reactivity of the cerebral vessels. It has been used by infusion to maintain anaesthesia during neurosurgery.

*Methohexitone*

Methohexitone reduces CBF and ICP and has also been used by infusion to maintain anaesthesia during neurosurgery.

*Etomidate*

Etomidate reduces $CMRO_2$, CBF and ICP. CPP is usually well maintained (Moss et al., 1979) and the carbon dioxide reactivity of the cerebral circulation is preserved (Cold et al., 1985). EEG activity is depressed as the brain concentration of etomidate increases (Cold et al., 1986) but convulsions have occurred after a short general anaesthetic in which only etomidate was used (Hansen and Drenck, 1988).

*Propofol*

Propofol reduces $CMRO_2$, CBF (Stephan et al., 1987) and ICP (Herregods et al., 1989), but CPP may be reduced due to a reduction in MAP (Herregods, 1988). Propofol also reduces the pressure under the brain retractor during intracranial surgery, but careful attention to dosage is required to avoid excessive reduction in CPP. The reactivity of the cerebral vessels to changes in $PaCO_2$ is well maintained during propofol anaesthesia and EEG activity is depressed (Stephan et al., 1987) but spikes and slow waves have been demonstrated on electrocorticography in patients undergoing temporal lobectomy (Hodkinson et al., 1987) and a grand mal convulsion has been reported after propofol anaesthesia in a patient who had never had a fit before (Victory and Magee, 1988). Animal work has demonstrated that anaesthetic doses of propofol have an anticonvulsant effect (Lowson et al., 1990) and the duration of convulsions during electroconvulsive therapy is reduced by propofol (Simpson et al., 1988). Lowson and his colleagues (personal communication) have demonstrated that propofol does not have proconvulsant properties but when its administration is stopped, the blood level falls more quickly than that of thiopentone, so its anticonvulsant properties terminate rapidly. This may allow convulsions to occur in susceptible patients.

*Ketamine*

Ketamine causes an increase in CBF and ICP but increases in $CMRO_2$ have only been demonstrated in animals. It increases the resistance to reabsorption of CSF (Mann et al., 1980). The reactivity of the cerebral circulation to $PaCO_2$ is not altered by ketamine. Ketamine has a similar potency to methohexitone as an anticonvulsant (Wardley-Smith et al., 1988).

**Opioid analgesics**

The narcotic analgesics have little effect on CBF and ICP provided that respiration is not depressed, causing an increase in $PaCO_2$. Thus if the $PaCO_2$ remains constant morphine has no effect on CBF or ICP. Cerebrovascular autoregulation is unaffected by fentanyl and morphine.

*Phenoperidine*

When given in combination with droperidol at constant $PaCO_2$, phenoperidine causes small changes in CSF pressure which can be in either direction and there is no effect on CBF (Barker et al., 1968). Phenoperidine has been widely used in patients with head injury for sedation and to prevent them straining against the ventilator, but a recent report indicates that phenoperidine may increase ICP in such patients, perhaps by causing cerebral vasodilation and precipitating A waves (Grummitt and Goat, 1984).

*Pentazocine*

At constant $PaCO_2$ pentazocine produces small decreases in ICP in patients undergoing intracranial surgery but when given to patients with brain trauma who are breathing spontaneously, the ICP and $PaCO_2$ increase (Barker et al., 1972).

*Fentanyl*

In man fentanyl, when given with droperidol does not affect $CMRO_2$ or CBF. In the absence of droperidol fentanyl causes small changes in ICP which may be in either direction (Moss et al., 1978b) and it decreases the resistance to absorption of CSF (Artru, 1984). When given to dogs anaesthetised with nitrous oxide in oxygen it causes a reduction in $CMRO_2$ and CBF (Michenfelder and Theye, 1971). Fentanyl increases cerebral vascular reactivity to carbon dioxide (Vernhiet et al.,

1977). Grand mal convulsions have occurred following the administration of fentanyl, mostly after large doses of opioids but in one report only 100 μg of fentanyl had been given (Hoien, 1984).

*Alfentanil*

There is little information on the effects of alfentanil on CBF and ICP but there is one report which suggests that it causes cerebral vasodilation even when the $PaCO_2$ is controlled (Marx et al., 1988). An increase in ICP associated with an increase in CVP has also been demonstrated in rats during alfentanil induced rigidity (Benthuysen et al., 1988). Large doses of alfentanil do not alter cerebral reactivity to changes in $PaCO_2$, $PaO_2$ or MAP (McPherson, 1985) but reduce cerebrovascular resistance. This change was probably secondary to a decrease in MAP in the presence of normal cerebral autoregulation leading to compensatory vasodilation of the cerebral vessels. When given in combination with midazolam to patients with raised ICP, alfentanil reduced ICP to a greater extent than fentanyl (Hoffman, 1987). It seems likely that alfentanil does not affect CBF and ICP in the absence of a change in $PaCO_2$ but further investigations are required to confirm this. Alfentanil causes an increase in the delta-activity, a reduction in the higher frequency components and less sychronisation of the EEG than do fentanyl or sufentanil. Spindle activity on the EEG is prominent following alfentanil administration (Bovill et al., 1983).

*Sufentanil*

Sufentanil is a cerebral vasodilator (Marx et al., 1988) and would be expected to cause an increase in ICP.

**Muscle relaxants**

None of the muscle relaxants have been shown to alter CBF or ICP in man.

*Suxamethonium*

Suxamethonium increases lumbar CSF pressure, an effect which is probably caused by muscle fasciculations leading to an increase in intra-abdominal, intrathoracic and central venous pressures. The author was unable to demonstrate any significant increase in ICP when suxamethonium was given to patients already paralysed with *d*-tubocurarine (Moss, unpublished observations). Lanier and colleagues (1986) did demonstrate an increase in CBF following the administration of suxamethonium to dogs lightly anaesthetised with halothane but they attributed this increase to afferent muscle spindle activity and a secondary rise in $PaCO_2$ consequent upon muscle fasciculations.

### *Non-depolarising muscle relaxants*

Sondergard (1961) found that *d*-tubocurarine had no effect on ICP provided that $PaCO_2$ was not allowed to increase. However, Tarkkanen and colleagues (1974) showed an increase in ICP following *d*-tubocurarine 0.6 mg/kg which they attributed partly to histamine causing cerebral vasodilation. They allowed the patients to breathe spontaneously for between 1 and 2 min after the administration of the *d*-tubocurarine and the $PaCO_2$ increased by 0.6 kPa which was sufficient to account for an increase in ICP of about 20%. In addition, the patients were either sedated or only very lightly anaesthetised and some of the increase in ICP could have been due to an arousal effect as $PaCO_2$ increased and respiration became more difficult. *d*-Tubocurarine in doses of 15 or 20 mg in adults does not increase ICP (Moss, unpublished observations). *d*-Tubocurarine is a useful agent for neurosurgery because of its ganglion blocking properties which help in the control of arterial pressure.

*Pancuronium* has no effect on ICP during induction of anaesthesia but has the disadvantage of causing arterial hypertension, which can cause problems during some intracranial operations.

*Alcuronium, vecuronium* and *atracurium* have no effect on ICP.

## Other agents

### *Lignocaine*

Lignocaine 1.5 mg/kg reduces ICP in patients with head injury and prevents increases in ICP associated with intubation in patients with cerebral tumours (Bedford et al., 1980). In animals a dose of 3 mg/kg reduces $CMRO_2$ but much larger doses are required to reduce CBF (Sakabe et al., 1974).

### *Diazepam*

Diazepam reduces $CMRO_2$ and CBF but has no effect on ICP in neurosurgical patients (Tateishi et al., 1981). Nitrous oxide increases the effect of diazepam on CBF and $CMRO_2$ (Carlsson et al., 1976). Diazepam has no effect on the carbon dioxide reactivity of the cerebral vessels (Cotev and Shalit, 1975).

### *Lorazepam*

Lorazepam reduces $CMRO_2$ and CBF and increases cerebral vascular resistance in primates (Rockoff et al., 1980). There was no change in cerebral metabolism indicative of cerebral hypoxia or ischaemia.

*Midazolam*

Midazolam reduced CBF and increased cerebral vascular resistance in human volunteers (Forster et al., 1982) but did not reduce ICP in patients with brain tumours and did not abolish increases in ICP associated with laryngoscopy and intubation (Griffin et al., 1984), but these authors also found that thiopentone had no effect on ICP in a similar group of patients and this finding casts doubt on the validity of their results with midazolam. Large doses of midazolam reduce $CMRO_2$ in dogs providing greater protection against hypoxia than diazepam but less than thiopentone (Nugent et al., 1982).

*Droperidol*

Droperidol reduces CBF in dogs but has no effect on $CMRO_2$ (Michenfelder and Theye, 1971). It appears to have little effect on ICP in man (Misfeldt et al., 1976).

## ADVANTAGES OF TOTAL INTRAVENOUS ANAESTHESIA FOR INTRACRANIAL SURGERY

From the foregoing account of the effects of anaesthetic agents on the cranial contents it is reasonable to conclude that intravenous anaesthetic agents have properties which make them suitable for intracranial surgery. The advantages which they offer for this type of surgery are a reduction in CBF and thus brain bulk, reducing the chance of brain shift or cerebral ischaemia when the cranium is intact, and reducing trauma to the brain and improving surgical access when brain retractors are applied. The depression of $CMRO_2$ may be useful in protecting against ischaemic damage to the brain but, except when large doses of thiopentone and possibly etomidate are used, this has yet to be demonstrated.

Total intravenous anaesthesia has the additional advantage that it avoids the use of nitrous oxide which is a cerebral vasodilator and a cerebral stimulant. Avoidance of nitrous oxide reduces atmospheric pollution with anaesthetic gases and the detrimental effects of nitrous oxide on vitamin $B_{12}$ metabolism. During posterior fossa surgery in the sitting position, air embolism is common and nitrous oxide diffuses into the air pocket causing it to expand, which worsens the effects of the embolism on the circulation. Nitrous oxide may also diffuse into the collection of air which sometimes forms under the cranial vault during exploration of the posterior fossa in the sitting position and this may cause pressure effects after the dura is closed. So the avoidance of nitrous oxide during surgery in the sitting position is advantageous. It is clear that the use of nitrous oxide is reducing in parts of the U.S.A. but it is important that it is not replaced by a more toxic alternative.

With the exception of ketamine, the intravenous anaesthetic agents and analgesics have little or no effect on the rate of CSF production or absorption. Intravenous anaesthetics are the only suitable agents for induction of anaesthesia for neurosurgery (Moss, 1989) and during maintenance of anaesthesia they help to avoid recall of intra-operative events, help to prevent sudden large increases in arterial pressure and attenuate the increase in intracranial pressure associated with intubation.

The infusion of intravenous agents also has advantages during the period when the muscle relaxant is reversed and the patient is extubated. This period of recovery from the anaesthetic can lead to marked increases in ICP. The residual sedative effects of propofol, in particular, tend to prevent the patient from coughing at the time when spontaneous respiration returns and pharyngeal suction and extubation is performed. In contrast, volatile agents have a tendency to sensitise the larnyx to stimulation by secretions and coughing is likely to occur.

## DISADVANTAGES OF TOTAL INTRAVENOUS ANAESTHESIA FOR INTRACRANIAL SURGERY

As with all invasive procedures used in medicine there are disadvantages to weigh against the advantages. Many intravenous anaesthetic or sedative drugs have a prolonged action which is not desirable after intracranial surgery because early assessment of conscious level and neurological signs is required in the post-operative period. This is necessary in order to detect treatable post-operative complications before they cause permanent damage. Drugs administered intravenously can precipitate an anaphylactic reaction whereas inhaled anaesthetics do not. Acute toxic effects caused by overdosage are more likely to occur when the drugs are given intravenously, rather than by inhalation, because the absorption into the circulation by the latter route is limited by the physical characteristics of the alveolar capillary membrane.

Most anaesthetists find that intravenous anaesthesia is technically more difficult to administer than inhalation anaesthesia because they have been trained in and are used to maintaining anaesthesia by inhalation. Special equipment is required to administer the drugs and anaesthetists need to become as familiar with it as they are with their anaesthesia machines, vaporisers and ventilators. The equipment is expensive and financial restrictions may limit the number of infusion pumps available to anaesthetists. The infusion devices create problems in themselves in that malfunction can lead to the administration of too much or too little anaesthetic. The infusion may leak into the tissues which will lead to inadequate blood levels of anaesthetic with the risk of awareness as well as causing tissue damage. Another practical difficulty lies in ventilating the lungs during total intravenous anaesthesia. It is generally accepted that 100% oxygen should not be administered routinely because it causes atelectasis but many modern anaesthetic ventilators will not entrain air and require a compressed air supply which is not always readily available.

Opioid analgesics cause respiratory depression which may extend into the post-operative period, whereas the analgesic effect of nitrous oxide can be continued up until the end of surgery without danger of post-operative respiratory depression. Intravenous anaesthetics tend to reduce MAP and thus will tend to reduce CPP, but this is not necessarily a problem during intracranial surgery provided that cerebral autoregulation is intact. Conversely, the hypotensive effect of these agents may not be sufficient to control the arterial pressure adequately during some intracranial operations and hypotensive agents may be needed to reduce MAP to the desired level.

Finally a reduction in $CMRO_2$ and CBF is desirable during intracranial surgery, but if the CBF is reduced more than the $CMRO_2$ the supply to demand ratio for oxygen will be worsened. There is some evidence that propofol reduces $CMRO_2$ to a lesser extent than CBF (Stephan et al., 1987) but studies of the arterial to jugular venous difference for oxygen during the administration of propofol are required to clarify the situation.

## AGENTS SUITABLE FOR USE IN TOTAL INTRAVENOUS ANAESTHESIA

Total intravenous anaesthesia for intracranial surgery requires the use of a balanced anaesthetic technique. This requires a hypnotic, an analgesic and a muscle relaxant. Benzodiazepines are appropriate agents for preoperative medication because they do not depress respiration significantly and diazepam has anticonvulsant properties.

### Choice of hypnotic

Intravenous infusions of anaesthetic agents to maintain anaesthesia during intracranial surgery were first used by Hunter (1972a) who used thiopentone and methohexitone. It is generally accepted that the pharmacokinetic properties of these agents make them unsuitable for use by infusion during prolonged operations because cumulation occurs.

Cold and colleagues (1985) demonstrated that etomidate infusions produced dose dependent reductions in $CMRO_2$ and CBF in patients with supratentorial tumours and it appeared that this agent would be suitable. However, its lack of hypotensive effects meant that control of arterial pressure was not always satisfactory and many neuroanaesthetists formed a clinical impression that there was an increased incidence of vomiting after craniotomy when etomidate infusions had been used. Etomidate was incriminated in an increase in mortality in multiple trauma patients admitted to an intensive therapy unit and this problem was later linked to adrenocortical suppression due to inhibition of 11 beta-hydroxylation, 17 alpha-hydroxylation and other intramitochondrial hydroxylation reactions. This agent is no longer recommended for use other than for induction of anaesthesia. If it is used by infusion steroids must be administered for the duration of the infusion and for at least 24 h after the infusion.

These problems with etomidate meant that neuroanaesthetists were again searching for an intravenous agent suitable for maintaining anaesthesia and for sedation of neurosurgical patients in the intensive therapy unit. Midazolam has useful effects on $CMRO_2$ and CBF and has been used extensively for sedation during intensive care. It has also been used for induction and maintenance of anaesthesia for a variety of surgical procedures (Nilsson et al., 1988) but there are no reports of its use during neurosurgical operations. Its duration of action is longer than etomidate and it causes quite prolonged sedation post-operatively. This is a disadvantage in neurosurgery because neurosurgeons like their patients to wake up quickly after intracranial surgery in order to assess their neurosurgical state. The sedation can be reversed by flumazenil which does not alter CBF (Forster et al., 1987) but it is expensive and would need to be given by infusion because of its short half-life. In the author's opinion, this technique using midazolam followed by reversal with flumazenil seems unduly complicated and inappropriate for neurosurgical anaesthesia.

It is not surprising that when propofol was introduced many neuroanaesthetists soon started using it in situations where they had previously used Althesin or etomidate. They have used it by infusion to maintain anaesthesia during craniotomy with or without nitrous oxide (Freedman and Levy, 1988; Wright and Murray, 1989). They have been convinced that the advantages of the technique to the patient are sufficient to use it outside the conditions of its product licence, which at the time of writing only allows its continuous infusion for up to 1 h. Propofol has pharmacokinetic properties which make it suitable for use by infusion to maintain as well as induce anaesthesia and it is known to reduce $CMRO_2$, CBF and ICP (see above). Many workers have used propofol and an analgesic as the main agents for total intravenous anaesthesia in patients breathing oxygen enriched air. An infusion of propofol starting with 12 mg/kg per h for 10 min then reducing to 6 mg/kg per h with bolus doses of fentanyl as required has been shown to provide satisfactory anaesthesia with no evidence of recall (Ledderose et al., 1988). When given in combination with alfentanil, propofol is a better anaesthetic for major surgery than methohexitone with fewer side effects (Kay, 1986). For total intravenous anaesthesia in patients undergoing craniotomy ventilated with 35% oxygen in air, Merckx and colleagues (1988) used an infusion of propofol 21 mg/kg per h for 5 min, then 12 mg/kg per h for 10 min and 6 mg/kg per h thereafter, supplemented with an infusion of alfentanil 0.025 to 0.1 mg/kg per h. The recovery of the patients was satisfactory and brain relaxation, as assessed by the surgeons, was good. Satisfactory operating conditions during propofol infusions with and without nitrous oxide have also been reported by other authors (Freedman and Levy, 1988; Galletly and Short, 1988; Wright and Murray, 1989). Propofol reduces the hypertensive response to intubation but does not abolish it. Propofol may be more effective than thiopentone in this respect.

Propofol reduces the incidence of post-operative nausea and vomiting and does not suppress adrenocortical function significantly, having a similar effect to thiopentone on adrenal steroidogenesis. However, propofol infusions do depress the ventilatory response to carbon dioxide and increasing the dose increases this depression (Goodman et al., 1987). This property is not important to neuroanaesthetists during the operation because ventilation is controlled, but it presents a problem during recovery from anaesthesia when respiratory depression may lead to cerebral congestion. There is evidence that respiration returns more quickly when alfentanil is used for analgesia during propofol infusions than when fentanyl is given (Fragen et al., 1983).

Ketamine is another intravenous agent which has been used by infusion during intracranial surgery (Barker, personal communication). Its effect on cerebral metabolism and CBF make it necessary to give it in combination with drugs, such as benzodiazepines or lignocaine, which obtund these effects. After the infusion is discontinued recovery can take up to 2 h, which is far from ideal following neurosurgery. Ketamine is a non-competitive antagonist of NMDA receptors and, as brain damage associated with anoxia, stroke, hypoglycaemia and epilepsy is thought to be at least partially caused by excessive activation of NMDA receptors, it may offer some cerebral protection against ischaemia. However, the case for ketamine in this situation is not proven and only enthusiasts would use it during neurosurgical operations.

### Choice of muscle relaxant

In order to facilitate tracheal intubation and avoid coughing on the tracheal tube or straining against the ventilator during total intravenous anaesthesia for neurosurgical operations, good muscle relaxation is required. Many neuroanaesthetists prefer to use suxamethonium to provide good conditions for tracheal intubation, whereas others prefer the non-depolarising relaxants which avoid the short-lived increase in ICP associated with the administration of suxamethonium. The non-depolarising relaxants also allow the establishment of hypocapnia before intubation which may help to prevent an increase in ICP associated with laryngoscopy and intubation (Moss et al., 1978a). All the non-depolarising muscle relaxants, with the exception of gallamine which causes tachycardia, are suitable for use during intracranial surgery. However, pancuronium can cause an increase in heart rate and arterial pressure which is undesirable during surgery on the brain when autoregulation may be impaired. Vecuronium and atracurium are shorter acting agents which can be given by infusion during long operations maintaining a stable level of muscle relaxation. The muscle relaxation should be monitored with a nerve stimulator. They are both easily reversed at the end of the procedure provided the infusion is discontinued in good time.

Atracurium is rapidly metabolised to metabolites which have very weak relaxant properties, but one of the metabolites, laudanosine, is a cerebral stimulant. However, during anaesthesia for most intracranial procedures plasma concentrations of laudanosine which can cause convulsions are unlikely to be reached. Vecuronium and atracurium have small cardiovascular effects whereas *d*-tubocurarine, and to a lesser extent alcuronium, cause a reduction in arterial pressure which can be useful during intracranial operations.

### Choice of analgesic

With the exception of sufentanil, the opioid analgesics have no effect on CBF and ICP if pulmonary ventilation is controlled, so any opioid or opiate would suffice during total intravenous anaesthesia for neurosurgery. However, post-operative respiratory depression is undesirable after intracranial surgery and the shorter acting opioids, such as fentanyl or alfentanil, are therefore preferable to longer acting agents because their respiratory depressant effects are less likely to continue after the end of the anaesthetic.

After comparing the actions of fentanyl, alfentanil and sufentanil on CSF pressure in patients with cerebral tumours, Marx and colleages (1988) concluded that fentanyl is the preferred opioid in patients with compromised intracranial compliance. Sufentanil is a cerebral vasodilator and alfentanil may also increase CBF and ICP. Although fentanyl (5 μg/kg) has been used successfully to attenuate the haemodynamic and ICP response to intubation, it seems that this response cannot be blocked completely by fentanyl (Wynands et al., 1984). High dose fentanyl (100 μg/kg followed by increments of 250 μg as required) has produced satisfactory anaesthesia with cardiovascular stability for posterior fossa operations in the sitting position (Shupak et al., 1983) but the fentanyl had to be reversed by naloxone at the end of the procedure. For this reason high dose fentanyl is not a useful or practical anaesthetic technique for intracranial surgery. However, fentanyl has been tried and tested in neuroanaesthesia and is very widely used in total doses of approximately 5 to 6 μg/kg.

Alfentanil 10 μg/kg prevents the increase in heart rate and arterial pressure associated with tracheal intubation and the increase in plasma adrenaline concentration after intubation, but larger doses (40 μg/kg) cause profound hypotension and bradycardia. Infusions of alfentanil are superior to bolus administration for producing smooth anaesthesia with stable cardiovascular parameters. Infusion rates of 7.5 μg/kg per min up to 10 μg/kg per min for 10 min followed by 0.75 to 1 μg/kg per min for the rest of the procedure have been recommended. The data sheet recommends a loading dose of 50 to 100 μg followed by an infusion of 0.5 to 1 μg/kg per min. The loading dose should be reduced by up to one-third in the elderly because they have a prolonged elimination half-life. The loading dose can be given as a bolus of 75 to 100 μg/kg but hypotension and bradycardia are less likely if the same dose is given by fast infusion. However, these doses are too large for neuroanaesthesia because of the profound respiratory depression they will cause. A dose of 20 μg/kg per h has been shown to give analgesia compatible with spontaneous respiration (Chamberlain, 1985) and such dosage is more appropriate. The pharmacokinetics of alfentanil with its short half-life and small volume of distribution make it an attractive agent for use by infusion during neuroanaesthesia, but there are considerable interindividual differences in its pharmacokinetics which make the dosage requirements unpredictable. The elimination half-life and the plasma clearance of alfentanil is greater in children than in adults, so consideration should be given to increasing the infusion rate in children. There is a good correlation between respiratory depression and plasma alfentanil concentration. One worrying reports is that of Jaffe and Coalson (1989), who found that patients who have had alfentanil may wake up initially but then relapse into somnolence and respiratory depression. Therefore, it is important to keep a close watch on these patients for some time after they initially regain consciousness. Further investigations into the effects of alfentanil on CBF and ICP are required before alfentanil can be considered to be the opioid of choice for patients in whom intracranial compliance is compromised.

## INDICATIONS FOR TOTAL INTRAVENOUS ANAESTHESIA IN NEUROSURGERY

Total intravenous anaesthesia could be used for any neurosurgical procedure but has specific advantages for certain operations. It is theoretically an ideal technique for intracranial surgery and infusions of agents such as propofol are preferable to volatile anaesthetic agents when the intracranial compliance is reduced. Therefore, total intravenous anaesthesia should be considered for patients with acute head injury, large intracranial mass lesions such as tumours or haematomata or in patients undergoing shunt procedures for raised ICP. Infusion of propofol reduces brain bulk and the pressure under the brain retractor, so it gives better operating conditions and reduces the risk of brain trauma during operations for cerebral aneurysms or arteriovenous malformations. For carotid endarterectomy the cerebral depressant effects of intravenous anaesthetics may be of benefit, but the hypotension caused by thiopentone or propofol may have detrimental effects on cerebral perfusion. Repeated short periods of intravenous anaesthesia with short acting agents have been used for thermocoagulation of the trigeminal nerve for trigeminal neuralgia. Following induction of anaesthesia the needle is inserted into the foramen ovale, then the patient is allowed to wake up and the needle is stimulated to identify whether it is correctly placed. The process is repeated until the needle is sited in the right division of the nerve. Then anaesthesia is induced once more and maintained whilst a coagulating current is applied to the nerve. For spinal surgery total intravenous anaesthesia has no theoretical or clinical advantages when compared with conventional anaesthetic techniques.

## PRACTICAL ASPECTS

The author believes that the best agents presently available for use in total intravenous anaesthesia for intracranial operations are propofol as the hypnotic, atracurium and/or tubocurarine as the muscle relaxant and either fentanyl or alfentanil as the analgesic. When propofol was first introduced for maintenance of anaesthesia by infusion it was often used with 67% nitrous oxide in oxygen and many anaesthetists still use it in this way. This is intravenous anaesthesia but not total intravenous anaesthesia. The author has personal experience of the use of propofol infusions used to supplement nitrous oxide, opioid and relaxant anaesthesia in over 100 patients undergoing intracranial operative procedures and uses the following technique. Following premedication with an oral benzodiazepine (diazepam 10 mg or temazepam 20 mg,) fentanyl 2.5 μg/kg is administered intravenously followed immediately by induction of anaesthesia with propofol (1.5 to 2.5 mg/kg) titrated to effect and atracurium 0.5 mg/kg. An infusion of propofol at a rate of 12 mg/kg per h is commenced and the patient is intubated at least 2 min after the administration of the atracurium. The lungs are mechanically ventilated with 67% nitrous oxide in oxygen to maintain a $PaCO_2$ of 3.5 to 4 kPa. Whilst the venous and arterial lines and the bladder catheter are being inserted, the arterial pressure is carefully monitored and the infusion rate of propofol is adjusted to maintain the arterial pressure near to the patient's normal value. If there is arterial hypertension, additional doses of fentanyl up to a total dose of 5 μg/kg are given. Additional fentanyl is usually required to prevent a haemodynamic response to the application of the Mayfield skull clamp. During the procedure the infusion rate is adjusted to maintain a stable heart rate and arterial pressure, and additional doses of fentanyl are given as required, but a total dose of fentanyl of 5 μg/kg is rarely exceeded. The most painful parts of a craniotomy are the reflection of the scalp flap and resuturing the scalp at the end of the procedure. It is inappropriate to give intravenous analgesics within 30 min of the end of the surgery, although small bolus doses of alfentanil can be used with good effect if marked fluctuations in arterial pressure occur. It follows that it is appropriate to give most of the fentanyl before the scalp flap is reflected. It is the author's experience that if the propofol infusion is continued up until the last skin suture or staple has been inserted, the arterial pressure changes are usually well controlled. The maintenance dose of propofol usually required is 6 mg/kg per h reducing to 3 mg/kg per h over the last 10—15 min of the procedure. Muscle relaxation is maintained with *d*-tubocurarine given in doses of 15 to 20 mg as the atracurium wears off. These doses of *d*-tubocurarine do not cause the profound hypotension which larger doses can cause, but help to avoid surges in arterial pressure during the procedure. The neuromuscular block is monitored using a nerve stimulator.

During the procedure the patient is monitored clinically and these observations are supplemented by additional electronic monitoring equipment. The electrocardiogram, oxygen saturation, the inspired concentration of oxygen, the end-tidal carbon dioxide concentration, radial artery pressure, nasopharyngeal and skin temperature, urine output and ventilation pressures are routinely monitored, and central venous pressure monitoring and the Doppler ultrasound are used when indicated. Two 14 or 16 s.w.g. intravenous cannulae are inserted to allow rapid replacement of blood loss, if necessary, and to act as a route for infusion of hypotensive agents. A bladder catheter is passed once the patient is asleep because diuretics are routinely used to reduce brain bulk.

The infusion of propofol is discontinued when the last suture or staple has been inserted into the skin. The muscle relaxation is reversed with neostigmine and atropine or glycopyrrolate and the nitrous oxide is discontinued. Pulmonary ventilation is reduced over the last few minutes of the procedure allowing the $PaCO_2$ to return to normal with early restoration of spontaneous respiration, usually within 2 to 3 min. When spontaneous respiration has returned, the pharynx is cleared of secretions and the patient is extubated carefully to avoid coughing. The patient is transferred to the recovery room and carefully observed for at least an hour before return to the neurosurgical ward. The patients usually open their eyes and respond to commands about 10 min after the propofol infusion is stopped. Once they had awoken none of the patients who were managed in this way became resedated and respiration was always clinically adequate. Arterial blood gases have been measured in the recovery room as part of a continuing investigation in the author's hospital and, with one exception, the $PaCO_2$ values have all been within the normal range 5 min after extubation. All the $PaCO_2$ values have been normal at 30 min later, but too few patients have been studied to draw firm conclusions at present.

Alfentanil is a suitable alternative to fentanyl and is effective when given as a loading dose of 15 to 30 $\mu$g/kg either by bolus injection or preferably by rapid infusion over a 5-min period, followed by infusion at a rate of 0.5 $\mu$g/kg per min. If the alfentanil is discontinued at least 30 min before the end of surgery this dosage regime is unlikely to produce significant respiratory depression post-operatively. If respiratory depression does occur it may be reversed with naloxone.

Thiopentone may be used instead of propofol for induction of anaesthesia allowing a reduction in the total dose of propofol. A second dose of thiopentone, of about 25% of the dose required for induction, is given approximately 30 s before intubation provided that the patient is not hypotensive. This supplementary dose of thiopentone has been shown to reduce the increase in ICP associated with intubation (Shapiro et al., 1972c) but it must be allowed to circulate before intubation is attempted. If thiopentone is used, provided that the patient is not hypotensive, the propofol infusion is started at a rate of 12 mg/kg per h once intubation has been performed. Lignocaine 1.5 mg/kg can also be given to reduce the ICP response to intubation.

The author has less experience with true total intravenous anaesthesia with propofol but has used both etomidate and propofol in combination with fentanyl for maintenance of anaesthesia in patients breathing oxygen enriched air. Anaesthesia can be satisfactorily maintained using propofol and an opioid. The disadvantage of avoiding nitrous oxide lies with the loss of its analgesic properties. The analgesic properties of nitrous oxide last until its administration is stopped, when it is rapidly excreted through the lungs and its action is terminated. Intravenous analgesics rely first on redistribution and then on metabolism and excretion for the termination of their effects. Therefore with these agents it is easy to cause post-operative respiratory depression, which is unwanted after intracranial surgery and, in the absence of nitrous oxide, larger doses of analgesics will be required to compensate for the loss of its analgesic properties.

Provided that alfentanil does not cause cerebral vasodilation it is probably the most suitable agent for use during total intravenous anaesthesia with propofol because, after discontinuation, respiratory depression is less prolonged than with fentanyl. The author prefers to use nitrous oxide unless the operation involves a risk of air embolism or the compliance of the cranial contents is considerably reduced. In the presence of these conditions the avoidance of the cerebral vasodilator effect of nitrous oxide is advantageous. Nitrous oxide is also best avoided in patients with multiple trauma undergoing repeated anaesthetics (Nunn, 1988). In these situations anaesthesia is induced and maintained with propofol 6 to 15 mg/kg per h and alfentanil 15 to 30 $\mu$g/kg followed by 0.5 $\mu$g/kg per min and the patient is ventilated with oxygen enriched air. Muscle relaxation is achieved initially with atracurium and maintained with *d*-tubocurarine. The alfentanil is discontinued 30 min before the end of surgery and the propofol is stopped when the last skin suture or staple has been inserted. Fentanyl can be used instead of alfentanil but should not be given within an hour of the end of surgery. When the head frame has been removed and the wound dressed the muscle relaxation is reversed and spontaneous respiration restored.

## Recovery from anaesthesia

After intracranial surgery recovery from anaesthesia should be smooth, to avoid marked surges in MAP and ICP, and rapid to allow early neurological assessment. There should be minimal depression of respiration to avoid increases in $PaCO_2$ and CBF. In the recovery room the neurological and cardiorespiratory status should be carefully monitored and recorded at regular intervals. In addition to clinical observations, the cardiovascular and respiratory status can be monitored using pulse oximetry, ECG and automatic non-invasive blood pressure monitoring. Oxygen is administered for at least 12 h post-operatively and codeine phosphate 30 to 60 mg is given intramuscularly or orally for analgesia. Anticonvulsants are administered if post-operative fits occur and nausea and vomiting are treated symptomatically as they occur. Vomiting is only common after posterior fossa operations.

There is no evidence that recovery from anaesthesia after long operations is any quicker following total intravenous anaesthesia than following the use of volatile agents, but it is the author's opinion that recovery is smoother when an infusion of propofol is used. Also there is no information available to indicate whether respiratory depression is more likely to occur following the use of propofol or volatile anaesthetics.

## INTRAVENOUS SEDATION FOR NEUROSURGICAL PATIENTS

Intravenous sedation has been used in neurosurgical patients for a variety of different purposes. In the past, restless patients with head injury have been sedated with phenothiazines or benzodiazepines to prevent further injury, and patients undergoing biopsy of an intracranial tumour through a burr hole have been made more comfortable and cooperative using intravenous benzodiazepines or neuroleptanalgesia. Nowadays sedation for specific purposes is usually confined to neuroradiological procedures such as CT scan, nuclear magnetic resonance imaging and cerebral angiography. Sedation, usually with benzodiazepines, is still used for restless patients with head injury and intravenous infusions of these agents, hypnotics and opioids are used for sedation of neurosurgical patients on controlled ventilation. Intravenous benzodiazepines are also used as the first line of treatment for convulsions following brain damage due to head injury or surgery.

### Neuroradiology

#### *CAT scanning*

This procedure is not uncomfortable or painful but the patient is required to lie perfectly still. Sedation is usually only required in very small children who are unable to cooperate or adult patients who are confused or restless. Any patient with a raised ICP who is restless or uncooperative, including patients with severe head injury, should be given a general anaesthetic with controlled ventilation but, in the absence of raised ICP, sedation with a benzodiazepine or phenothiazine is usually very effective.

A variety of sedative regimes have been described for children including a mixture of pethidine, promethazine and chlorpromazine for children over 2 months and less than 20 kg body weight and trimeprazine 4 mg/kg for older children, given 1.5 to 2 h before scanning. Quinalbarbitone 7.5 to 10 mg/kg given orally 2 h before scanning has been used with good effect in the author's hospital in children from 6 months to 5 years. If quinalbarbitone is not effective trimeprazine is used. If the children will not lie still with or without sedation the only alternative is a general anaesthetic. However, because modern CAT scanners are much faster than the original machines, sedation and anaesthesia is needed much less frequently now than previously.

*Nuclear magnetic resonance imaging (MRI)*

During this investigation the patient is inserted into the cylindrical scanner, which can be frightening for children and patients who suffer from claustrophia. As for CAT scanning the patient is required to lie still and sedation or general anaesthesia may be required occasionally. The MRI scanner presents problems for the anaesthetist because metal connectors are attracted by the powerful magnets and monitoring equipment is also affected. ECG monitors are affected by the magnetic field but pulse monitoring using photoelectric devices has been found to be satisfactory during MRI scanning. Sedation techniques similar to those used for CAT scanning should be suitable.

*Cerebral angiography*

There has always been debate amongst neuroanaesthetists as to whether general anaesthesia or sedation is most appropriate for making the patient comfortable and cooperative during cerebral angiography. In the past the contrast media tended to cause quite severe discomfort at the time of injection, particularly when external carotid angiography was being performed. The introduction of non-ionic contrast media has reduced this discomfort to little more than a feeling of warmth, so light sedation in the cooperative patient is all that is required for most studies including external carotid angiography. There are still some patients who are better managed under general anaesthesia and these include young children, patients who are restless or uncooperative due to cerebral pathology, patients with cerebral tumours who have reduced intracranial compliance and raised ICP and those in whom very high quality images are required. Hyperventilation slows the transit time for the contrast so that it is maintained in the vessels giving much better definition of vessels on the radiograph. Conversely, sedation tends to cause respiratory depression, particularly if opioids are used, so that CBF is increased and the transit time for the contrast decreases.

The neuroradiologist requires the sedated patient to be relaxed but able to obey commands. Excessive respiratory depression or snoring due to excessive sedation leads to poor quality films, but it is necessary for the patient to be sufficiently comfortable to lie still for the duration of the procedure, which may last from 45 min to 2 h. The radiologist infiltrates the area around the femoral artery with local anaesthetic before the only painful part of the procedure which is the initial cannulation of the fermoral artery.

Many different combinations of drugs have been used intravenously for sedation in these circumstances. It is important to stress that, when intravenous sedation is used, a medically qualified person should be responsible for monitoring its effects on respiration and the circulation. The radiologist should not give intravenous sedation and carry out the angiography. For many years neurolept-analgesia was used with a variety of opioids administered in combination with droperidol.

The most popular opioids were phenoperidine and fentanyl. Using these drug combinations the patients would lie still and often sleep through the procedure, but would wake and obey commands if necessary. In recent years different combinations of sedative and analgesic drugs have been used. An oral benzodiazepine such as diazepam or temazepam can be used to relieve anxiety in the hour before the procedure followed by further intravenous doses of diazemuls as necessary. Fentanyl is the most commonly used analgesic because of its short half-life which avoids prolonged respiratory depression. Midazolam has become a very popular alternative to diazemuls and is the author's choice of sedative for cerebral angiography. It can be administered with fentanyl and if carefully titrated to effect, provides a comfortable and cooperative patient. Recently, nalbuphine has been used on its own and in combination with midazolam. The patient is well sedated, comfortable and cooperative, and the respiratory depression with nalbuphine reaches a plateau after which increasing the dose does not increase the respiratory depression. Lyons (personal communication) has used a continuous infusion of nalbuphine of 0.073 mg/kg per h following a loading dose of 0.3 mg/kg as the only sedation during cerebral angiography with good effect. There is a low incidence of nausea and vomiting with this technique and the arterial blood gases remain within the normal range.

When sedation for cerebral angiography is requested the author gives either diazepam 10 mg or temazepam 20 mg orally 90 or 60 min respectively before the procedure. The patient is positioned on the X-ray table and connected to an ECG monitor, a pulse oximeter and non-invasive blood pressure monitor. An 18 or 19 s.w.g. venous cannula is inserted so that intravenous fluids can be administered if necessary to maintain an acceptable arterial pressure. Midazolam 1 mg is administered intravenously followed by fentanyl 50 $\mu$g or nalbuphine 5 mg. When the effect of these doses has been assessed, further increments of midazolam and analgesic are administered as necessary to produce the desired level of sedation. It is important that sedation is not excessive because snoring can cause poor quality radiographs and oversedated patients can become restless and uncooperative. Fentanyl is given to a maximum dose of 1.5 $\mu$g/kg and nalbuphine 0.15 mg/kg to avoid excessive depression of respiration. Midazolam is given in 1-mg increments with at least 2-min intervals between them, because the responses of individual patients are variable and in some patients quite small doses can induce unconsciousness. The haemoglobin saturation often falls once a satisfactory level of sedation is established but rapidly returns to normal when oxygen 4 l/min is administered through a Hudson or MC mask.

With the newer contrast media it is possible to do cerebral angiography with no sedation at all. If the patient is not unduly anxious and the examination is unlikely to be prolonged, local infiltration with lignocaine around the femoral artery is all that is required. It seems likely that the demand for sedation for this procedure will decline, particularly with the more widespread use of digital vascular imaging which reduces the amount of contrast media used and the duration of the study.

*Interventional neuroradiology*

This involves the selective catheterisation of arteries and their embolisation with suitable materials, either to treat cerebral arteriovenous malformations or aneurysms which are technically difficult for the surgeon and, thereby, carry a greater risk for the patient from surgical intervention, or to reduce the vascularity of cerebral tumours before surgical removal. The neuroradiologist prefers the patient to be conscious and cooperative for these procedures so that neuroradiological assessment can be performed at regular intervals during the procedure. This allows for the early recognition of neurological deterioration and rapid treatment of the cause. However, these procedures are often prolonged and the patient has to lie still for many hours, so some sedation is desirable to make the patient more comfortable. Similar drug combinations to those described for cerebral angiography are suitable for interventional neuroradiology, and repeated increments of the drugs are required during prolonged procedures.

**Intravenous sedation for neurosurgical intensive therapy**

Most neurosurgical patients who require admission to the intensive therapy unit for intermittent positive pressure ventilation have severe brain trauma either secondary to intracranial surgery or head injury. Many of these patients will have raised ICP and if this exceeds 30 mmHg for more than 15 min continuously the prognosis is poor (Moss et al., 1983b). The aim of sedation in these patients is to avoid coughing and straining against the ventilator which will increase cerebral congestion and ICP, to relieve pain and to keep ICP wihtin the normal range if possible, but at least less than 25 mmHg. However, it is important that the CPP is maintained at an acceptable level so that a compromise has to be reached between the optimum reduction in ICP and maintenance of MAP at an acceptable level. Arterial hypertension must also be avoided because, it may increase cerebral oedema. There is debate amongst anaesthetists about whether to use opioids or muscle relaxants to prevent straining against the ventilator. The author believes that muscle relaxants are more reliable and should always be used to settle patients with brain trauma and avoid increases in CVP. However, muscle relaxants should not be used on their own but need to be given in combination with sedative agents. The agents available for this purpose include benzodiazepines, opioids and low concentrations of intravenous anaesthetic agents. Nitrous oxide should not be used for long term sedation because it depresses the bone marrow and increases ICP.

*Benzodiazepines*

The benzodiazepines reduce $CMRO_2$ and CBF (see above). The half-life of diazepam leads to prolonged sedation which interferes with neurological assessment and is not suitable for neurosurgical patients. Midazolam has a much shorter half-life, making it much more suitable for use in this situation either by intermittent bolus injection or by infusion. However, recovery from its effect is still prolonged and reversal with flumazenil may be necessary for neurosurgical assessment. It is relevant that midazolam has a more prolonged duration of action in 6% of the population who are slow metabolisers of this drug. (Dundee et al., 1986).

*Opioids*

In the ventilated patient the opioid analgesics, except for sufentanil, have no effect on $CMRO_2$, CBF or ICP but they do reduce the sympathetic and cerebral responses to painful stimulation and have an important place in the management of patients with head injury, both during surgery and on the intensive therapy unit. Alfentanil has been shown to be an effective sedative for ventilated patients (Cohen and Kelly 1987) and has been infused in a dose of 0.4 to 1 μg/kg per min after a loading dose of 0.67 μg/kg per min for 20 min. Similar doses have proved effective when administered to patients with head injury and its pharmacokinetics allow early assessment of neurological function after it is stopped. However, there is some evidence that alfentanil may be a cerebral vasodilator and Marx and colleagues (1988) believe that fentanyl is the preferred opioid in patients with compromised intracranial compliance. On the other hand, Hoffman (1987) found that a combination of alfentanil and midazolam caused a greater reduction in ICP than fentanyl and midazolam. There may be little to choose between the speed of recovery following fentanyl and alfentanil when they are administered for 2 h or more (Sold and Weis,1987) and there is evidence that some patients may be slow metabolisers of alfentanil leading to a more prolonged effect (McDonnell et al., 1982).

The opiates, such as morphine or papaveretum and diamorphine have sedative and mood elevating effects as well as analgesic properties and these drugs are also useful for analgesia in patients on controlled ventilation after brain trauma. These agents have a longer duration of action requiring a longer period between the last dose and assessment of neurological function. Morphine or papaveretum are usually given intravenously in 2.5 mg increments or by infusion and diamorphine is infused at a rate of 1 to 2 mg/kg per h following a loading dose of 2.5 to 5 mg given as a bolus. There is a large interpatient variation in morphine requirements for adults with the effective dose ranging from 2 to 20 mg/h (Dodson, 1982).

It must be stressed that there is a difference between analgesia and sedation. Analgesics should be given for the relief of pain whereas hypnotics and anxiolytics are required for relieving anxiety and promoting sleep.

*Intravenous anaesthetic agents*

Intravenous anaesthetic agents reduce $CMRO_2$, CBF and ICP and are helpful in the treatment of vasogenic cerebral oedema (see above). The barbiturates pentobarbitone and thiopentone have been given to patients with head injury to control ICP but their duration of action is prolonged with the result that there is a long wait after the last dose before neurological examination can be performed. Barbiturates also cause cardiovascular depression leading to a reduced cardiac output and hypotension. However, in the U.S.A. pentobarbitone is commonly used for the treatment of head injured patients with high ICP. The objective is to reduce ICP with increased CPP aiming to keep ICP below 20 mmHg and MAP in excess of 70 mmHg and a suitable dosage regime is described by Shapiro (1985). As with total intravenous anaesthesia, Etomidate has been used by infusion for sedation in patients with brain trauma but has been associated with an increased mortality in patients with multiple trauma requiring intensive therapy, linked to suppression of adrenocortical function (see above). It must also be remembered that infusions of any anaesthetic agent may reduce CPP.

Propofol infusion of 1 to 3 mg/kg per h has been shown to reduce ICP in patients with head injury to a greater extent than infusions of fentanyl (Herregods et al., 1989) and others have confirmed that infusion of propofol 3 mg/kg per h controls ICP without reducing CPP in such patients (Mangez et al., 1987). Agitation may occur with propofol sedation unless analgesia is given concurrently, and Harper and colleagues (1989) recommend that an infusion of alfentanil 0.25 $\mu$g/kg per min is given during propofol sedation.

There is a danger of fluid overload if propofol is infused for more than 7 days (Foster and Buckley, 1989). Propofol infusions used for sedation during intensive therapy do not affect steroidogenesis, but the critically ill are particularly sensitive to the cardiovascular depressant effects of propofol.

*Gamma hydroxybutyrate*

Sodium gamma hydroxybutyrate reduces CBF and $CMRO_2$ with little effect on arterial pressure. Recovery is faster than after barbiturates but it may cause hypernatraemia and hypokalaemia during prolonged continuous infusions.

**Alternative sedative agents**

*Inhalation anaesthetics*

Low concentrations of inhalation anaesthetics have been used for sedation as alternatives to intravenous agents. Nitrous oxide was used as a postoperative analgesic and sedative until its effects on the bone marrow became apparent. 0.1% to 0.6% isoflurane in an air/oxygen mixture has recently been used for sedation of critically ill patients in an intensive therapy unit (Kong et al., 1989). It may be useful for sedation in general intensive therapy but the cerebral vasodilation which it causes makes it unsuitable for use in patients with reduced intracranial compliance. This precludes its use in patients who require controlled ventilation following head injury or intracranial surgery.

**Management of status epilepticus**

Some intravenous sedatives have anticonvulsant properties which make them useful in the treatment of convulsions and status epilepticus following intracranial surgery. Intravenous diazepam is a well established immediate treatment for epileptic fits. In status epilepticus, when the convulsions are not adequately controlled with conventional doses of diazepam, intravenous infusions of anaesthetics such as thiopentone, etomidate or propofol can be very effective in controlling the fits until the longer acting convulsants such as phenytoin, sodium valproate or phenobarbitone take effect. Propofol or etomidate are preferred in this situation because their effects wear off quickly when the infusion is stopped. In the patient who has been treated for status epilepticus this allows rapid weaning from the ventilator and return to the neurosurgical ward once the longer acting convulsants are effective. Weaning takes longer if thiopentone is used to control the convulsions because the sedation takes longer to wear off. EEG activity is monitored during infusion of these agents, using a cerebral function monitor or cerebral function analysing monitor, to check that the convulsions are adequately controlled.

## SUMMARY

In order to make a rational choice of anaesthetic agents for neurosurgical operations it is necessary to have a thorough understanding of the physiology and pathophysiology of the cranial contents. It is also necessary to consider the conditions required by the surgeon during the operation and know about the effects of anaesthetic agents on the contents of the cranium. The effects of intravenous anaesthetic agents on the cranial contents give them definite advantages over the volatile anaesthetic agents. The intravenous agents cause a reduction in $CMRO_2$, cerebral vasoconstriction and a reduction in brain bulk, whereas the volatile anaesthetics cause cerebral vasodilation and an increase in brain bulk despite reducing $CMRO_2$. Therefore, infusions of intravenous anaesthetics have advantages when the intracranial compliance is reduced, for example in patients with large cerebral tumours or haematomata and where there is gross cerebral oedema after head injury, and should be used in these situations. However, when intracranial compliance is relatively normal low concentrations of enflurane or isoflurane can be safely used to supplement a relaxant anaesthetic technique and, because of their convenience and predictable effects, are likely to remain popular for elective intracranial surgery.

Propofol is the only intravenous anaesthetic presently available with pharmacological properties which make it suitable for maintenance of anaesthesia by continuous infusion. It is the agent of choice for total intravenous anaesthesia for neurosurgery and has also proved useful for sedation and control of ICP in patients with severe head injury. Despite the tendency for neuroanaesthetists to stop using nitrous oxide, the author considers that it still has properties which are useful in the maintenance of anaesthesia for intracranial surgery. The incidence of awareness with subsequent amnesia may be reduced by the use of nitrous oxide during the continuous infusion of propofol, so the author prefers to supplement propofol infusions with nitrous oxide unless the intracranial compliance is low. However, if the patient is at the right hand end of the pressure volume curve (Fig. 13.1) the vasodilator properties of nitrous oxide may have adverse effects and should be avoided. A propofol infusion with supplementation by alfentanil is the ideal anaesthetic under these circumstances, and the patient is ventilated with oxygen enriched air.

Intravenous benzodiazepines supplemented, if necessary, with small doses of analgesics have proved useful for sedation during neuroradiological procedures such as cerebral angiography, interventional neuroradiology and nuclear magnetic resonance imaging. The use of these agents often obviates the need for a general anaesthetic. Oral sedation with quinalbarbitone or trimeprazine is usually satisfactory for CT scanning in small children.

A variety of intravenous sedative and analgesic agents have been used for sedation of neurosurgical patients during intensive therapy. Intravenous benzodiazepines, opioids and intravenous infusions of propofol are the most suitable agents for use in this situation. Infusion of intravenous anaesthetic agents can also be of use in the immediate managment of status epilepticus whilst conventional anticonvulsants take effect.

## REFERENCES


Artru, A.A. (1984) Effects of halothane and fentanyl anesthesia on resistance to reabsorption of CSF. *J. Neurosurg.* 69, 252—256

Artru, A.A. (1988) Dose-related changes in the rate of cerebrospinal fluid formation and resistance to reabsorption of cerebrospinal fluid following administration of thiopental, midazolam and etomidate in dogs. *Anesthesiology* 69, 541—546.

Barker, J., Harper, A.M., McDowall, D.G., Fitch, W. and Jennett, W.B. (1968) Cerebral blood flow, cerebrospinal fluid pressure and EEG activity during neuroleptanalgesia induced with dehydrobenzperidol and phenoperidine. *Br. J. Anaesth.* 40, 143—144

Barker, J., Miller, J.D. and Johnston, I.H. (1972). The effect of pentazocine on pupillary size and intracranial pressure. *Br. J. Anaesth.* 44, 197—202.

Bedford, R.F., Winn, H.R., Tyson, G., Park, T.S. and Jane, J.A. (1980) Lidocaine prevents increased I.C.P. after endotracheal intubation. In: *Intracranial Pressure IV.* Editors: K. Shulman, A. Marmarou, J.D. Miller, D.P. Becker, G.M. Hochwald and M. Brock, Springer-Verlag, Berlin, pp. 595—598.

Benthuysen, J.L., Kein, N.D. and Quam, D.D. (1988) Intracranial pressure increases during alfentanil-induced rigidity. *Anesthesiology* 68, 438—440.

Bovill, J.G., Sebel, P.S., Wauquier, A., Rog, P. and Schuyt, H.C. (1983) Influence of high-dose alfentanil anaesthesia on the encephalogram: correlation with plasma concentrations. *Br. J. Anaesth.* 55, 199S—209S.

Carlsson, C., Hagerdal. M., Kaasik, A.E. and Siesjo, B.K. (1976) The effects of diazepam on cerebral blood flow and oxygen consumption in rats and its synergistic interaction with nitrous oxide. *Anesthesiology* 45, 319—325.

Chamberlain, M.E. and Bradshaw, E.G. (1985) The "wake up test". A new approach using drug infusions. *Anaesthesia* 40, 780—782.

Christensen, M.S., Broderson, P., Olesen. J. and Paulson, O.B. (1973) Cerebral apoplexy (stroke) treated with or without prolonged artificial hyperventilation: 2. Cerebrospinal fluid acid-base balance and intracranial pressure. *Stroke* 4, 620—631.

Christys, A.R., Moss E. and Powell, D. (1989) Retrospective study of early postoperative convulsions after intracranial surgery with isoflurane or enflurane anaesthesia. *Br. J. Anaesth.* 62, 624—627.

Cohen, R.J., Alexander, S.C. and Wollman, H. (1968) Effects of hypocarbia and of hypoxia with normocarbia on cerebral blood flow and metabolism in man. *Scand. J. Clin. Lab. Invest.* Suppl. 102 IV A.

Cohen, A.T. and Kelly, D.R. (1987) Assessment of alfentanil by intravenous infusion as a long term sedative in intensive care. *Anaesthesia* 42, 545—548.

Cold, G.E., Eskesen, V., Eriksen, H. Amtoft, D. and Madsen. J.B. (1985) CBF and $CMRO_2$ during continuous etomidate infusion with nitrous oxide and fentanyl in patients with supratentorial tumour. A dose response study. *Acta Anaesthesiol. Scand.* 29, 490—494.

Cold, G.E., Eskesen, V., Eriksen, H. and Blatt-Lyon, B. (1986) Changes in $CMRO_2$, E.E.G. and concentration of etomidate in serum and brain tissue during craniotomy with continuous etomidate supplemented with nitrous oxide and fentanyl. *Acta Anaesthesiol. Scand.* 10, 159—163.

Cotev, S. and Shalit, M.N. (1975) Effects of diazepam on cerebral blood flow and oxygen uptake after head injury. *Anaesthesiology* 43, 117—122.

Dodson, M.E. (1982) A review of methods for relief of post-operative pain. *Ann. R. Coll. Surg. Eng.* 64, 324—327.

Drummond, J.C., Scheller, M.S. and Todd, M.M. (1987) The effect of nitrous oxide on cortical cerebral blood flow during anaesthesia with halothane and isoflurane, with and without morphine, in the rabbit. *Anesth. Analg.* 66, 1083—1089.

Dundee, J.W., Collier, P.S., Carlisle, R.J.T. and Harper, K.W. (1986) Prolonged midazolam elimination half-life. *Br. J. Clin. Pharmacol.* 21, 425—429.

Eger, E.I. (1981) Isoflurane: A review. *Anesthesiology* 55, 559—576.

Forster, A., Juge, O. and Morel, D. (1982) Effects of midazolam on cerebral blood flow in human volunteers. *Anesthesiology.* 56, 453—455.

Forster, A., Juge, O., Louis, M. and Nahory, A. (1987) Effects of specific benzodiazepine antagonist (RO 15—1788) on cerebral blood flow. *Anesth. Analg.* 66, 309—313.

Foster, S.J. and Buckley, P.M. (1989) A retrospective review of two year's experience with propofol in one intensive care unit. *J. Drug Dev.* 2 (Suppl. 2), 73—74.

Fragen, R.J., Hanssen, E.H.J.H., Denissen. P.A.E., Booij. L.H.D.J. and Crul. J.F. (1983) Disoprofol (ICI 35868) for total intravenous anaesthesia. *Acta Anaesthesiol. Scand.* 27, 113—116.

Freedman, M. and Levy, E.R. (1988) Propofol intravenous anaesthesia for neurosurgery. *S. Afr. Med. J.* 74, 10—12.

Galletly, D.C. and Short, T.G. (1988) Total intravenous anaesthesia using propofol infusion — 50 consecutive cases. *Anaesth. Intensive Care* 16, 150—157.

Gelb, A.W., Boisvert, D.P., Tang, G., Lam, A.M., Marchak, B.E., Dowman, R. and Mielke. B.W. (1989) Primate brain tolerance to temporary focal cerebral ischaemia during isoflurane — or sodium nitroprusside — induced hypotension. *Anesthesiology* 70, 678—683.

Gomez-Sainz, J.J., Elexpurucamiruaga, J.A., Fernadez Cano, F. and De La Herran, J.L. (1988) Effects of isoflurane on intraventricular pressure in neurosurgical patients. *Br. J. Anaesth.* 61. 347—349.

Goodman, N.W., Black, A.M.S. and Carter, J.A. (1987) Some ventilatory effects of propofol as sole anaesthetic agent. *Br. J. Anaesth.* 59, 1497—1503.

Griffin, J.P., Cottrell, J.E., Shwiry, B., Hartung, J., Epstein, J. and Lim, K. (1984) Intracranial pressure, mean arterial pressure and heart rate following midazolam or thiopental in humans with brain tumors. *Anesthiology* 60, 491—494.

Grummitt, R.M. and Goat, V.A. (1984) Intracranial pressure after phenoperidine. *Anaesthesia* 39, 565—567.

Hansen, H.C. and Drenck, N.E. (1988) Generalized seizures after etomidate anaesthesia. *Anaesthesia*, 43, 805—806.

Hansen, T.D., Warner, D.S., Todd, M.M. and Vust, L.J. (1989) Effects of nitrous oxide and volatile anaesthetics on cerebral blood flow. *Br. J. Anaesth.* 63, 290—295.

Harper, A.M., Deshmukh, V.D., Rowan, J.O. and Jennett, W.B. (1972) The influence of sympathetic nervous activity on cerebral blood flow. *Arch. Neurol.* 27, 1—6.

Harper, J., Buckley, P.M., and Carr, K. (1989) A study of the utility of continuous infusions of propofol and alfentanil in ventilated intensive care patients. *J. Drug Dev.* 2 (Suppl. 2.) 75—76.

Hatano, Y., Nakamura, K., Moriyama, S., Mori, K. and Todd, N. (1989) The contractile responses of isolated dog cerebral vessels and extracerebral arteries to oxybarbiturates and thiobarbiturates. *Anesthesiology* 71, 80—86.

Herregods, L., Verbeke, J. Rolly, G. and Colardyn, F. (1988) Effects of propofol on elevated intracranial pressure. Preliminary results. *Anaesthesia* 43, (Suppl.), 107—109.

Herregods, L., Mergaert, C., Rolly, G. and Colardyn, F. (1989) Comparison of the effects of 24 h propofol or fentanyl infusion on intracranial pressure. *J. Drug Dev.* 2 (Suppl. 2) 99—100.

Hodkinson, B.P., Frith, R.W. and Mee, E.W. (1987) Propofol and the electroencephalogram. *Lancet* 2, 518.

Hoffman. P. (1987) Continuous infusions of fentanyl and alfentanil in intensive care (abstract). *Eur. J. Anaesthesiol.* 4 (Suppl. 1) 71—75.

Hoien, A.O. (1984) Another case of grand mal seizure after fentanyl administration (letter). *Anesthesiology* 60, 387—388.

Horsley, J.S. (1937) The intracranial pressure during barbital narcosis. *Lancet* 1, 141—143.

Hunter, A.R. (1972a) Thiopentone supplemented anaesthesia for neurosurgery. *Br. J. Anaesth.* 44, 506—510.

Hunter, A.R. (1972b) Methohexitone as a supplement to nitrous oxide during intracranial surgery. *Br. J. Anaesth.* 44, 1188—1190.

Jaffe, R.S. and Coalson, D. (1989) Recurrent respiratory depression after alfentanil administration. *Anesthesiology* 70, 151—153.

Kay, B. (1986) Propofol and alfentanil infusion. A comparison with methohexitone and alfentanil for major surgery. *Anaesthesia* 41, 589—595.

Kong, K.L., Willatts, S.M. and Prys-Roberts, C. (1989) Isoflurane compared with midazolam for sedation in the intensive care unit. *Br. Med. J.* 298, 1277—1280.

Lanier, W.L., Milde, J.H. and Michenfelder, J.D. (1986) Cerebral stimulation following succinylcholine in dogs. *Anesthiology* 64, 551—559.

Lassen, N.A. and Agnoli, A. (1972) The upper limit of autoregulation of cerebral blood flow — on the pathogenesis of hypertensive encephalopathy. *Scand. J. Clin. Lab. Invest.* 30, 113—116.

Ledderose, H., Rester, P., Carlsson, P. and Peter, K. (1988) Recovery times and side effects after propofol infusion and after isoflurane during ear surgery with additional infiltration anaesthesia. *Anaesthesia* 43, (Suppl.). 89—91.

Lowson, S. Goodchild, C.S. and Gent, J.P. (1990) Convulsive threshold in mice during the recovery phase from anaesthesia induced by propofol, thiopentone, methohexitone and etomidate. *Br. J. Anaesth.*, in press.

McDonnell, T.E., Bartowski, R.R., Bonilla, F.A., Henthorn, T.K. and Williams, J.J. (1982). Nonuniformity of alfentanil pharmacokinetics in healthy adults. *Anesthesiology* 57, A236.

McDowall, D.G. (1974) In: *Scientific Foundations of Anaesthesia;* 2nd. Edn., Editors: C. Scurr and S. Feldman, William Heinemann, London p. 151.

McDowall, D.G. (1966) Interrelationships between blood oxygen tensions and cerebral blood flow. In: *Oxygen Measurements in Blood and Tissues.* Editors: J.P. Payne and D.W. Hill, Churchill, London, pp. 205—219.

McPherson, R.W., Brian, J.E. and Traystman, R.J. (1989) Cerebrovascular responsiveness to carbon dioxide in dogs with 1.4% and 2.8% isoflurane. *Anesthesiology* 10, 843—850.

McPherson, R.W., Krempasanka, E., Eimerl, D. and Traystman, R.J. (1985) Effects of alfentanil on cerebral vascular reactivity in dogs. *Br. J. Anaesth.* 57, 1232—1238.

Mangez, J.F., Menguy, E. and Roux, P. (1987). Constant rate propofol sedation in the head injured patient. Preliminary data. *Ann. Fr. Anaesthesiol. Reanim.* 6, 336—337.

Mann, J.D., Cookson, S.L. and Mann. E.S. (1980) Differential effects of pentobarbital ketamine hydrochloride and enflurane anaesthesia on CSF formation rate and outflow resistance in the rat. In: *Intracranial Pressure IV.* Editors: K. Shulman, A. Marmarou, J.D. Miller, D.P. Becker, G.M. Hochwald and M. Brock, Springer-Verlag. Berlin, Heidelberg, New York, pp 466—471.

Marx, W., Shah, N., Long, C., Arbit, E., Galicich, J., Mascott, C., Mallya, K. and Bedford, R. (1988) Sufentanil, alfentanil and fentanyl impact on CSF pressure in patients with brain tumours. *Anesthesiology* 69, A627.

Merckx, L., Van Hemelrijck, J., Van Aken, H., Plets, C. and Goffin, J. (1988) Total intravenous anesthesia using propofol and alfentanil infusion in neurosurgical patients. *Anesthesiology* 69, A576.

Michenfelder, J.D. and Theye, R.A. (1971) Effects of fentanyl, droperidol, and Innovar on canine cerebral metabolism and blood flow. *Br. J. Anaesth.* 43, 630—636.

Michenfelder, J.D. and Theye, R.A. (1975) In vivo toxic effects of halothane on canine cerebral metabolic pathways. *Am. J. Physiol.* 229, 1050—1055.

Miller, J.D., Stanek, A.E. and Langfitt, T.W. (1973) Cerebral blood flow regulation during experimental brain compression *J. Neurosurg.* 39, 186—196.

Misfeldt, B.B., Jorgensen, P.B. and Rishoj, M. (1974) The effect of nitrous oxide and halothane upon the intracranial pressure in hypocapnic patients with intracranial disorders. *Br. J. Anaesth.* 46. 853—858.

Misfeldt, B.B., Jorgensen, P.B., Spotoft, H. and Ronde, F. (1976) The effects of droperidol and fentanyl on intracranial pressure and cerebral perfusion pressure in neurosurgical patients. *Br. J. Anaesth.* 48, 963—968.

Moss, E. (1989) Volatile anaesthetic agents in neurosurgery *Br. J. Anaesth.* 63, 4—6.

Moss, E., Powell, D., Gibson, R.M. and McDowall, D.G. (1979) Effect of etomidate on intracranial pressure and cerebral perfusion pressure. *Br. J. Anaesth.* 51, 347—352.

Moss, E., Powell, D., Gibson, R.M. and McDowall, D.G. (1978a) The effects of tracheal intubation on intracranial pressure following induction of anaesthesia with thiopentone or althesin in patients undergoing neurosurgery. *Br. J. Anaesth.* 50, 353—360.

Moss, E., Powell, D., Gibson, R.M. and McDowall, D.G. (1978b) Effects of fentanyl on intracranial pressure and cerebral perfusion pressure during normocapnia. *Br. J. Anaesth.* 50, 779—784.

Moss, E. and McDowall, D.G. (1979) ICP increases with 50% nitrous oxide in oxygen in severe head injuries during controlled ventilation. *Br. J. Anaesth.* 51, 757—760.

Moss, E., Dearden, N.M. and McDowall, D.G. (1983a) Effects of 2% enflurane on intracranial pressure and cerebral perfusion pressure *Br. J. Anaesth.* 55, 1083—1088.

Moss, E., Gibson, J.S., McDowall, D.G. and Gibson, R.M. (1983b) Intensive management of severe head injuries. A scheme of intensive management of severe head injuries. *Anaesthesia* 38, 214—225.

Newberg, L.A., Milde, J.H. and Michenfelder, J.D. (1983) The cerebral metabolic effects of isoflurane at and above concentrations that suppress cortical activity. *Anesthesiology* 59, 23—28.

Nilsson, A., Persson, M.P., Hartvig, P. and Wide, L. (1988) Effect of total intravenous anaesthesia with midazolam/alfentanil on the adrenocortical and hyperglycaemic response to abdominal surgery. *Acta Anaesthesiol. Scand.* 32, 379—382.

Nugent, M., Artru, A.A. and Michenfelder, J.D. (1982) Cerebral, metabolic, vascular and protective effects of midazolam maleate. *Anesthesiology* 56, 172—176.

Nunn, J.F. (1988) Clinical relevance of B12/nitrous oxide interaction. A report of a seminar. *Anaesthesia* 43, 587—589.

Ravussin, P., Guinard. J.P., Ralley, F. and Thorin, D. (1988) Effect of propofol on cerebrospinal fluid pressure and cerebral perfusion pressure in patients undergoing craniotomy. *Anaesthesia* 43, (Suppl.) 37—41.

Rockoff, M.A., Naughton, K.V.H., Shapiro, H.M., Ingvar, M., Ray, K.F., Gagnon, R.L. and Marshall, L.F. (1980) Cerebral circulatory and metabolic responses to intravenously administered lorazepam. *Anesthesiology* 53, 215—218.

Sakabe, T., Maekawa, T., Ishikawa, T and Takeshita, H. (1974) The effect of lidocaine on canine cerebral metabolism and circulation related to the encephalogram. *Anesthesiology* 40, 433—441.

Scheller, M.S., Tateishi, A., Drummond, J.C. and Zornow, M.H. (1988) The effects of sevoflurane on cerebral blood flow, cerebral metabolic rate for oxygen, intracranial pressure and the electroencephalogram are similar to those of isoflurane in the rabbit. *Anesthesiology* 68, 548—551.

Shapiro, H.M. (1985) Barbiturates in brain ischaemia. *Br. J. Anaesth.* 57, 82—95.

Shapiro, H.M., Wyte, S.R., Harris, A.B. and Galindo, A. (1972) Acute intraoperative intracranial hypertension in neurosurgical patients: mechanical and pharmacological factors. *Anesthesiology* 37, 399—405.

Shupak, R.C., Harp, J.R., Stevenson-Smith, W., Rossi, D. and Buchheit, W.A. (1983) High dose fentanyl for neuroanesthesia. *Anesthesiology* 58, 579—582.

Simpson, K.H., Halsall, P.J., Carr, C.M.E. and Stewart, K.G. (1988) Propofol reduces seizure duration in patients having anaesthesia for electroconvulsive therapy. *Br. J. Anaesth.* 61, 343—344.

Sold, M. and Weis, K.-H. (1987) Alfentanil or fentanyl for anaesthetic procedures of two hours duration? A double-blind study. *Eur. J. Anaesthesiol.* 4, 337—344.

Sondergard, W. (1961) Intracranial pressure during general anaesthesia. *Dan. Med. Bull.* 8, 18—25.

Steegers, P.A. and Foster, P.A. (1988) Propofol in total intravenous anaesthesia without nitrous oxide. *Anaesthesia* 43 (Suppl.), 94—97.

Stephan, H., Sonntag, H., Schenk, H.D. and Kohlhausen, S. (1987) Effect of disoprovan on cerebral blood flow, cerebral oxygen consumption and cerebral vascular reactivity. *Anaesthesist* 36, 60—65.

Tarkkanen, L., Laitinen, L. and Johansson, G. (1974) Effects of *d*-tubocurarine on intracranial pressure and thalamic electrical impedance. *Anesthesiology* 40, 247—251.

Tateishi, A., Maekawa, T., Takeshita, H. and Wakuta, K. (1981) Diazepam and intracranial pressure. *Anesthesiology* 54, 335—337.

Thoresen, M. and Walloe, L. (1980). Changes in cerebral blood flow in humans during hyperventilation and $CO_2$ breathing. *J. Physiol.* (Lond.), 298. 53P—54P.

Todd, M.M. and Drummond, J.C. (1984) A comparison of the cerebro-vascular and metabolic effects of halothane and isoflurane in the cart. *Anesthesiology* 60, 276—282.

Van Aken, H., Fitch, W., Graham, D.L., Brussel, T. and Themann, N. (1986) Cardiovascular and cerebrovascular effects of isoflurane-induced hypotension in the baboon. *Anesth. Analg.* 65, 565—574.

Vernhiet, J., Macrez, P., Renou, A.M., Constant, P., Billery. J. and Caille, J.M. (1977) The effects of large doses of morphinomimetics (fentanyl and fentathienyl) on the cerebral circulation in the normal subject. *Ann. Anaesthesiol. Fr.* 18, 803—810.

Victory, R.A.P. and Magee, D. (1988) A case of convulsions after propofol anaesthesia (letter). *Anaesthesia* 43, 904.

Wardley-Smith, B., Little, H.J., and Halsey, M.J., (1988) Lack of correlation between the anaesthetic and anticonvulsant potencies of Althesin, ketamine and methohexitone. *Br. J. Anaesth.* 60, 140—145.

Wright, P.J. and Murray, R.J. (1989) Penetrating craniocerebral airgun injury. Anaesthetic management with propofol infusion and review of recent reports. *Anaesthesia* 44, 219—221.

Wynands, J.E., Wong, P., Townsend, G.E., Sprigge, J.S. and Whalley, D.G. (1984) Narcotic requirements for intravenous anesthesia. *Anesth. Analg.* 63, 101—105.

# 14

# *Intravenous anaesthesia and sedation for regional anaesthesia*

Neil Mackenzie

## INTRODUCTION

Regional anaesthesia is assuming an increasingly important role in modern anaesthetic practice as more and more anaesthetists recognise the limitations of general anaesthesia and the advantages conferred by local techniques in many situations. These include particularly the preservation of consciousness and protective reflexes, the beneficial influences on certain aspects of peri-operative morbidity and the provision of excellent postoperative analgesia. This current popularity has been aided by the publication of several large studies confirming the inherent safety of regional anaesthesia (Dripps and Vandam, 1954; Moore and Bridenbaugh, 1966; Phillips et al., 1969), the reformation of the American Society of Regional Anesthesia in 1976 followed by the founding of its European counterpart six years later, and the present availability of several local anaesthetic agents of low toxicity and variable spectrum of action together with specifically designed, high quality equipment for regional use.

Prolonged analgesia using continuous regional anaesthetic techniques is now relatively straightforward, normally involving the placement of a catheter either in the epidural space or alongside a peripheral nerve or plexus. This has become standard practice in obstetrical anaesthesia and analgesia and is being applied increasingly to the control of acute pain following major surgery or trauma and to the management of chronic intractable pain. Either local anaesthetic agents or opiates may be administered and further advances in this field are likely.

In addition to developments of local anaesthetic agents and equipment there have been many advances in the related field of peri-operative sedation, resulting in the wide range of supplementary drugs and techniques currently available to aid patient acceptance of and management during regional blockade. This has been a major factor in convincing patients and surgeons alike that regional anaesthesia is a genuine alternative to general anaesthesia and has contributed significantly to its advancement.

## PATIENT MANAGEMENT DURING REGIONAL ANAESTHESIA

In many respects this is the most challenging aspect of regional anaesthesia and must never be neglected. The nerve block is only part of the total anaesthetic management of the patient and should not preclude the concurrent administration of other anaesthetic techniques and agents as appropriate. Most patients expect to be asleep while undergoing surgery and this must always be borne in mind by the anaesthetist. Only if the supplementary sedation is as carefully chosen and administered as the local block itself will the full potential of the technique be realised thus ensuring ultimate patient benefit and satisfaction.

### Pre-operative assessment

Adequate preparation of the patient for surgery under regional anaesthesia is fundamental to its success. The pre-operative visit with establishment of good doctor-patient rapport is vital and indeed constitutes the start of the sedation process. The anaesthetist can assess the patient's general health and psychological make-up. He can discuss the nature of the proposed block and decide on the degree of supplementary sedation required. Any questions can be answered and possible fears or misconceptions allayed. The understandable wishes of many patients to be asleep during surgery and not to see the actual operation being performed can be guaranteed, relieving much of the pre-operative anxiety. On the other hand, that smaller number of patients who express a fear of 'going to sleep' and who specifically want to remain awake during the operation can also be accommodated and reassured.

### Premedication

Once the patient has been assessed the need for premedication must be considered. Some anaesthetists, particularly in the United States, advocate heavy premedication with intramuscular opiates to avoid any physical or psychological discomfort associated with carrying out the nerve block. This may be useful if the patient is in pain as, for example, following a fracture, or if the anaesthetist is inexperienced or teaching a junior colleague. The effects, however, are often unpredictable and may interfere with patient co-operation particularly if this is essential to performance of the block, or may cause postural hypotension, nausea and vomiting, respiratory depression or delayed gastric emptying. For these reasons many anaesthetists prefer premedication with a short-acting benzodiazepine and rely primarily on the pre-operative establishment of patient confidence to relieve anxiety. Gjessing and Tomlin (1977) have demonstrated the value of diazepam premedication in improving the quality of subsequent intra-operative sedation produced with intravenous diazepam. The greater sedative, anxiolytic and amnesic effects of midazolam compared to diazepam when given by intramuscular injection as premedication for regional anaesthesia may be advantageous but only if given within an hour of the anticipated procedure (Reinhart et al., 1985).

In certain circumstances, particularly with elderly patients, premedication may be omitted completely. This is also true for the increasing number of patients undergoing day case procedures under regional anaesthesia. However, if the unacceptably high incidence of vaso-vagal attacks which McClure and colleagues (1983) found while performing spinal analgesia in unpremedicated young patients is to be avoided, intravenous supplementation is advisable.

Anticholinergic drugs have no place in routine premedication and should be reserved for situations where excessive secretions might prove troublesome as, for example, in intra-oral or airway surgery. Administration of a long-acting non-steroidal anti-inflammatory drug orally before major operations is often useful in counteracting the pain and stiffness which many patients experience during a long period of immobility on the operating table (Charlton, 1987).

## Peri-operative sedation

A wide range of supplementary methods are available from simple forms of distraction therapy through increasing depths of inhalational or intravenous sedation to full general anaesthesia. The appropriate method and level of sedation must be chosen for each patient individually, taking into account such variables as the nature of surgery, the type of regional block, the general health and temperament of the patient and the experience and attitude of both the surgeon and anaesthetist.

### *Distraction*

Often regional anaesthesia is chosen for a particular patient specifically to avoid rendering him or her unconscious as, for example, in the presence of upper airway obstruction, a full stomach or general debility. In this situation anything other than the lightest of sedation is inappropriate and should be avoided. Similarly, in operative obstetrics sedative agents may obtund protective reflexes and consciousness in the mother and will cross the placenta readily, causing fetal depression and negating the advantages of the regional technique. In all of these situations verbal support and simple distraction therapy are indicated, including the playing of pre-recorded music through personal headphones or even watching television.

The importance of a calm, quiet theatre environment remains just as crucial in this respect as it did in Gaston Labat's day (1922) when regional anaesthesia was in its infancy.

> 'In certain hospitals music is brought to the operating room either by victrola or radio. Music tends to take the patient's attention away from the operating room, if it does not divert the surgeon. The radio head-piece is the most convenient because it does not disturb the silence which is so urgently needed in the operating room. Every noise should be avoided or softened, particularly that made by throwing instruments in metal or enamelled basins. Making remarks or in any way discussing the operation is not permitted, since many a word may be erroneously interpreted and harmful suspicions aroused.'

Nonetheless most patients appreciate and will benefit from more formal pharmacological methods of sedation, enabling them to rest quietly or sleep lightly during operation.

*Sedation*

Light sedation provides a calm and relaxed patient without depression of consciousness. This ensures that protective reflexes are adequate, that the patient will maintain an unobstructed airway and that he or she maintains verbal contact with the operator. This level of sedation is often employed in out-patient dental practice and is commonly termed 'conscious sedation'. It controls restlessness and anxiety, not pain, and is often carried out by the operator himself.

Deeper sedation, however, will inevitably involve some degree of reduced consciousness and therefore the risk of obtunding protective reflexes and losing airway control. Although the patient may be rousable to command or mild stimulation, spontaneous verbal communication is lost and this state may merge imperceptibly into light general anaesthesia with resultant loss of consciousness and airway control. Incremental techniques of intravenous sedation may cause the patient to fluctuate between the two. Thus heavy sedation or hypnosis and light general anaesthesia should always be administered by an independent practitioner, preferably an anaesthetist, who is fully trained in airway management and resuscitation. The patient must be closely monitored if circulatory and respiratory depression are to be detected and treated effectively and rapidly. The use of pulse oximetry is invaluable in this respect and supplementary oxygen should always be administered unless measured tissue oxygen saturation is shown to be satisfactory.

It can therefore be seen that verbal contact is the crucial factor in drawing the dividing line between the two very different entities of conscious sedation and deep sedation/anaesthesia and this must always be stressed, particularly to non-anaesthetists who are involved in performing procedures under regional anaesthesia in sedated patients.

As a general rule, distraction with or without light sedation is appropriate for short, relatively stress-free procedures up to about 1 h duration in co-operative adults. This would include most minor and intermediate types of gynaecological, urological and general surgical procedures in the lower abdomen and simple orthopaedic or plastic surgery on the limbs, also the majority of day-case and dental operations. For longer, more invasive surgery, particularly if it involves awkward or uncomfortable positioning of the patient on the operating table, a deeper level of sedation is advisable to avoid patient distress. Examples include major orthopaedic joint replacement surgery, amputations, peripheral vascular and major plastic operations, also intra-abdominal and intrathoracic procedures. This applies also to patients with pre-existing arthritis where pain and stiffness in the affected joints can cause considerable discomfort while lying on a hard operating table.

## PHARMACOLOGICAL METHODS OF SEDATION

Sedation may be delivered by the inhalational or intravenous routes.

## INHALATIONAL SEDATION

Light levels of inhalational sedation are often used in dental practice in the technique of relative analgesia where the patient breathes low to moderate concentrations of nitrous oxide in oxygen through a nasal mask to provide sedation as an adjunct to dental surgery under local anaesthesia. This has been shown to alleviate fear, reduce pain and improve patient co-operation, (Langa 1968; Roberts, 1983). Constant verbal assurance and semi-hypnotic suggestion on the part of the operator is essential to the success of the method and most subjects will assume the desired level of sedation with 20—35% nitrous oxide. At this level the incidence of side effects is low and no impairment of airway reflexes has been demonstrated. At higher levels, however, this may not apply and incompetence of laryngeal closure has been demonstrated in 20% of volunteers breathing 50% nitrous oxide in oxygen (Rubin et al., 1977). Subanaesthetic concentrations of volatile anaesthetic agents are also used to supplement regional anaesthesia, particularly for ambulatory procedures and in dental practice (Philip, 1985; Parbrook et al., 1989).

All inhalational techniques, however, necessitate the use of close-fitting masks or mouthpieces to ensure adequate drug intake and reduce environmental pollution and many patients find this unpleasant or uncomfortable. More importantly, there is always the risk of obtunding protective reflexes and constant vigilance must be exercised at all times to avoid unintentional general anaesthesia. It is often preferable to aim for general anaesthesia from the outset, particularly for intra-abdominal and intrathoracic surgery under central neural blockade. Indeed, the term 'balanced anaesthesia' was introduced in 1942 by Lundy to describe just this situation. General anaesthesia is conventionally provided by the inhalational route using nitrous oxide in oxygen with a small concentration of volatile agent, but an intravenous infusion of propofol is a good alternative to the volatile agent (Mackenzie, 1988).

Children provide another group where the combination of regional and general anaesthesia is particularly appropriate and rewarding. With young children explanation is difficult and co-operation unlikely, so the block is best performed once the child is anaesthetised. The depth of anaesthesia can then be lightened during the operation providing a rapid and most importantly pain-free recovery (Armitage, 1987; Lloyd-Thomas, 1990).

## INTRAVENOUS SEDATION

Intravenous supplementation of regional anaesthesia is more suited to routine use than the inhalational route and is much more extensively practised. It is easier to administer, does not involve the use of bulky and expensive equipment, is free from environmental pollution and is much more acceptable to the patient. It should always be delivered in a slow, carefully controlled manner, either by incremental bolus or continuous infusion, titrating dose to effect for each individual patient. The ideal intravenous sedative agent has been defined thus, 'it would provide reliable sedation or sleep with airway maintenance and minimal effect on the circulation or respiration and recovery would be rapid with no residual drowsiness' (McClure et al., 1983). In addition, it should be compatible with other anaesthetic drugs, non-toxic, free of hypersensitivity problems and, if possible, water soluble and stable in solution.

Three main drug groups are used in an attempt to meet these criteria, namely, tranquillisers, intravenous anaesthetic agents and opioids.

**Tranquillisers**

The benzodiazepines provide the main drugs in this group although the Vitamin $B_1$ derivative chlormethiazole may be a useful alternative.

**Benzodiazepines**

All benzodiazepines possess anxiolytic, hypnotic, anticonvulsant, muscle relaxant and amnesic properties. They act on specific receptor sites throughout the central nervous system, the density of which is greatest in the cerebral cortex, hippocampus and cerebellum, and produce their effects by potentiating inhibitory interneurones which use gamma-amino-butyric acid (GABA) as a neurotransmitter. Their clinical use is related more to their pharmacokinetic profiles and pharmaceutical preparation than to different pharmacodynamic effects and they will all cause dose-related cerebral depression ranging from sedation to drowsiness, sleep, and finally narcosis.

Of the 30 or so benzodiazepines which have been used clinically the majority are only available as oral preparations marketed as hypnotics for night sedation, day time anxiolytics and sedatives. Several are popular in anaesthetic practice as premedicants but only four are commonly administered by the intravenous route in the related fields of anaesthesia and sedation. Diazepam and midazolam are administered most frequently while flunitrazepam and lorazepam are used to a much lesser extent, although there is some degree of variability in usage patterns between different countries.

Table 14.1 illustrates the different pharmacokinetic parameters of these four injectable benzodiazepines.

*Diazepam*

First introduced into clinical practice in the mid 1960s, diazepam rapidly became the mainstay of intravenous sedation. It revolutionised dental practice (Main, 1968),

TABLE 14.1

Pharmacokinetics of the injectable benzodiazepines (from Kanto and Klotz, 1982)[a]

| | $t_{1/2\alpha}$ (min) | $V1$ (l/kg) | $t_{1/2\beta}$ (h) | $Vd_{\beta}$ (l/kg) | $Cl$ (ml/min) |
|---|---|---|---|---|---|
| Diazepam | 9—130 | 0.31—0.41 | 31.3—46.6 | 0.9—1.2 | 26—35 |
| Lorazepam | 3—10 | 0.30—0.72 | 14.3—14.6 | 1.14—1.30 | 1.05—1.10 (ml/kg per min) |
| Midazolam | 3—38 | 0.17—0.44 | 2.1—2.4 | 0.8—1.14 | 202—324 |
| Flunitrazepam | 15 ± 8 | 0.61 ± 0.36 | 25 ± 11 | 3.6 ± 1.3 | 94 ± 37 |

[a]$t_{1/2\alpha}$, distribution half life; $V1$, volume of central compartment; $t_{1/2\beta}$, eliminiation half life; $Vd_{\beta}$, apparent volume of distribution; $Cl$, total plasma clearance.

removing much of the need for general anaesthesia and replacing the less satisfactory intravenous sedative techniques then in vogue, such as intermittent methohexitone sedation, or the pentobarbitone, pethidine and hyoscine technique popularised by Jorgensen (1961), with their fine dividing line between sedation and general anaesthesia.

Diazepam has many of the desirable features of an intravenous sedative. It provides good sedation and amnesia, is relatively undisturbing to the cardiovascular and respiratory systems, and is a good anticonvulsant increasing protection against local anaesthetic toxicity. Gjessing and Tomlin (1977) found that a small intravenous dose of 2.5—5 mg improved sedation in patients undergoing surgery under regional blockade when compared to placebo, particularly if no premedication had been given. Anterograde amnesia is produced in 50% and 90% of patients, respectively, after 5 mg or 10 mg i.v. This comes on within 1 min, peaks at 2—3 min and lasts for approximately 30 min (Dundee and Pandit, 1972). Retrograde amnesia has been reported but this is an inconsistent feature (Dundee and Wyant, 1988a).

Although diazepam may be administered in large doses i.v., up to 2 mg/kg, to induce anaesthesia, much less is given to sedate patients for surgery under regional anaesthesia. Conventional practice is to titrate small intravenous doses over several minutes to produce the required level of sedation. A typical starting bolus would be 2.5—5 mg followed by increments of approximately 50% of the initial dose at 30-s to 1-min intervals. A typical sedative dose is 0.1 mg/kg to 0.3 mg/kg and in this range very little physiological disturbance is seen.

Thus Pearce (1974a) found no significant changes in $PaCO_2$ in a series of elderly male patients undergoing lower abdominal surgery under central neural blockade following an average sleep dose of 20.7 mg diazepam i.v. after 10 mg intramuscularly as premedication. Catchlove and Kafer (1971a), in contrast, observed a 19% rise in $PaCO_2$ in a younger group of patients following 0.14 mg/kg diazepam i.v. Their patients, however, were not premedicated and had low $PaCO_2$ values to start with, rising during sedation to a normal mean value of 40.5 mmHg, suggesting that a degree of hyperventilation was present prior to anaesthesia. They demonstrated a depression of the slope of the ventilatory response to carbon dioxide in over half their patients indicating some respiratory depresssion, although not of clinical importance in normal patients. A smaller number of patients with obstructive lung disease were given a reduced dose of diazepam (0.11 mg/kg) and showed a small rise in $PaCO_2$ and reduced response to carbon dioxide, but again of no clinical significance (Catchlove and Kafer, 1971b).

Stovner and Endresen (1966) reported a 20—30% reduction in respiratory minute volume following diazepam 15—20 mg i.v. but this followed a morphine and hyoscine premedication, and Hellewell (1968) also cautions against its use in aged patients who have had opiate premedication. In another study there was no evidence of significant respiratory depression at doses of up to 0.27 mg/kg diazepam i.v. (Cohen et al., 1969). Dixon and colleagues (1973) showed no difference in oxygen saturation between unsedated controls and patients sedated with incremental diazepam (mean dose of 0.25 mg/kg) for dental surgery under local anaesthesia, apart from one patient who fell asleep and obstructed his airway. The importance of respiratory obstruction as the most significant respiratory effect of sedative doses of diazepam is emphasised by Healy and co-workers (1970). They found no significant changes in $PaO_2$ or $PaCO_2$ in patients sedated with diazepam 0.2 mg/kg i.v. by an incremental technique. However, in a preliminary study where the same total dose was given more rapidly all subjects went to sleep and there was a high incidence of sub-clinical respiratory obstruction. They also demonstrated a degree of laryngeal incompetence in some patients during the first 5 min of sedation.

Cardiovascular stability is a feature of diazepam. With marked sedation or loss of consciousness there is the usual peripheral vasodilatation with a slight drop in cardiac output and peripheral vascular resistance (Dundee and Wyant, 1988a), but this is of little clinical significance. Some caution should be exercised, however, if the patient is upright or semi-upright in the dental chair or where they are already markedly vasodilated from a spinal or epidural block.

Dalen and colleagues (1969) administered 5—10 mg diazepam i.v. to 15 patients undergoing cardiac catheterisation and found no significant changes in heart rate, systemic and pulmonary vascular resistance and stroke volume. There were minimal falls in diastolic and mean blood pressures. Systolic pressure remained unchanged in 6 patients, increased in one and fell by 12—25 mmHg in 8. These changes were asymptomatic and required no treatment, being comparable to observations during normal sleep (Khatri and Freis, 1967). Again, Healy and colleagues (1970a) found no significant changes in the haemodynamic status of their patients given 0.2 mg/kg diazepam i.v. for dental sedation apart from a transient tachycardia during injection and confirmed this in a larger interdisciplinary study (1970b). Similarly Pearce (1974a) could find no circulatory changes attributable to diazepam 0.32 mg/kg in his series of elderly male patients.

Diazepam does, however, have several important disadvantages as an intravenous sedative, including pain on injection with subsequent thrombophlebitis, wide biological variations in patient response and delayed recovery.

TABLE 14.2

Local venous sequelae to i.v. injection of the three forms of diazepam (from Schou-Olesen and Huttel, 1980)

Results are numbers (and percentages) out of 197 patients.

| | Diazemuls (emulsion) $n = 67$ | Stesolid M R (Cremophor) $n = 66$ | Stesolid (propylene glycol) $n = 64$ |
|---|---|---|---|
| Pain on injection | 1 (1) | 25 (38) | 50 (78) |
| Local redness/tenderness and induration | 2 (3) | 2 (3) | 11 (17) |
| Thrombophlebitis | 4 (6) | 6 (9) | 31 (48) |
| No pain or reaction | 64 (96) | 37 (49) | 9 (14) |

Diazepam, like most benzodiazepines, is insoluble in water and the original intravenous preparation was solubilised in propylene glycol, ethanol and sodium benzoate in benzoic acid as Valium. This preparation causes a high incidence of pain on injection with subsequent venous damage, particularly when small veins are used. Alternative solvents have been introduced in an attempt to overcome this problem. Thus Cremophor EL was used in the preparation of Stesolid M R. This led to a significant decrease in venous complications but was implicated in severe anaphylactoid reactions (Schou-Olesen and Huttel, 1978) and withdrawn for this reason. Reformulation in a soya bean emulsion as Diazemuls has virtually eliminated the venous problem, however, with no alteration in therapeutic effect (Thorn-Alquist, 1977) and this is now the preparation of choice for intravenous administration. Table 14.2 summarises these findings.

Delayed recovery and patient variation in response remain the major problems with diazepam no matter how formulated. The drug has a long elimination half-life of between 20 and 70 h (Dundee and Wyant, 1988a) and there is a second peak effect some 4—6 h after initial intravenous administration due to the enterohepatic recirculation of drug excreted in the bile and reabsorbed by the intestinal mucosa. This may cause a degree of resedation (Baird and Hailey, 1972). The ingestion of food but not water within 5 h of injection will influence the remobilisation of diazepam, with an increase in serum levels and evidence of significant impairment of psychomotor skills (Korttila et al., 1976). Diazepam is metabolised in the liver to desmethyldiazepam which itself is pharmacologically active, having an elimination half-life greater than that of the parent compound (more than 100 h). This may be of great clinical importance following repeated use. Many investigators have found clinical evidence of delayed recovery. Pearce (1974a) states that his patients usually fell asleep 4—6 h after initial recovery following diazepam 0.32 mg/kg i.v. Anterograde amnesia was marked and lasted from 1—3 days in some patients. Gale (1976) found that diazepam 0.31 mg/kg produced a more prolonged recovery period than conventional general anaesthesia and was incomplete after 3 h when measured by a battery of 11 psychomotor tests. Brown and Dundee (1968) showed persistent ataxia in 30% of patients 24 h after a larger dose of diazepam (0.6 mg/kg). Other workers have produced evidence of a dose-related impairment of recovery. Grove-White and Kelman (1971) demonstrated critical flicker fusion threshold changes 90 min following diazepam 0.05 mg/kg. Gale showed psychomotor impairment 3 h after 0.31 mg/kg with ataxia persisting for 90 min, and Brown and Dundee 24 h after twice the dose. Korttila and Linnoila (1975) gave intravenous doses of diazepam 0.15 mg/kg, 0.3 mg/kg or 0.45 mg/kg to healthy volunteers and investigated their effects on psychomotor function with particular respect to driving skills. They found significant impairments 2, 6 and 8 h later and also a large inter-patient variation in serum diazepam concentration with each dose level. Their conclusion was that patients should not drive or operate machinery for at least 6 h after 0.15 mg/kg and for 10 h after the larger doses.

Dixon and Thornton (1973) also demonstrated delayed recovery in patients undergoing dental sedation and advised that all such patients should be accompanied home and desist from driving for 24 h. Similar advice is given by O'Neil and colleagues (1970).

The clinically obvious between-patient variability in dose response to diazepam is a feature of all the benzodiazepines and is thought to be due to high plasma protein binding (Bond et al., 1977). Of diazepam in the blood, 98% is bound to albumin (Greenblatt et al., 1982), therefore small changes in protein binding will markedly alter the concentration of free drug available. This emphasises the importance of titrating small intravenous increments of drug over several minutes to produce the desired effect for each individual patient. Thus Barker and his coworkers (1986) found a six-fold variation in dose requirement in young, fit patients undergoing dental sedation to produce the same clinical effect, namely 0.08 mg/kg to 0.47 mg/kg.

Elderly patients often demonstrate an increased sensitivity to diazepam (Klotz et al., 1975). Kanto and colleagues (1979) showed that all of the major determinants of diazepam pharmacokinetics (elimination half-life, volume of distribution and total plasma clearance) were altered with advancing age in patients given the drug in conjunction with spinal anaesthesia. They conclude that in patients over 60 the dose should be reduced by a half to a quarter as compared to younger subjects. Kanto and Klotz (1982) comment that incremental administration of intravenous benzodiazepines is difficult and long-lasting in geriatric patients and that reduced doses of the orthodox induction agents give more predictable results.

### *Midazolam*

This imidazobenzodiazepine derivative offers several distinct advantages over the conventional benzodiazepines and in many respects is the best intravenous supplement for regional anaesthesia currently available. The fused imidazole ring (Fig. 14.1) makes the drug highly basic and therefore water soluble and also allows rapid

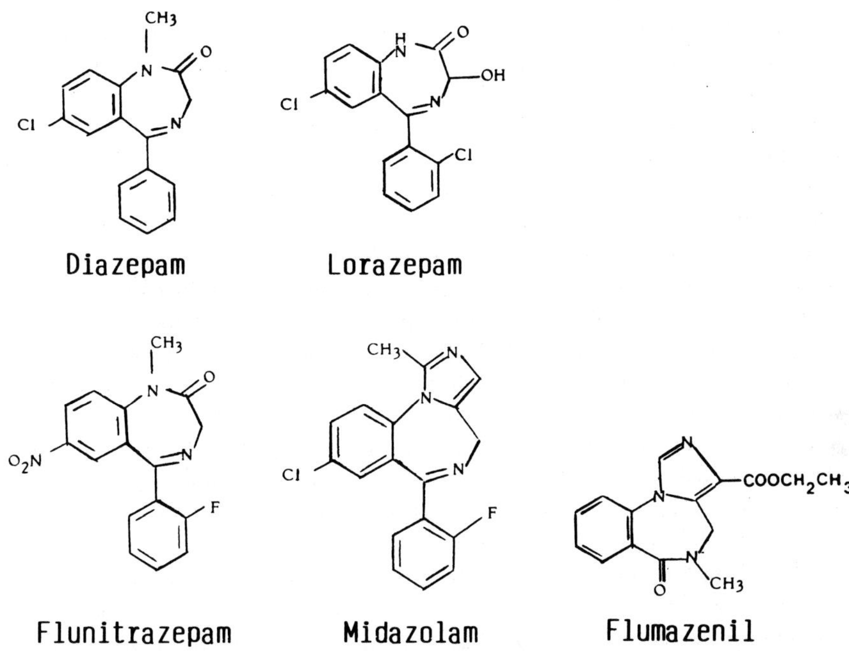


Fig. 14.1. Chemical structures of the injectable benzodiazepines.

hepatic metabolism. Midazolam has an elimination half-life some twenty times shorter than diazepam (approximately 2 h) and is cleared about 10 times more rapidly from plasma (Table 14.1). There is no evidence of enterohepatic recirculation or of pharmacologically active metabolites. It is highly protein bound (96—97%) (Greenblatt et al, 1984) and the free drug has approximately twice the affinity for benzodiazepine receptors as diazepam (Mohler and Okada, 1977) Clinically, it is approximately one and a half to two times as potent as diazepam (Whitwam et al., 1983). Its high lipophilicity at body pH produces a rapid onset of action and its pharmacokinetic profile a short duration of effect.

Being water soluble midazolam is relatively free from venous irritation. Pain on injection is rare, and there is a low incidence of thrombophlebitis. The overall incidence is similar to thiopentone (Berggren and Eriksson, 1981). Midazolam produces some respiratory depression. In healthy volunteers 0.15 mg/kg i.v. reduced the ventilatory response to carbon dioxide and the maximum decrease in minute ventilation is similar to that produced by an equivalent dose of diazepam (0.3 mg/kg) (Forster et al., 1980). In patients with chronic obstructive lung disease, respiratory depression is evident sooner and is more prolonged than in normal patients after 0.2 mg/kg i.v. (Morel et al., 1982). A lower sedative dose of 0.075 mg/kg does not affect the ventilatory response to carbon dioxide (Power et al., 1983), suggesting that at these levels of sedation clinically important respiratory depression is unlikely.

Concurrent administration of opioids or other CNS depressants may produce additive respiratory depression, however, and similarly apnoea is more likely to occur after intravenous midazolam in patients premedicated with opioids (Kanto et al., 1982).

Midazolam 0.15 mg/kg i.v. has been shown to reduce systolic and diastolic blood pressure slightly and to increase heart rate (Forster et al., 1980). Compared to diazepam, there is a greater decrease in blood pressure and slightly greater fall in systemic vascular resistance when these agents are used for induction of anaesthesia (Samuelson et al., 1981). However, in sedative doses cardiorespiratory depression is normally insignificant. Thus McClure and colleagues (1983) gave either midazolam 0.19 mg/kg or diazepam 0.42 mg/kg to sedate patients undergoing surgery under spinal anaesthesia. They found only small insignificant decreases in mean systolic blood pressure and slight increases in heart rate and respiratory rate with no evidence of respiratory obstruction. Similarly Al-Khudhairi and colleagues (1982), giving smaller doses of midazolam (0.1 mg/kg) or diazepam (0.15 mg/kg) for gastroscopy, found no evidence of significant cardiorespiratory depression. The only change of note was a 10—-15% fall in systolic blood pressure, no more than might be expected in response to the sedation of an anxious group of patients. Similar findings were reported with midazolam 0.05 mg/kg versus diazepam 0.15 mg/kg (Berggren et al., 1983), and with midazolam 0.07 mg/kg or diazepam 0.15 mg/kg (Whitwam et al., 1983). Caution must be exercised, however, when opioids are given concurrently. Magni et al. (1983) administered pethidine 50 mg with hyoscine i.v. together with midazolam 0.11 mg/kg or diazepam 0.17 mg/kg, again for upper gastrointestinal endoscopy. Although they showed no clinically significant alteration in arterial pressure or heart rate in either group, three patients (one midazolam and two diazepam) suffered from respiratory depression severe enough to require naloxone reversal.

Many comparative studies have been carried out with midazolam and diazepam for sedation. Procedures include surgery under spinal, epidural and brachial plexus blockade, upper gastrointestinal endoscopy, and dental surgery under local anaesthesia. All have shown that midazolam provides equivalent or better quality of sedation, with an average dose requirement of approximately 0.1 mg/kg. Most studies demonstrate faster onset of sedation and a significantly greater amnesic effect following midazolam (Berggren et al., 1983; Whitwam et al., 1983; Aun et al., 1984; Barker et al., 1986). The amnesia is present 2 min after injection and declines over the ensuing 20—40 min, (Dundee and Wilson, 1980), correlating well with clinical sedation and anxiolysis. Thus Barker and colleagues (1986) demonstrated significant differences in peri-operative recall in a cross-over study of 50 patients undergoing dental sedation (Fig. 14.2). This did not apply to later events such as leaving hospital and returning home. This ability to produce a short period of anterograde amnesia forms part of the basis of the efficacy of midazolam and diazepam as sedatives for endoscopy and dental practice where patients have little or no recall of the unpleasant passage of the endoscope or injection of local anaesthetic. The quick recovery allows the patient to maintain control of the air

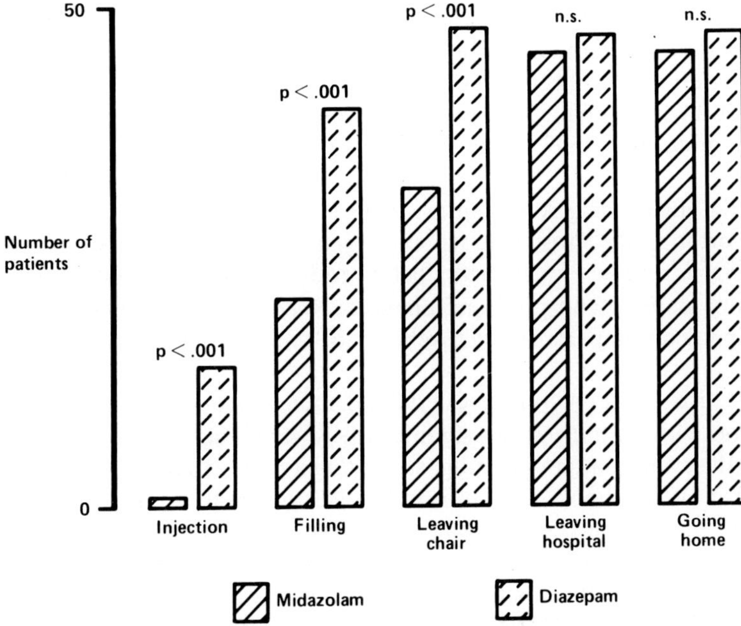


Fig. 14.2. Patient recall. Midazolam versus diazepam sedation for conservative dentistry. From Barker et al. (1986).

way and other vital functions while remaining quietly sedated for the remainder of the procedures and capable of returning home safely postoperatively (Dundee and Wyant, 1988a). Patient acceptability of operative sedation is very good with midazolam and there is significant preference for midazolam over diazepam in Magni's study (1983). Similarly Barker (1986) found that more patients preferred midazolam to diazepam in his cross-over study.

Although midazolam is short acting in comparison to diazepam there may be no differences in time to complete recovery when sedative doses of the two drugs are given. Berggren (1983) showed no difference in return of normal psychomotor function 2 h after sedation for endoscopy. Similarly, Magni (1983) demonstrated impaired sensorimotor performance at 2 h in both his endoscopy groups. Whitwam (1983) also found similar results in gross recovery parameters (orientation, walking ability and Romberg steadiness), both groups being ready for discharge home 75 min after injection.

When used to supplement regional blockade Dixon and coworkers (1984) found no differences in Trieger test results 4 and 6 h after surgery with equipotent sedative doses of midazolam and diazepam although drowsiness was commoner in the postoperative period with the latter. McClure et al. (1983) also failed to show any differences in Trieger testing 3 h after sedation despite observing that the midazolam group were more alert. Similarly Korttila and Tarkkanen (1985) found no difference in recovery of psychomotor function between midazolam 0.1 mg/kg and diazepam 0.2 mg/kg given for sedation to cover bronchoscopy under local anaesthesia. The incidence of side effects has been shown to be greater in the later postoperative period (up to 30 h) in out-patients receiving diazepam 0.15 mg/kg compared to those receiving midazolam 0.07 mg/kg for gastroscopy sedation (Sanders et al., 1989).

Midazolam has also been given by intravenous infusion to provide deep sedation for major orthopaedic surgery under spinal anaesthesia (Wilson et al., 1988, 1990). A mean infusion rate of 0.26 mg/kg per h produced excellent sedation with cardiorespiratory stability and profound amnesia. Recovery, however, was prolonged, with significant impairment of psychomotor function 3 h after the end of infusion.

In dental practice Aun and colleagues (1984) demonstrated similar immediate recovery features with both drugs but significantly fewer midazolam patients felt drowsy during the evening after operation, suggesting a more rapid total recovery. Similarly, Barker (1986) showed a significantly faster return to normal activities once the patient had returned home following midazolam sedation.

As with all the benzodiazepines, there is great inter-patient variability in midazolam dose requirements making careful titration of drug to effect essential. For example, there was a five-fold difference in dose requirement (0.05 mg/kg to 0.27 mg/kg) in Barker's study (1986) to produce the same level of dental sedation.

Elderly patients have a more consistent response to a given dose of midazolam (Brophy et al., 1982), but a reduced sensitivity to the drug. The elimination half-life is prolonged, approximately doubling in patients over 50 compared to younger subjects (Harper, 1985).

### *Flunitrazepam*

This intravenous benzodiazepine is not available in some countries including the United Kingdom, but is used commonly in others, particularly Continental Europe. It is prepared in an organic solvent similar to diazepam in a 1 mg/ml concentration and is approximately ten times as potent (Dundee et al., 1976a,b). Maximum effects appear 90—120 s after injection and are long lasting. There is a low incidence of venous sequelae following its administration compared to diazepam and it produces less pain on injection than methohexitone.

Cardiovascular and respiratory effects are similar to those produced by equipotent doses of diazepam. Pearce (1974b) however found that 0.024 mg/kg flunitrazepam as sedation for elderly men undergoing lower abdominal surgery under spinal anaesthesia produced relaxation of the lower jaw muscles such that all required jaw support to prevent respiratory obstruction. In his patients this dose produced sleep of 45 min average duration with everyone awakening and reacting normally by 90 min. He found no adverse circulatory effects but Haldeman and colleagues (1977) demonstrated that elderly patients were susceptible to a fall in blood pressure even after a small intravenous dose.

Small doses of flunitrazepam have more amnesic effect than corresponding doses of diazepam (Kortilla and Linnoila, 1976; Kortilla et al., 1978) but recovery is more prolonged, with impairment of coordination 6 h after 0.01 mg/kg and 10 h after 0.02 mg/kg and 0.03 mg/kg. This corroborates the demonstration of behavioural impairment 12 h, and EEG alteration 18 h after 1—2 mg of the drug orally (Bond and Lader, 1975), and supports Kortilla's recommendation that patients should not drive or operate machinery for 6 h after 0.01 mg/kg and for 24 h after larger doses.

Thornton and Martin (1976) showed that flunitrazepam 1 mg i.v. produced good sedation for dental procedures with a dense anterograde amnesic effect and no significant cardiorespiratory depression.

*Lorazepam*

This injectable benzodiazepine has a long duration of effect and is not indicated for out-patients although its prolonged amnesic effect may be useful for longer procedures. It is produced in an organic solvent in a strength of 4 mg/ml, 2.5 mg being roughly equivalent to 10 mg of diazepam (Dundee et al., 1979). Venous problems are rare following injection.

The duration of action is some three to four times greater than diazepam despite its short half-life of approximately 12 h (Dundee et al., 1979). This is because it is less extensively distributed than the other benzodiazepines (George and Dundee, 1977). There is delayed onset of effect after injection. Peak levels are achieved after 1—4 h and significant concentrations persist for 24 h and decrease slowly over the next 24 h (Elliott, 1976). This may be due to slow penetration of the blood-brain barrier with resultant delayed uptake into CSF because of its low lipophilicity. Its pharmacokinetics make it unsuitable for induction of anaesthesia but useful for intravenous premedication. It is also particularly suited to preventing the psychotomimetic effect of ketamine if given 30—60 min beforehand (Lilburn et al., 1976).

Amnesia is of slower onset but longer duration than sedation (Heisterkamp and Cohen, 1975) and there is no correlation between plasma levels of the drug and amnesic as opposed to sedative effects (Blitt et al., 1976). Lorazepam 2 mg and 4 mg i.v. produce good, long-lasting sedation of 3 and 4 h, respectively. Amnesia, however, lasts for less than 30 min with a latency of 30 min after 2 mg as opposed to 4—6 h with a shorter latency following 4 mg. Heisterkamp and Cohen (1975) have shown amnesia of up to 6 h duration following intravenous administration. Lorazepam is also the only benzodiazepine with significant amnesic effects at low dosages following oral administration (McKay and Dundee, 1980), one of the reasons for its popularity as an oral premedicant prior to major surgery under regional anaesthesia.

*Flumazenil*

This imidazobenzodiazepine derivative (Fig. 14.1) acts as a specific benzodiazepine antagonist and reverses the behavioural, neurological and electrophysiological effects of all benzodiazepines by competition for receptor sites in the central nervous system (Hunkeler et al., 1981). Several studies have shown this to be a safe and effective procedure following benzodiazepine-supplemented regional anaesthesia (Brogden and Goa, 1988).

Thus Ricou and colleagues (1986) administered a large dose of flumazenil 0.1 mg/kg or placebo at the end of surgery to two groups of patients undergoing urological surgery under spinal anaesthesia supplemented with midazolam. Sedation was completely reversed within 5 min of injection and remained less than in the control group for 30 min. Anterograde amnesia was also suppressed for 60 min. Five patients out of the 31 who received flumazenil, however, became anxious although this was manageable with simple reassurance.

Similarly, Sage and colleagues (1987) studied 65 patients undergoing prostatic surgery under spinal anaesthesia, again sedated with midazolam using a mean dose of 16 mg. Their patients were given flumazenil or placebo in the recovery room by an an incremental technique of 0.2 mg initially followed by 0.1 mg supplements if required. The average dose of flumazenil required was 0.36 mg and this produced dramatic, immediate improvement in patients' ability to comprehend and obey commands, in their orientation and in anterograde amnesia. The changes remained significant when compared to the placebo group for 1 h. There was no effect on heart rate, blood pressure or respiratory rate and no anxiety states were seen. After the initial complete awakening, however, sedation increased gradually in the flumazenil group whereas there was a slow steady improvement in sedation scores and cognitive function in the placebo group. They conclude that flumazenil is safe and effective in reversing sedation, disorientation and amnesia but that mild resedation can occur after 1 h, in keeping with the different elimination half-lives of the drugs involved (49—58 min for flumazenil; 2.1—2.4 h for midazolam) (Klotz et al., 1984).

Geller et al. (1985) also showed complete reversal of sedation and amnesia with a mean dose of 0.31 mg flumazenil in patients undergoing lower abdominal surgery under epidural anaesthesia with diazepam premedication and intra-operative midazolam sedation. Short and Galletly (1989), however, found evidence of residual psychomotor deficit 2 h after reversal of midazolam (10 mg) sedation with flumazenil 1 mg and 1 h after 4 mg, despite rapid reversal of hypnotic and amnesic effects. They also showed evidence of resedation occurring 35 min after flumazenil and caution against early discharge of out-patients following benzodiazepine reversal.

Sage (1988) has reviewed seven studies of flumazenil reversal of benzodiazepine sedation in regional anaesthesia. Flunitrazepam, diazepam and midazolam were variously used as sedatives. In no instance was there any pain on injection and there was a general lack of cardiorespiratory effects. Patient and environmental factors determine whether there will be a calm, relaxed emergence from sedation. Anxiety is high following its use in post cardiac surgery intensive care (Louis et al., 1984), and in neurosurgery (Chiolero et al., 1986). In regional anaesthesia the most important factor is flumazenil dosage. Small doses of less than 1 mg probably leave some residual anxiolysis, whereas high doses have an unacceptably high incidence of post-reversal anxiety.

Flumazenil gives clinicians the ability to titrate safely and reliably the reversal of benzodiazepine sedation accompanying regional anaesthesia. It allows correction of excessive sedation or the occasional unwanted benzodiazepine-induced paradoxical excitement. The practice of routinely abolishing sedation in hospitalised patients is questionable, however, especially when midazolam sedation is itself short-lived and inherently safe. A recent study where patients acted as their own controls for dental procedures under local anaesthesia with midazolam sedation revealed that most patients preferred to remain unreversed (Rodrigo and Rosenquist, 1987). The high cost of flumazenil is another factor militating against its widespread usage, although it may have potential benefits in day-case surgery, always bearing in mind the risk of resedation. In contrast to naloxone, additional subcutaneous injection of flumazenil does not eliminate resedation (Luger et al., 1990).

An entirely different approach to reversal of diazepam sedation is provided by the use of aminophylline (Arvidsson et al., 1984). Patients undergoing genito-urinary surgery under regional anaesthesia were heavily sedated with diazepam (approximately 0.6 mg/kg) and then given aminophylline 60—120 mg by slow intravenous injection at the end of the operation. All but one patient showed a rapid reversal of sedation persisting for the 2 h of the study as compared to a control group. There were no cardiovascular side effects attributable to aminophylline and no anxiety emergence phenomena. The effect is thought to be mediated through adenosine. Diazepam is known to potentiate the depressant effects of adenosine in the brain and aminophylline is an adenosine antagonist (Phillips, 1979).

**Chlormethiazole**

This thiamine derivative with sedative, hypnotic and anti-convulsant properties is well established in the treatment of alcohol withdrawal states, pre-eclampsia and status epilepticus. It is normally given intravenously by 0.8% infusion in 5% glucose as higher concentrations predispose to thrombophlebitis. After short duration infusions wakening is rapid due to redistribution but recovery may be delayed following more prolonged administration, due to cumulation. It has a long half-life of 3.5—12 h (Moore et al., 1975; Scott et al., 1980) although total body clearance is high. It had little effect on blood pressure or cardiac output but does produce tachycardia (Wilson et al., 1969).

Several studies have demonstrated chlormethiazole's value in providing sedation for regional anaesthesia. Most recommend a two stage infusion of the standard 0.8% solution in the form of a rapid initial rate followed by a slower maintenance rate once sleep supervenes. Schweitzer (1978) gave a rapid infusion of 20 ml/min over 3 min, reducing to 125 ml/h for the next hour and 50 ml/h thereafter to supplement epidural blockade and Marley and Ward (1980) gave a similar 1—3 min rapid infusion reducing to a slower maintenance rate thereafter. Mather and Cousins (1980) and Seow and colleagues (1981) administered a loading dose of 60 or 50 mg/min over 25 or 30 min followed by a maintenance infusion of 10 mg/min. All investigators comment on the smooth quality of sedation produced and the easy rousability of patients. There was a general lack of cardiovascular and respiratory side effects, apart from an increase in heart rate which was of clinical benefit in counteracting the cardiovascular depression produced by central neural blockade. This cardiovascular stability was confirmed in a later study using a higher loading dose of 30—40 ml/min (Sinclair et al, 1985). Depth of sedation was easily controlled in all studies and awakening rapid, even in the elderly, provided the dose had been reduced to avoid cumulation. Most patients regained consciousness within 10 min of stopping infusion. The drug also produced excellent amnesia for the period of administration.

Apart from the problem of the relatively large fluid volume required to deliver the drug and the need for careful dose adjustment to avoid cumulation, also side-effects such as nasal itching or irritation, it is difficult to argue with Mather and Cousin's statement (1980) that chlormethiazole 'appears close to being an ideal sedative to supplement neural blockade'.

## Intravenous induction agents

Any of the intravenous anaesthetic agents may be given in reduced doses either intermittently or by infusion to provide sedation as an adjunct to regional anaaesthesia. Their different pharmacological features, however, make some more suitable than others (Table 14.3).

### *Barbiturates*

Pharmacokinetically these drugs are not ideal for this form of administration. Despite this, thiopentone is often given in sub-anaesthetic doses to produce hypnosis at the start of a procedure under regional anaesthesia (Vindhya et al., 1987) or

TABLE 14.3

Pharmacokinetics of the intravenous induction agents (from Goat, 1985)

| | $t_{1/2\alpha}$ (min) | $t_{1/2\beta}$ (h) | $Vd_{ss}$ (l/kg) | $Cl$ (ml/kg per min) |
|---|---|---|---|---|
| Thiopentone | 2.4—6.8 | 5.1—11.9 | 1.4—2.3 | 2.1—4.3 |
| Methohexitone | 5.6 | 1.6—3.9 | 1.1—2.2 | 10.9—12.1 |
| Althesin | 1.6—2.8 | 0.5—1.5 | 0.7—2.2 | 16.9—21 |
| Etomidate | 2.6—3.9 | 1—5.4 | 2.2—4.5 | 11.6—26.1 |
| Ketamine | 8.7—17 | 2.5—3.1 | 2.3—3.1 | 17.5—20 |
| Propofol | 2.5 | 0.9 | 4.6 | 59.6 |

to allow positioning of the patient if this is likely to be awkward or uncomfortable. It is inexpensive, freely available and familiar, but the long elimination half-life (up to 12 h), cumulative properties and dose-related cardiovascular and respiratory depression preclude its prolonged administration. A small dose of thiopentone, however, will induce sleep smoothly and rapidly and recovery will be reasonably rapid due to the initial redistribution. This may be valuable as a standby measure. A sedative dose of 2—3 mg/kg in healthy volunteers followed by an infusion of 0.1—0.3 mg/kg per min produced light sedation with no alteration in any aspects of ventilatory control (hypoxic ventilatory reflex and responses to carbon dioxide and doxapram) (Knill et al., 1978). In a higher anaesthetic dose of 4—6 mg/kg followed by an infusion of 0.2—0.4 mg/kg per min, all of these parameters are depressed.

Methohexitone, with its faster elimination, has been used more extensively as supplementation for regional anaesthesia. Its elimination half-life is some three times shorter than thiopentone and its clearance three times greater (Hudson et al., 1983), so that when given by intermittent injection or infusion it is much less cumulative. Side effects including pain on injection, excitatory phenomena with involuntary movement, and airway problems are often seen.

It is particularly useful as a sub-anaesthetic bolus given immediately before performing a painful or distressing nerve block; for example, in head and neck surgery (Gilbert et al., 1987), but can also be given over longer periods of up to approximately 2 h. Thus Mackenzie and Grant (1985) gave 1.5 mg/kg i.v. followed by repeated increments of one-quarter to one-third of the induction dose to maintain light general anaesthesia in patients undergoing orthopaedic surgery under spinal block. The technique was clinically acceptable but there was a high incidence of pain on injection, spontaneous movement, twitching and hiccough. The mean dose requirement of 5.4 mg/kg per h produced little effect on blood pressure or respiratory rate, although heart rate was consistently increased. Patients regained consciousness and orientation approximately 9 min after the last bolus but psychomotor impairment persisted for 3 h. Grounds and colleagues (1985) produced similar effects with a slow induction bolus of 1.5 mg/kg followed by a continuous infusion (mean of 6.2 mg/kg per h) for anaesthesia to cover operations under spinal or epidural blockade. Both these studies involved comparison with propofol which proved superior in terms of quality of anaesthesia, lack of side-effects and speed of recovery.

Intermittent methohexitone was previously popular in out-patient dental practice as an adjunct to local anaesthesia. Proponents held that the technique was safe if properly carried out and produced sedation rather than anaesthesia. The dividing line is fine, however, and clinically undetected respiratory obstruction, depression of laryngeal reflexes and arterial hypoxaemia were demonstrated in practice especially if cumulative doses in excess of 200 mg were administered (Wise et al., 1969). The advent of safer methods of sedation have led to the virtual demise of the technique in modern practice.

*Etomidate*

This agent is pharmacokinetically attractive for intravenous infusion and not cumulative when given by intermittent injection. It also produces excellent cardiovascular stability. The problem of adrenocortical suppression following prolonged administration, however, has led to its withdrawal from use in this way (Owen and Spence, 1984). Previous work had indicated its potential in supplementing regional anaesthesia, particularly in respect of its rapid recovery and lack of cardiovascular side effects.

Birks et al. (1983) gave a two-stage infusion of 60 μg/kg per min reducing to a maintenance level of 5—7 μg/kg per min over the next 10 min to patients undergoing hip replacement under epidural anaesthesia. Patients remained drowsy but responsive to commands at this level, corresponding to plasma concentrations of 175—200 μg/l. All cardiovascular and respiratory parameters remained remarkably stable, but there was a high incidence (40%) of muscle twitching.

Incremental etomidate has been used in out-patient dental surgery under local anaesthesia (Ward and Rose, 1982). A combination of etomidate 0.1 mg/kg with diazepam 0.1 mg/kg followed by increments of etomidate for further sedation gave the best results in terms of reduced involuntary muscle movement without respiratory problems when compared to etomidate alone or along with pentazocine. Pain on injection was a problem with small veins. Again, there was good cardiovascular stability but the margin between sedation and anaesthesia was small with frequent loss of verbal contact, making constant supervision essential. Recovery was rapid, with patients walking 4—7 min after the end of the procedure.

*Ketamine*

The sedative, analgesic and dissociative properties of this phencyclidine derivative have encouraged its use as an adjunct to regional anaesthesia both to provide sedation and to overcome inadequate blocks. It is particularly useful where positioning the patient or performing the nerve block is likely to cause pain as in fracture surgery. Here its lack of respiratory depression is a distinct advantage over the opioids. Ketamine is usually administered with a benzodiazepine in an attempt to attenuate the unpleasant psychic side effects which constitute one of the major disadvantages of the drug.

Austin (1980) gave ketamine 20 mg with diazepam 2.5 mg i.v. prior to turning patients with fractured necks of femur for spinal anaesthesia. Sedation was supplemented by further small doses of the drugs if necessary. A mean dose of ketamine 3.9 mg and diazepam 4.7 mg produced a trance-like state from which the patient was easily rousable.

Thompson and Moore (1971) found that ketamine 2 mg/kg i.v. produced excellent sedation and patient acceptance for inter-costal nerve block in contrast to diazepam 20 mg i.m. and 20 mg i.v. or a droperidol/fentanyl mixture (Thalamonal)

2 ml i.m. and 3 ml i.v., both of which failed to sedate over 50% of patients adequately. Ketamine did, however, produce a 10% incidence of unpleasant dreams.

Sub-anaesthetic doses of ketamine have provided analgesia and sedation for postoperative surgery (Ito and Ichiyanagi, 1974) and for superficial surgical interventions (Slogoff et al., 1974). Korttila and Levanen (1978) compared similar analgesic/sedative doses of ketamine and diazepam to anaesthetic doses for the supplementation of epidural and brachial plexus blocks. The analgesic group received ketamine 0.5 mg/kg with diazepam 0.15 mg/kg i.v. and had no more side-effects or need for postoperative care and supervision than unsedated controls who received a block alone. The anaesthetic groups who received 1.5 mg/kg or 3 mg/kg ketamine with 0.15 mg/kg or 0.3 mg/kg diazepam respectively, had significantly more postoperative confusion, anxiety and visual disturbances and needed considerably more supervision.

Low dose ketamine with benzodiazepine prior to local anaesthetic injection is particularly popular in out-patient plastic and cosmetic surgery, where patients appear to be comfortable, co-operative and satisfied with the combination (Rothe and Schorer, 1980; Beekhuis and Kahn, 1978). White and colleagues (1982) recommend a loading dose of 0.2—0.75 mg/kg i.v. over 2—3 min followed by a continuous infusion of 5—20 $\mu$g/kg per min for sedative purposes.

Emergence phenomena, involuntary movement and hypertension, however, militate against its widespread use, certainly in anaesthetic doses, and ketamine is best reserved for selected cases where its unique features outweigh its disadvantages.

### *Propofol*

This recently introduced induction agent has already proved its value in supplementing regional anaesthesia either by repeated bolus administration or preferably by continuous infusion. Advantages include the rapidity and excellent quality of recovery and ease of dose adjustment to provide an appropriate level of sedation, ranging from light sleep through to full general anaesthesia (Mackenzie and Grant, 1987). Pharmacokinetically the drug is ideal for prolonged administration with rapid redistribution and elimination half-lives and very high clearance in excess of liver blood flow (Kay et al., 1985).

Propofol causes dose-related cardiovascular depression, mainly by an effect on systemic vascular resistance, but has little effect on heart rate. It also depresses respiration in a dose-dependent manner. Despite formulation in a soya bean oil emulsion, there is an appreciable incidence of pain on injection, especially when using small veins. There is no evidence for suppression of adrenal responsiveness (Langley and Heel, 1988). Drug clearance is reduced significantly in the elderly making them more sensitive to a given dose (Dundee et al., 1986).

Mackenzie and Grant (1985) and Jessop and colleagues (1985) gave propofol either by intermittent bolus or continuous infusion to provide light general anaesthesia for patients undergoing surgery under central neural block and compared this to methohexitone. Mean administration rates of 7.8 mg/kg per h and 6.1 mg/kg per h, respectively, produced smooth anaesthesia and few excitatory side effects. As would be anticipated from a continuous intravenous technique, the total dose was less and recovery faster in Jessop's study. Patients opened their eyes and repeated their dates of birth 4.1 min and 6.3 min after stopping the propofol infusion as compared to 9.6 min and 15.4 min after methohexitone. A deeper level of anaesthesia is necessary to provide endotracheal tube toleration (De Grood et al., 1987). Rates as high as 12 mg/kg per h following an induction bolus of 2.5 mg/kg may be insufficient to provide good anaesthetic conditions in intubated patients undergong surgery under central neural or brachial plexus block.

Lighter levels of sedation are more appropriate for most regional procedures and Mackenzie and Grant (1987) described the sub-anaesthetic infusion of propofol to provide sedation rather than anaesthesia for patients undergoing orthopaedic surgery under spinal blockade. A mean infusion rate of 3.8 mg/kg per h produced a state of light sleep with easy rousability, although this was very much age-dependent. Patients over 65 required significantly less than younger patients at 3.0 and 4.1 mg/kg per h, respectively. The technique was devoid of the cardiovascular or respiratory depression seen with larger doses and recovery was extremely rapid and pleasant. In some cases surgery encroached outwith the analgesic field of the regional block and sedation was simply converted to general anaesthesia by increasing the infusion rate and supplementing with nitrous oxide.

Other investigators have since confirmed these findings. Dubois and colleagues (1988) gave a mean infusion rate of 4.3 mg/kg per h following a slow induction bolus of 1.76 mg/kg for sedation during endoscopy. Recovery was rapid with complete amnesia for the procedure and 99% of patients had good or adequate sedation.

As sedation for inguinal hernia repair under field block, a mean infusion rate of 4.9 mg/kg per h was required to abolish the eyelash reflex and spontaneous movement (Janssen et al., 1988). Recovery was again rapid.

Nolte and Dertwinkel (1988) gave low dose infusions of 1, 1.5 and 2 mg/kg per h after an induction bolus of 1 mg/kg and opiate premedication to patients having surgery under epidural anaesthesia. This produced excellent sedation and the authors considered the technique superior to other available drugs.

Comparative studies with midazolam have shown the superiority of propofol in respect of predictability of effect, control of sedation, and rapidity and quality of recovery. Thus Wilson and colleagues (1990) administered propofol or midazolam by infusion to provide a similar deep level of sedation in patients undergoing major orthopaedic surgery under spinal anaesthesia. A mean infusion rate of 3.6 mg/kg per h and 0.26 mg/kg per h were required, respectively. Quality of sedation was comparable in both groups but recovery was significantly faster following propofol both in respect of immediate indices of recovery and subsequent restoration of higher mental function. Patients opened their eyes and repeated their dates of birth at approximately 2 min in contrast to 10 min after midazolam. Similarly, choice reaction time testing was impaired for up to 3 h after midazolam as opposed to

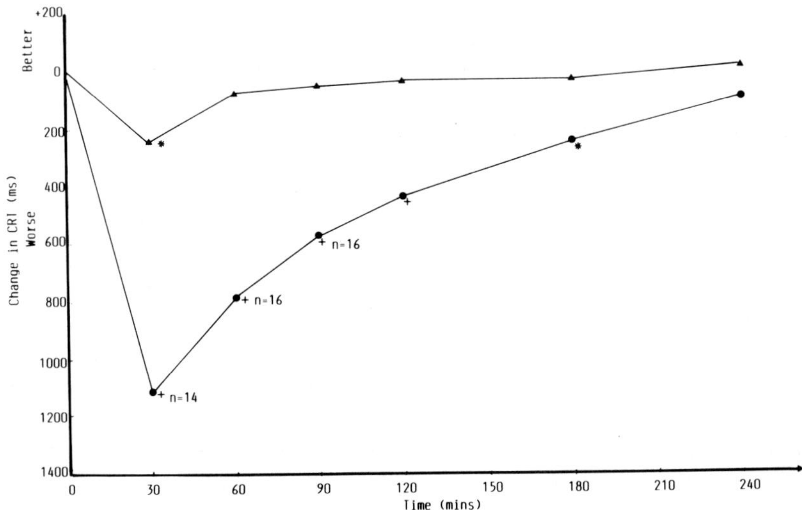


Fig. 14.3. Mean choice reaction time changes from pre-test baseline, $n$ = 20 unless otherwise stated. ● = midazolam ▲ = propofol. *$P < 0.05$; †$P < 0.005$. From Wilson et al. (1986).

30 min after propofol (Fig. 14.3). Postoperative amnesia was significantly more profound after midazolam. Negus and White (1988) administered broadly similar infusions of the two agents to maintain sleep with easy rousability during regional anaesthesia. Again, they demonstrated more rapid recovery with propofol but greater amnesia with midazolam.

Fanard and co-workers (1988) compared a sub-anaesthetic infusion of propofol of only 1.74 mg/kg per h following an induction bolus of 1.5 mg/kg with boluses of midazolam to produce light sleep during epidural anaesthesia. The dose of midazolam required was much less predictable than that of propofol and recovery much slower after midazolam. Twenty-five percent of patients had still not fully recovered after 2 h compared to complete recovery after 15 min with propofol.

Propofol may also be used in dental sedation, Valtonen et al. (1989). A slow infusion was titrated to produce ptosis or slurring of speech and then adjusted according to clinical requirements. This was compared to diazepam (as Diazemuls), again titrated to response. A mean infusion rate of propofol 4.2 mg/kg per h equated to diazepam 0.28 mg/kg. Quality of sedation was equally good in both groups and there were no cardiorespiratory problems or other significant side-effects apart from discomfort on injection following propofol. Recovery was faster and amnesia better at the time of tooth extraction with propofol and most patients preferred this drug to midazolam.

Propofol, especially if given by infusion, therefore appears to be an eminently suitable drug for supplementing regional blocks, in respect of its predictability of effect, quality of sedation and rapidity of recovery. Loach (1989) states that it 'might form the perfect complement to regional anaesthesia', sentiments endorsed by Blake and colleagues (1988) following haemodynamic studies with the drug in animals. Computer controlled infusion devices may simplify propofol administration in the future (White and Kenny, 1989). These deliver a variable rate infusion to maintain a predicted blood level necessary for the appropriate clinical effect. For sedation this is normally within the region of 0.5—1.5 μg/ml as opposed to 3—5 μg/ml for anaesthesia.

## Opioids

Small intravenous doses of opioids are frequently administered as supplementary sedation during regional anaesthesia. Given alone they are of limited value as they only address the additional analgesic needs of the patient and have little effect on the control of amnesia and wakefulness (Bridenbaugh, 1988). They may be useful if administered prior to performing a regional block if this is likely to cause pain, or to relieve the non-specific distress that many patients experience when undergoing prolonged procedures despite perfectly adequate local analgesia, and some obstetrical anaesthetists advocate their administration immediately after delivery in patients undergoing Caesarean section under epidural anaesthesia (Moir and Thorburn, 1986).

A useful concept is that of balanced regional anaesthesia as proposed by Tomlin and Gjessing (1978). In a review of a wide variety of operations performed under different regional blocks, they discovered that many patients were distressed intra-operatively despite anatomically perfect blocks with good sensory analgesia. This applied particularly to operations on the trunk as opposed to more peripheral sites, also where the patient was placed in an abnormal position on the operating table, e.g., prone or lateral. Discomfort was related to a strong desire to change position and was, in their view, due to a disturbance of sensory input produced by the regional block. They advocate a triad of balanced regional anaesthesia involving local anaesthetics for relief of the surgical pain, tranquillisers for relief of anxiety and opiates for the non-specific distress caused by the disturbed central proprioreception.

### *Pure agonists*

All of the pure opioid agonists have been used to supplement regional anaesthesia, normally in conjunction with an intravenous tranquilliser of the benzodiazepine or butyrophenone group. The synthetic piperidine derivates and more recently the structurally related fentanyl and alfentanil are most popular in this respect (Table 14.4).

TABLE 14.4

Pharmacokinetics of the pure opioid agonists (from Dundee and Wyant, 1988b and Willatts and Kong, 1989)

| | $t_{½\alpha}$ (min) | $t_{½\beta}$ (h) | $Vd_{ss}$ (l/kg) | $Cl$ (ml/kg per min) |
|---|---|---|---|---|
| Morphine | 25 | 1.5—4 | 3.4 | 2.3 |
| Pethidine | 7 | 3—6.5 | 4.4 | 7.7 |
| Fentanyl | 3 | 2—5 | 4.0 | 12.6 |
| Alfentanil | 3 | 1.5—3.5 | 0.7 | 5.1 |

### *Pethidine*

This, the original synthetic opioid, has been used extensively for intra-operative sedation for many years. It has been particularly investigated in endoscopy. In one study pethidine 50 mg was given intravenously along with either diazepam 0.17 mg/kg or midazolam 0.11 mg/kg (Magni et al., 1983). Sedation was satisfactory and operating conditions good. There was, however, significant impairment in psychomotor performance persisting for 2 h post-operatively and three patients experienced respiratory depression severe enough to warrant naloxone reversal. In an attempt to obviate this problem, Boldy and colleagues (1984) gave naloxone 0.4 mg i.v. to a group of patients sedated with pethidine 50 mg or 75 mg and diazepam 10 mg and compared the technique to another group receiving diazepam alone (mean dose of 30 mg). The opioid/benzodiazepine combination produced significantly better co-operation for the endoscopist but both groups accepted sedation equally well. Following naloxone administration at the end of the procedure there was no difference in sedation between the two groups. The routine prophylactic use of naloxone, however, with its attendant risks, cannot be endorsed especially in out-patients who have received a long-acting opioid and remain at risk of resedation once the effects of the shorter acting antagonist have worn off.

The structurally related compounds fentanyl and alfentanil are more suitable than pethidine in respect of their potency, faster onset and shorter duration of effect, although they possess less sedative effect.

### *Fentanyl*

Following intravenous administration, subjective response begins within 1 min and lasts 45—60 min (McClain and Hug, 1980). The redistribution half-life is 13 min and virtually all of the injected dose is cleared from the plasma in 60 min. The elimination half-life is, however, quite prolonged at around 200 min which can lead to delayed recovery after repeated administration. Elimination is also prolonged in the elderly (Bentley et al., 1982). These rapid early drug kinetics illustrate why fentanyl has become the most widely used opioid drug to supplement ambulatory procedures under regional anaesthesia. Increments of 25—50 μg may be given to achieve the desired analgesic effect with an initial dose of 50—200 μg. The elderly require reduced doses.

Fentanyl, in common with all opioids, has several important disadvantages, including nausea and vomiting and most importantly dose-related respiratory depression. A small intravenous bolus of 1.3 μg/kg caused equivalent depression of the carbon dioxide ventilatory response slope to 0.12 mg/kg morphine and this persisted for 4 h (Rigg and Goldsmith, 1976). Delayed respiratory depression postoperatively has been reported following small intravenous doses intraoperatively (Becker et al., 1976; Adams and Pybus, 1978). This biphasic respiratory depression may be due to secondary peaks in plasma fentanyl concentration during the elimination phase as a result of enterohepatic recirculation, or release of active drug from muscle body stores with increased patient activity during recovery. Whatever the reason, Adams and Pybus clearly demonstrated that somnolence, respiratory depression requiring ventilatory support and respiratory arrest can occur from 30 min to 4 h after apparent recovery from fentanyl.

Fentanyl may be given by continuous infusion rather than by intermittent injection. This may reduce significantly the total dose of drug required and produce faster recovery with less postoperative somnolence or respiratory depression. This has usually been done, however, in conjunction with general anaesthesia or in the postoperative period and it is difficult to extrapolate to surgery under regional anaesthesia. Here there are often rapid changes in the degree and frequency of noxious stimuli which necessitate rapid action, usually by bolus drug injection. If this is done on top of a continuous infusion, greater doses of drug might conceivably be delivered causing more unwanted side-effects.

Fentanyl is frequently combined with droperidol. For example, Erwin and colleagues (1980) described a series of patients undergoing carotid artery surgery under cervical plexus block. They were sedated with 150—200 μg of fentanyl and 5—10 mg of droperidol i.v. and given further 25 μg doses of fentanyl if required during surgery. The technique allowed testing for motor function during carotid clamping and avoided the extra hazard of shunt insertion in the majority of cases. The fentanyl-droperidol combination provided excellent sedation and patient cooperation. Without the droperidol the authors felt that considerably more fentanyl would have been required and that this would have produced unacceptable respiratory depression.

The combination of fentanyl and droperidol may be particularly useful in operations known to have a high incidence of postoperative emesis such as ophthalmic or gynaecological surgery provided the dose of droperidol is small. Larger doses can cause prolonged and excessive sedation, hypotension, extrapyramidal symptoms and apprehension. Korttila and Linnoila (1974) demonstrated evidence of prolonged sedation following doses of 0.04 mg/kg droperidol or more, with significant impairment of psychomotor function and tiredness persisting for more than

10 h in 50% of subjects. Concurrent administration of fentanyl 200 μg did not affect these results.

In a large series of over 6000 cases of regional anaesthesia, a combination of small doses of fentanyl 20 μg, droperidol 1 mg and either midazolam 1.5—3 mg or flunitrazepam 0.2—0.4 mg i.v. provided good sedation and amnesia with little change in cardiovascular or respiratory parameters (Van Steenberge et al., 1987). Midazolam was given for procedures of up to 90 min duration and flunitrazepam for longer operations.

*Alfentanil*

Alfentanil is some four times less potent than fentanyl with a more rapid onset of action and approximately one-third its duration (Kay, 1982). It has a short redistribution half-life of 11.6 min and elimination half-life of 94 min (Bovill et al., 1982). In contrast to fentanyl, termination of effect depends primarily on hepatic metabolism rather than redistribution (Stanski and Hug, 1982), so that cumulation and prolongation of action after repeated doses should not occur. Recovery is rapid if appropriate doses are used (Rosow et al., 1983; Patrick et al., 1983). The pharmacokinetics of alfentanil suggest that it may best be used to supplement regional anaesthesia by continuous infusion. Patients can be given a loading dose of 250—500 μg, followed by an infusion of 40—70 μg/min (Coe et al., 1983). This will reduce significantly the total dose compared to a 250 μg bolus administration and hasten time to awakening and ambulation.

*Mixed agonist-antagonists*

These drugs with a spectrum of agonist and antagonist activity at the different opiate receptors are frequently administered during regional anaesthesia. They are usually given in combination with tranquillisers or hypnotics in an attempt to provide analgesia without some of the side effects of the pure opioid agonists, particularly the respiratory depression.

*Pentazocine*

This older drug is approximately one quarter as potent as morphine. Its main disadvantages are psychotomimetic side effects and its deleterious effects on systemic vascular resistance, pulmonary artery pressure and myocardial workload (Jewitt et al., 1971). Pentazocine has largely been replaced in clinical practice by newer agents with less side effects, but doses of 15—30 mg i.v. had been shown to be of value in dental sedation with diazepam (Murray-Lawson and Milne, 1981), increasing subjective patient comfort and allowing smaller doses of sedative to be given.

*Butorphanol*

This is approximately four times as potent as morphine. Butorphanol 2 mg causes equivalent respiratory depression to 10 mg morphine, but thereafter there is a ceiling effect with no further depression following doses of over 4 mg (Nagashima et al., 1976). A similar ceiling effect is seen with analgesia (Murphy and Hug, 1982). It has a subjectively pleasant slightly sedative effect with rapid onset and long duration of action but like pentazocine may cause psychotomimetic effects, increased pulmonary pressure and cardiac work.

*Nalbuphine*

In low doses nalbuphine is approximately equipotent with morphine but a ceiling of analgesic activity and respiratory depression is reached above 0.4 mg/kg (Romagnoli and Keats, 1980). Unlike pentazocine and butorphanol, it does not increase cardiac workload or pulmonary artery pressure. It is long acting and causes less nausea and vomiting and psychotomimetic effects than pentazocine (Errick and Heel, 1983).

Several studies have investigated nalbuphine-benzodiazepine combinations in the provision of sedation. In conjunction with midazolam 0.05 mg/kg, nalbuphine in doses of 0.05, 0.1 or 0.2 mg/kg caused a mild degree of respiratory depression in volunteers evidenced by a slight increase in expired carbon dioxide concentration and a 25% decrease in the carbon dioxide ventilatory response gradient, maximal 3—30 min after injection (Sury and Cole, 1988a). Sedation was pleasant and there were no cardiovascular side effects. There was, however, a 33% incidence of movement-related nausea during recovery.

Nalbuphine 0.2 mg/kg and midazolam 0.05 mg/kg was compared with midazolam 0.05 mg/kg alone to provide sedation for out-patient bronchoscopy. Patients receiving nalbuphine had slightly higher arterialised venous carbon dioxide levels, but otherwise cardiorespiratory changes were similar in both groups. The opioid-benzodiazepine combination markedly increased patient comfort during bronchoscopy, but again at the expense of nausea, dizziness and prolonged recovery. Furthermore two patients had obstructive apnoea (Sury and Cole, 1988b). The authors conclude that the combination should be reserved for prolonged painful procedures where benzodiazepines alone are inadequate and that full resuscitative facilities should be available.

In dental surgery, nalbuphine 10 mg and diazepam 11 mg i.v. produced equivalent sedation and pain relief to fentanyl 50 $\mu g$ and diazepam 11 mg, with less peri-operative amnesia (Dolan et al., 1988). Nalbuphine and midazolam were compared to pentazocine and midazolam, again for dental surgery under local anaesthesia (Hook and Lavery, 1988). Nalbuphine 0.2 mg/kg and pentazocine 0.5 mg/kg both produced significant reductions in mean midazolam dosage with no adverse circulatory or respiratory effects. Both drug combinations provided excellent operating conditions with a high degree of patient acceptability but significantly more nalbuphine patients were pain-free 2 h postoperatively, and the authors therefore recommend this combination.

Combined with methohexitone in doses of 0.1 mg/kg and 0.5 mg/kg, respectively, nalbuphine produces safe, reliable sedation for cataract surgery, under retrobulbar and facial nerve block (Gilbert et al., 1987). This is more profound and longer lasting than a fentanyl-midazolam combination titrated to produce the required sedative effect.

A nalbuphine and droperidol combination also appears well suited to local anaesthetic sedation (Klein, 1983). Droperidol 2.5 mg given 5 min after nalbuphine 30 mg i.v. produces good sedation with easy patient rousability and minimal respiratory depression. With the small dose of droperidol, dysphoria is prevented.

It must always be remembered that opioid supplementation of regional anaesthesia, while increasing patient comfort, will increase the frequency of side effects, most importantly that of respiratory depression. Respiratory depression following a diazepam-opiate combination is much greater than would be expected after administration of the drugs individually. Apnoea following midazolam is much more likely to occur in patients premedicated with opiates (Kanto et al., 1982), and recovery will be delayed if opioid-benzodiazepine combinations are used (Korttila and Linnoila, 1974).

Opioid drugs all decrease ventilatory responsiveness to carbon dioxide and to hypoxia. Great care must be exercised in administering them to spontaneously breathing, pain-free patients and adequate respiratory monitoring must be provided, preferably involving pulse oximetry. Keats (1988) emphasises the role of surgical stimulation, pain, noise and movement in antagonising the decreased carbon dioxide responsiveness produced by opiates and questions the role of spinal anaesthesia in modifying this response by its deafferentation and removal of facilitatory proprioreceptive input into the respiratory centre. A recent review of 14 cases of unexpected cardiac arrest with poor outcome in healthy young patients undergoing spinal anaesthesia is salutory (Caplan et al., 1988). A common feature in the series was the intra-operative use of sufficient sedation to produce a sleep-like state with no 'spontaneous verbalisation'. Twelve patients received at least one intravenous sedative and 9 two or more, the commonest being fentanyl with diazepam, droperidol or thiopentone. In no case was a large dose given but cyanosis often heralded the onset of cardiac arrest, suggesting that unappreciated respiratory insufficiency might have played an important aetiological role.

Ward-Booth (1986) also cautions against the administration of intravenous opioids with benzodiazepines for sedation in dentistry. He rightly questions the logic of adding opioid analgesia with its inherent risk of respiratory depression to patients who have already received one of the safest and most effective analgesics available, namely local anaesthesia.

Finally, the temptation to compensate for an inadequate regional block by increasing doses of intravenous opioid should always be resisted. It is infinitely better to repeat the local block or abandon it completely and convert to a fully controlled, conventional general anaesthetic.

## CONCLUSIONS

Interest in and practice of regional anaesthesia have increased considerably over the last decade. This branch of the specialty will undoubtedly continue to develop further as more and more anaesthetists, especially those in training, come to realise its advantages and develop the necessary expertise to carry it out routinely. The stimulation of enthusiastic proponents, specialist societies and their training programmes, improved equipment and drugs, continuing research and the expanding range of excellent textbooks on the subject are all important in this respect.

It is, however, vital not to overlook the patient's needs and expectations with this resurgence in popularity. Most patients expect and will benefit from some degree of peri-operative sedation. This will vary from patient to patient depending on their general condition and personality, the nature of surgery and regional block and the experience and attitude of both anaesthetist and surgeon. The aim should be to produce a calm, relaxed patient, co-operative if necessary, who is comfortable and capable of lying still on an operating table for differing lengths of time while surgery of a variable nature and complexity is being performed. In many ways this is the most challenging aspect of regional anaesthesia. As J.A. Lee, a doyen of the specialty says, 'it requires more skill and experience to manage the patient on the table than to perform the block itself' (1964).

Every patient must be well prepared beforehand and premedicated appropriatly. For short, relatively stress-free procedures this combined with reassuring verbal support and simple methods of distraction may be sufficient. In most instances, however, some degree of supplementary sedation is useful. This should be light enough not to obtund consciousness or verbal contact between operator and patient. The intravenous route is the best method of delivery and currently the benzodiazepines are the agents of choice. They should always be administered in a gradual, controlled manner, titrating dose to effect on an individual basis and in view of its superior pharmacokinetic profile midazolam is normally the preferred drug. For longer, more invasive surgery a deeper level of sedation is necessary, occasionally merging into full general anaesthesia. This may be provided by the intravenous or inhalational routes, but in many respects intravenous administration is preferable. Infusion techniques are particularly useful for this because of the smooth quality of sedation and ease of its control, and propofol is a particularly suitable agent in view of its versatility, predictability of effect and rapidity of recovery. When deeper levels of sedation are employed respiratory depression will occur and protective reflexes may be obtunded. This necessitates constant supervision with close patient monitoring and the provision of supplemental oxygen. With the prolonged effects of sedative drugs it is important to extend supervision into the post-operative period and assess recovery adequately, especially in the increasing number of day-case patients, prior to discharge.

## REFERENCES

Adams, A.P. and Pybus, D.A. (1978) Delayed respiratory depression after use of fentanyl during anaesthesia. *Br. Med. J.* 1, 278—279.

Al-Khudhairi, D., Whitwam, J.G. and McCloy, R.F. (1982) Midazolam and diazepam for gastroscopy. *Anaesthesia* 37, 1002—1006.

Armitage, E.N. (1987) Regional anaesthesia in children. In: *Principles and Practice of Regional Anaesthesia.* Editors: J.A.W. Wildsmith and E.N. Armitage, Churchill Livingstone, Edinburgh, pp. 176—183.

Arvidsson, S., Niemand, D., Martinall, S. and Ekstrom-Jodal, B. (1984) Aminophylline reversal of diazepam sedation. *Anaesthesia* 39, 806—809.

Aun, C., Flynn, P.J., Richards, J. and Major, E. (1984) A comparison of midazolam and diazepam for intravenous sedation in dentistry. *Anaesthesia* 39, 589—593.

Austin, T.R. (1980) Low dose ketamine and diazepam during spinal analgesia. *Anaesthesia* 35, 391—392.

Baird, E.S. and Hailey, D.M. (1972) Delayed recovery from a sedative. Correlation of the plasma levels of diazepam with clinical effects after oral and intravenous administration. *Br. J. Anaesth.* 44, 803—808.

Barker, I., Butchart, D.G.M., Gibson, J., Lawson, J.I.M. and Mackenzie, N. (1986) I.V. sedation for conservative dentistry. A comparison of midazolam and diazepam. *Br. J. Anaesth.* 58, 371—377.

Becker, L.D., Paulson, B.A., Muller, R.D., Severinghaus, J.W. and Eger, E.G. (1976) Biphasic respiratory depression after fentanyl-droperidol or fentanyl alone used to supplement nitrous oxide anesthesia. *Anesthesiology* 44, 291—296.

Beekhuis, G.J. and Kahn, D.L. (1978) Anesthesia for facial cosmetic surgery. Low dosage ketamine-diazepam anesthesia. *Laryngoscope* 88, 1709—1712.

Bentley, J.B., Borel, J.D. and Nenad, R.E. (1982) Influence of age on the pharmacokinetics of fentanyl. *Anesth. Analg.* 61, 171—172.

Berggren, L. and Eriksson, I. (1981) Midazolam for induction of anaesthesia in out-patients: a comparison with thiopentone. *Acta Anaesthesiol. Scand.* 25, 492—496.

Berggren, L., Eriksson, I., Mollenholt, P. and Wichbom, G. (1983) Sedation for fibreoptic gastroscopy: A comparative study of midazolam and diazepam. *Br. J. Anaesth.* 55, 289—296.

Birks, R.J.S., Edbrooke, D.L. and Mundy, J.V.B. (1983) Etomidate as a sedative agent in patients undergoing hip surgery under epidural anaesthesia. *Anaesthesia* 38, 295—296.

Blake, D.W., Jover, B. and McGrath, B.P. (1988) Haemodynamic and heart rate reflex responses to propofol in the rabbit. *Br. J. Anaesth.* 61, 194—199.

Blitt, D.C., Petty, W.C., Wright, W.A. and Wrights, B. (1976) Clinical evaluation of injectable lorazepam as a premedicant. The effect on recall. *Anesth. Analg.* 55, 522—528.

Boldy, D.A.R., English J.S.C., Lang, G.S. and Hoare, A.M. (1984) Sedation for endoscopy: A comparison between diazepam and diazepam plus pethidine with naloxone reversal. *Br. J. Anaesth.* 56, 1109—1111.

Bond, A.J. and Lader, M.H. (1975) Residual effects of flunitrazepam. *Br. J. Clin. Pharmacol.* 2, 143—150.

Bond, A.J., Hailey, D.M. and Lader, M.H. (1977) Plasma concentrations of benzodiazepines. *Br. J. Clin. Pharmacol.* 4, 51—56.

Bovill, J.G., Sebel, P.S., Blackburn, C.L. and Heykants, J. (1982) The pharmacokinetics of alfentanil (R39209): a new opioid analgesic. *Anesthesiology* 57, 439—443.

Bridenbaugh, P.O. (1988) Patient management for neural blockade. In: *Neural Blockade in Clinical Anesthesia and Management of Pain,* 2nd Edn. Editors: M.J. Cousins and P.O. Bridenbaugh, J.B. Lippincott, Philadelphia, pp. 191—210.

Brogden, R.N. and Goa, R.L. (1988) Flumazenil. A preliminary review of its benzodiazepine antagonist properties, intrinsic activity and therapeutic use. *Drugs* 35, 448—467.

Brophy, T.O'R., Dundee, J.W., Heazelwood, V., Kawar, P., Varghese, A. and Ward. M. (1982) Midazolam, a water soluble benzodiazepine for gastroscopy. *Anaesth. Intensive Care* 10, 344—347.

Brown, S.S. and Dundee, J.W. (1968) Clinical studies of induction agents. XXV: Diazepam. *Br. J. Anaesth.* 40, 108—112.

Caplan, R.A., Ward, R.J., Posner, K. and Cheney, F.W. (1988) Unexpected cardiac arrest during spinal anesthesia: A closed claims analysis of predisposing factors. *Anesthesiology* 68, 5—11.

Catchlove, R.F.H. and Kafer, E.R. (1971a) The effect of diazepam on the ventilatory response to carbon dioxide and on steady-state gas exchange. *Anesthesiology* 34, 9—13.

Catchlove, R.F.H. and Kafer, E.R. (1971b) The effects of diazepam on respiration in patients with obstructive pulmonary disease. *Anesthesiology* 34, 14—18.

Charlton, J.E. (1987) The management of regional anaesthesia. In: *Principles and Practice of Regional Anaesthesia.* Editors: J.A.W. Wildsmith and E.N. Armitage, Churchill Livingstone, Edinburgh, pp. 37—61.

Chiolero, R., Rauvussin, P., Chassot, P.G., Neff, R. and Freeman, J. (1986) RO 15-1788 for rapid recovery after craniotomy. *Anesthesiology* 65, A466.

Coe, V., Shafer, A. and White, P.F. (1983) Technique for administering alfentanil during outpatient anesthesia — a comparison with fentanyl. *Anesthesiology* 59, A347.

Cohen, R., Finn, H. and Steen, S.N. (1969) Effect of diazepam and meperidine, alone and in combination, on respiratory response to carbon dioxide. *Anesth. Analg.* 48. 353—355.

Dalen, J.E., Evans, G. L., Banas, J.S. Brooks, H. L., Paraskos, J.A. and Dexter, L. (1969) The hemodynamic and respiratory effects of diazepam. *Anesthesiology* 30. 259—263.

de Grood, P.M.R.M. Coenen, L.G.J., Van Egmond, J., Booij, H.D.J. and Crul, J.F. (1987) Propofol emulsion for induction and maintenance of anaesthesia. A combined technique of general and regional anaesthesia. *Acta Anaesthesiol. Scand.* 31. 219—223.

Dixon, R.A. and Thornton, J.A. (1973) Tests of recovery from anaesthesia and sedation: intravenous diazepam in dentistry. *Br. J. Anaesth.* 45, 207—215.

Dixon, R.A., Day, C.D., Eccersley, P.S. and Thornton, J.A. (1973) Intravenous diazepam in dentistry: monitoring results from a controlled clinical trial. *Br. J. Anaesth.* 45. 202—206.

Dixon, J., Power, S.J., Grundy, E.M., Lumley, J. and Morgan, M. (1984) Sedation for local anaesthesia. Comparison of intravenous midazolam and diazepam. *Anaesthesia* 39. 372—376.

Dolan, E.A., Murray, W.J., Immediata, A.R. and Gleason, N. (1988) Comparison of nalbuphine and fentanyl in combination with diazepam for outpatient oral surgery. *J. Oral Maxillofac. Surg.* 46, 471—473.

Dripps, R.D. and Vandam, L.D. (1954) Long-term follow-up of patients who received 10,098 spinal anesthetics. Failure to discover major neurological sequelae. *J. Am. Med. Assoc.* 156, 1486—1491.

Dubois, A., Balatoni, E., Peeters, J.P. and Baudoux, M. (1988) Use of propofol for sedation during gastrointestinal endoscopies. *Anaesthesia* 43 (Suppl.) 75—80.

Dundee, J.W. and Pandit, S.K. (1972) Anterograde amnesic effects of pethidine, hyoscine and diazepam in adults. *Br. J. Pharmacol.* 44, 140—144.

Dundee, J.W. and Wilson, D.B. (1980) Amnesic action of midazolam. *Anaesthesia* 35, 459—461.

Dundee, J.W. and Wyant, G.M. (1988a) The benzodiazepines. In: *Intravenous Anaesthesia,* 2nd Edn. Churchill Livingstone, Edinburgh, pp. 184—205.

Dundee, J.W. and Wyant, G.M. (1988b) The opioids in intravenous anaesthesia. In: *Intravenous Anaesthesia,* 2nd Edn. Churchill Livingstone, Edinburgh, pp. 206—247.

Dundee, J.W., Varadarajan, C.R., Gaston, J.H. and Clarke, R.S.J. (1976a) Clinical studies of induction agents. XLIII: Flunitrazepam. *Br. J. Anaesth.* 48, 551—555.

Dundee, J.W., George, K.A., Varadarajan, C.R., Clarke, R.S.J. and Nair S.K.G. (1976b) Anaesthesia and amnesia with flunitrazepam. *Br. J. Anaesth.* 48, 266—267.

Dundee, J.W., McGowan, W.A.W., Lilburn, J.K., McKay, A.C. and Hegarty, J.E. (1979) Comparison of the actions of diazepam and lorazepam. *Br. J. Anaesth.* 51, 439—446.

Dundee, J.W., Robinson, F.P., McCollum, J.S.C. and Patterson, S.C. (1986) Sensitivity to propofol in the elderly. *Anaesthesia* 41, 482—485.

Elliott, H.W. (1976) Metabolism of lorazepam. *Br. J. Anaesth.* 48, 1017—1023.

Errick, J.K. and Heel, R.C. (1983) Nalbuphine. A preliminary review of its pharmacological properties and therapeutic efficacy. *Drugs* 26, 191—211.

Erwin, D., Pick, M.J. and Taylor, G.W. (1980) Anaesthesia for carotid artery surgery. *Anaesthesia* 35, 246—249.

Fanard, L., Van Steenberge, A., Demeire, X. and Van der Puyl, F. (1988) Comparison between propofol and midazolam as sedative agents for surgery under regional anaesthesia. *Anaesthesia* 43 (Suppl.), 87—89.

Forster, A., Gardaz, J.P., Suter, P.M. and Gemperle, M. (1980) Respiratory depression by midazolam and diazepam. *Anesthesiology* 53, 494—497.

Gale, G.D. (1976) Recovery from methohexitone, halothane and diazepam. *Br. J. Anaesth.* 48, 691—697.

Geller, E., Niv, D., Matzkin, C., Silbiger, A., Nevo, Y., Cohen, F. and Braf, Z. (1985) The antagonism of midazolam sedation by RO 15-1788 in 50 post-operative patients. *Anesthesiology* 63, A369.

George, K.A. and Dundee, J.W. (1977) Relative amnesic actions of diazepam, flunitrazepam and lorazepam in man. *Br. J. Clin. Pharmacol.* 4, 45—50.

Gilbert, J., Holt, J.E., Johnston, J., Sabo, B.A. and Weaver, J.S. (1987) Intravenous sedation for cataract surgery under regional blockade. *Anaesthesia* 42, 1063—1069.

Gjessing, J. and Tomlin, P.J. (1977) Intravenous sedation and regional anaesthesia. *Anaesthesia* 32, 63—69.

Goat, V.A. (1985) Pharmacokinetics of intravenous induction agents. In: *Recent Advances in Anaesthesia and Analgesia* 15. Editors: R.S. Atkinson and A.P. Adams, Churchill Livingstone, Edinburgh, pp. 27—41.

Greenblatt, D.J., Shader, R.I. Abernethy, D.R., Ochs, H.R., Divoll, M. and Sellers, E.M. (1982) Benzodiazepines and the challenge of pharmacokinetic taxonomy. In: *Pharmacology of Benzodiazepines.* Editors: E. Usdin, P. Skolnick, J.F. Tallman, D. Greenblatt and S.M. Paul, Macmillan Press, London, pp. 257—269.

Greenblatt, D.J., Abernethy, D.R., Locniskar, A., Harmatz, J.S., Limjuco, R.A. and Shader, R.I. (1984) Effect of age, gender and obesity on midazolam kinetics. *Anesthesiology* 61, 27—35.

Grounds, R.M., Morgan, M. and Lumley, J. (1985) Some studies on the properties of the intravenous anaesthetic propofol — a review. *Postgrad. Med. J.* 61 (Suppl. 3), 90—95.

Grove-White, I.G. and Kelman, G.R. (1971) Critical flicker fusion frequency after small doses of methohexitone, diazepam and sodium 4-hydroxybutyrate. *Br. J. Anaesth.* 43, 110—116.

Haldemann, G., Hossli, G. and Schaer, H. (1977) Die anaesthesie mit Rohypnol (Flunitrazepam) und fentanyl beim geriatrischen patienten. *Anaesthesist* 26, 168.

Harper, K.W., Lowry, K.G., Elliott, P., Collier, P.S., Halliday, N.J. and Dundee, J.W. (1985) Age and nature of operation influence the pharmacokinetics of midazolam. *Br. J. Anaesth.* 57, 866—871.

Healy, T.E.J., Robinson, J.S. and Vickers, M.D. (1970a) Physiological responses to intravenous diazepam as a sedative for conservative dentistry. *Br. Med. J.* 3, 10—13.

Healy, T.E.J., Lautch, H., Hall, N., Tomlin, P.J. and Vickers, M.D. (1970b) Interdisciplinary study of diazepam sedation for outpatient dentistry. *Br. Med. J.* 3, 13—17.

Heisterkamp, D.V. and Cohen, J.P. 1975, The effect of intravenous premedication with lorazepam (Ativan), pentobarbitone or diazepam on recall. *Br. J. Anaesth.* 47, 79—81.

Hook, P.C.G. and Lavery, K.M. (1988) New intravenous sedative combinations in oral surgery: a comparative study of nalbuphine or pentazocine with midazolam. *Br. J. Oral Maxillofac. Surg.* 26, 95—106.

Hudson, R.J., Stanski, D.R. and Burch, P.A. (1982) Comparative pharmacokinetics of methohexital and thiopental. *Anesthesiology* 57, A240.

Hunkeler, W., Mohler, H., Pieri, L., Polc, P., Bonnetti E.P., Cumin, R., Schaffner, R. and Haefely, W. (1981) Selective antagonists of benzodiazepines. *Nature* 290, 514—516.

Ito, Y. and Ichiyanagi, R. (1974) Post-operative pain relief with ketamine infusion. *Anaesthesia* 29, 222—229.

Janssen, L.A., Opheide, J., Erperls, F.A. and Vermeyen, K.M. (1988) Propofol as a sedative for inguinal hernia repair under local anaesthesia. *Anaesthesia* 43 (Suppl.), 116.

Jessop, E., Grounds; R.M., Morgan, M. and Lumley, J. (1985) Comparison of infusions of propofol and methohexitone to provide light general anaesthesia during surgery with regional blockade. *Br. J. Anaesth.* 57, 1173—1177.

Jewitt, D.E., Maurer, B.J., Sonnenblick, E.J. and Shillingford, J.P. (1971) Pentazocine: effect on ventricular muscle and hemodynamic changes in ischaemic heart disease. *Circulation,* 44 (Suppl.) 118.

Jorgensen, N.B. and Leffingwell, F. (1961) Premedication in dentistry. *Dental Clinics of North America*, 5, 299.

Kanto, J. and Klotz, V. (1982) Intravenous benzodiazepines as anaesthetic agents: pharmacokinetics and clinical consequences. *Acta Anaesthesiol. Scand.* 26, 554—569.

Kanto, J., Maenpaa, M., Mantyla, R., Sellman, R. and Valovirta, E. (1979) Effect of age on the pharmacokinetics of diazepam given in conjunction with spinal anesthesia. *Anesthesiology* 51. 154—159.

Kanto, J., Sjovall, S. and Vuori, A. (1982) Effect of different kinds of premedication on the induction properties of midazolam. *Br. J. Anaesth.* 54, 507—511.

Kay, B. (1982) Alfentanil. *Br. J. Anaesth.* 54, 1011—1013.

Kay, N.H., Uppington, J., Sear, J.W., Douglas, E.J. and Cockshott, I.D. (1985) Pharmacokinetics of propofol as an induction agent. *Postgrad. Med. J.* 61 (Suppl. 3), 55—57.

Khatri, I.M. and Freis, E.D. (1967) Hemodynamic changes during sleep. *J. Appl. Physiol.* 22, 867.

Klein, D.S. (1983) Nalbuphine and droperidol combination for local standby sedation. *Anesthesiology* 58, 397.

Klotz, V., Avant, G.R., Hoyumpa, A., Schenker, S. and Wilkinson, G.R. (1975) The effects of age and liver disease on the disposition and elimination of diazepam in adult man. *J. Clin. Invest.* 55, 347—359.

Klotz, V., Ziegler, G. and Reimann, I.W. (1984) Pharmacokinetics of the selective benzodiazepine antagonist RO 15-1788 in man. *Eur. J. Clin. Pharmacol.* 27, 115—117.

Knill, R.L., Bright, S. and Manninen, P. (1978) Hypoxic ventilatory responses during thiopentone sedation and anaesthesia in man. *Can. Anaesth. Soc. J.* 25, 366—372.

Korttila, K. and Levanen J. (1978) Untoward effect of ketamine combined with diazepam for supplementing conduction anaesthesia in young and middle-aged adults. *Acta Anaesthesiol. Scand.* 22, 640—648.

Korttila, K. and Linnoila, M. (1974) Skills related to driving after intravenous diazepam, flunitrazepam or droperidol. *Br. J. Anaesth.* 46, 961—969.

Korttila, K. and Linnoila, M. (1975) Recovery and skills related to driving after intravenous sedation: dose-response relationship with diazepam. *Br. J. Anaesth.* 47, 457—463.

Korttila, K. and Linnoila, M. (1976) Amnesic action of and skills related to driving after intravenous flunitrazepam. *Acta Anaesthesiol. Scand.* 20, 160—168.

Korttila, K. and Tarkkanan, J. (1985) Comparison of diazepam and midazolam for sedation during local anaesthesia for bronchoscopy. *Br. J. Anaesth.* 57, 581—586.

Korttila, K., Saarnivaara, L., Tarkkanen, J., Himberg, J.J. and Hytonen, M. (1978) Comparison of diazepam and flunitrazepam for sedation during local anaesthesia for bronchoscopy. *Br. J. Anaesth.* 50, 281—287.

Langa, H. (1968) *Relative Analgesia in Dental Practice.* W.B. Saunders Co., Philadelphia.

Langley, M.S. and Heel, R.C. (1988) Propofol. A review of its pharmacodynamic and pharmacokinetic properties and use as an intravenous anaesthetic. *Drugs* 35, 334—372.

Lee, J.A. (1964) The management of the patient under peridural anesthesia. *Int. Anesthesiol. Clin.* 2, 499—505.

Lilburn, J.K., Dundee, J.W. and Moore, J. (1976) Lorazepam-ketamine: preliminary report. *Br. J. Anaesth.* 48, 1125.

Lloyd-Thomas, A.R. (1990) Pain management in paediatric patients. *Br. J. Anaesth.* 64, 85—104.

Loach, A. (1989) New views on local analgesia. In: *Recent Advances in Anaesthesia and Analgesia* No. 16. Editors: R.S. Atkinson and A.P. Adams, Churchill Livingstone, Edinburgh, pp. 65—81.

Louis, M., Foster, A., Suter, P.M. and Gemperle, M. (1984) Clinical and haemodynamic effects of a specific BZ antagonist (RO 15-1788) after open heart surgery. *Anesthesiology* 61, A61.

Luger, T.G., Morawetz, R.F. and Mitterschiffthaler, G. (1990) Additional subcutaneous administration of flumazenil does not shorten recovery time after midazolam. *Br. J. Anaesth.* 64, 53—58.

Lundy, J.S. (1942) *Clinical Anesthesia.* W.B. Saunders, Philadelphia.

McClure, J.H., Brown, D.T. and Wildsmith, J.A.W. (1983) Comparison of the I.V. administration of midazolam and diazepam as sedation during spinal anaesthesia. *Br. J. Anaesth.* 55, 1089—1093.

McKay, A.C. and Dundee, J.W. (1980) Effect of oral benzodiazepines on memory. *Br. J. Anaesth.* 52, 1247—1257.

Mackenzie, N. and Grant, I.S. (1985) Comparison of propofol with methohexitone in the provision of anaesthesia for surgery under regional blockade. *Br. J. Anaesth.* 57, 1167—1172.

Mackenzie, N. and Grant, I.S. (1987) Propofol for intravenous sedation. *Anaesthesia* 42, 3—6.

McClain, D.A. and Hug, C.C. (1980) Intravenous fentanyl kinetics. *Clin. Pharmacol. Ther.* 28, 106—114.

Magni, V.C., Frost, R.A., Leung, J.W.C. and Cotton, P.B. (1983) A randomised comparison of midazolam and diazepam for sedation in upper gastrointestinal endoscopy. *Br. J. Anaesth.* 55, 1095—1101.

Main, D.M.G. (1968) The use of diazepam in dental anaesthesia. In: *Diazepam in Anaesthesia.* Editors: P.F. Knight and C.G. Burgess, Wright, Bristol, pp. 85—87.

Marley, J.E. and Ward, S. (1980) Chlormethiazole as sleep cover for the elderly. Intravenous infusion during local analgesia. *Anaesthesia* 35, 386—390.

Mather, L.E. and Cousins, M.J. (1980) Low dose chlormethiazole infusion as supplement to central neural blockade: blood concentrations and clinical effects. *Anaesth. Intensive Care* 8, 421—425.

Mohler, H. and Okada, T. (1978) The benzodiazepine receptor in normal and pathological human brain. *Br. J. Psychiatry* 133, 261—268.

Moir, D.D. and Thorburn, J. (1986) The selection of anaesthesia. In: *Obstetric Anaesthesia and Analgesia,* 3rd Edn. Bailliere Tindall, London, pp. 305—355.

Moore, D.C. and Bridenbaugh, L.D. (1966) Spinal (subarachnoid) block. A review of 11,574 cases. *J. Am. Med. Assoc.* 195, 907—912.

Moore, R.G., Triggs, E.J. Shanks, C.A. and Thomas, J. (1975) Pharmacokinetics of chlormethiazole in humans. *Eur. J. Clin. Pharmacol.* 8, 353—357.

Morel, D. Forster, A., Bachmann, M. and Suter, P.M. (1982) Changes in breathing pattern induced by midazolam in normal subjects. *Anesthesiology* 57, A481.

Murphy, M.R. and Hug, C.C. (1982) The enflurane sparing effect of morphine, butorphanol and nalbuphine. *Anesthesiology* 57, 489—492.

Murray-Lawson, J.I. and Milne, M.R. (1981) Intravenous sedation with diazepam and pentazocine. A study in dosage. *Br. Dent. J.* 151, 379—380.

Nagashima, H., Karamanian, A., Malovany, R., Rodnay, P., Ang, M., Koerner, S. and Folder, F.F. (1976) Respiratory and circulatory effects of intravenous butorphanol and morphine. *Clin. Pharmacol. Ther.* 19, 738—745.

Negus, J.B. and White, P.F. (1988) Use of sedative infusions during local and regional anesthesia — a comparison of propofol and midazolam. *Anesthesiology* 69, (Supplement) 3A711.

Nolte, H. and Dertwinkel, R. (1988) Propofol for sedation during epidural anaesthesia. *Anesthesia* 43 (Supplement), 115—116.

O'Neil, R., Verrill, P.J., Aellig, W.H. and Laurence, D.R. (1970) Intravenous diazepam in minor oral surgery. *Br. Dent. J.* 128, 15—18.

Owen, H. and Spence, A.A. (1984) Etomidate. *Br. J. Anaesth.* 56, 555—557.

Parbrook, G.D., Still, D.M. and Parbrook, E.O. (1989) Comparison of I.V. sedation with midazolam and inhalational sedation with isoflurane in dental outpatients. *Br. J. Anaesth.* 63, 81—86.

Patrick, M., Eager, B., Toft, D.F. and Sebel, P.S. (1983) Alfentanil supplemented anesthesia for short procedures: a double blind comparison with fentanyl. *Anesthesiology* 59, A346.

Pearce, C. (1974a) The respiratory effects of diazepam supplementation of spinal anaesthesia in elderly males. *Br. J. Anaesth.* 46, 439—441.

Pearce, C. (1974b) A clinical trial of RO5-4200 (Flunitrazepam) used to supplement spinal anaesthesia in elderly patients. *Br. J. Anaesth.* 46, 877—880.

Philip, B.K. (1985) Supplemental medication for ambulatory procedures under regional anesthesia. *Anesth. Analg.* 64, 1117—1125.

Phillips, J.W. (1979) Diazepam potentiation of purinergic depression of central neurons. *Can. J. Physiol. Pharmacol.* 57, 432—435.

Phillips, O.C., Ebner, H., Nelson, A.T. and Black. M.H. (1969) Neurologic complications following spinal anesthesia with lidocaine: a prospective review of 10,440 cases. *Anesthesiology* 30, 284—289.

Power, S.J., Morgan, M. and Chakrabarti, M.R. (1983) Carbon dioxide response curve following midazolam and diazepam. *Br. J. Anaesth.* 55, 837—841.

Reinhart, K., Dallinger-Stiller, G., Dennhardt, R., Heinemeyer, G. and Eyrich, K. (1985) Comparison of midazolam, diazepam and placebo, I.M. as premedication for regional anaesthesia. *Br. J. Anaesth.* 57, 294—299.

Ricou, B. Forster, A., Bruckner, A., Chastonay, P. and Gemperle, M. (1986) Clinical evaluation of a specific benzodiazepine antagonist (RO 15-1788). *Br. J. Anaesth.* 58, 1005—1011.

Rigg, J.R.A. and Goldsmith, C.H. (1976) Recovery of ventilatory response to carbon dioxide after thiopentone, morphine and fentanyl in man. *Can. Anaesth. Soc. J.* 23, 370—382.

Roberts, G.J. (1983) Relative analgesia in clinical practice. In: *Anaesthesia and Sedation in Dentistry,* Monographs in Anaesthesiology 12. Editors: M.P. Coplans and R.A. Green, Elsevier, Amsterdam, pp. 231—279.

Rodrigo, M.R.C. and Rosenquist, J.B. (1987) The effect of RO 15-1788 (Anexate) on conscious sedation produced with midazolam. *Anaesth. Intensive Care* 15, 185—192.

Romagnoli, A. and Keats, A.S. (1980) Ceiling effect for respiratory depression by nalbuphine. *Clin. Pharmacol. Ther.* 27, 478—485.

Rosow, C.E., Latta, W.B., Keegan, C.R., Nozick, D.L., Murphy, A.L., Kimball, W.R. and Philbin, D.M. (1983) Alfentanil and fentanyl in short surgical procedures. *Anesthesiology* 59, A345.

Rothe, K.F. and Schorer, R. (1980) Ataranalgesia — an intravenous anaesthetic technique. Experience with 978 administrations. *Acta Anaesthesiol. Belg.* 31, 77—89.

Rubin, J., Brock-Utne, J.G., Greenberg, M., Bortz, J. and Downing, J.W. (1977) Laryngeal incompetence during experimental relative analgesia using 50% nitrous oxide in oxygen. *Br. J. Anaesth.* 49, 1005—1008.

Sage, D.J. (1988) Reversal of sedation with flumazenil in regional anaesthesia: a review. *Eur. J. Anaesthesiol.* Suppl. 2, 201—207.

Sage, D.J., Close, A. and Boas, R.A. (1987) Reversal of midazolam sedation with Anexate. *Br. J. Anaesth.* 59, 459—464.

Samuelson, P.N., Reves, J.G., Kouchoukos, N.T., Smith, L.R. and Dole, K.M. (1981) Haemodynamic responses to anesthetic induction with midazolam or diazepam in patients with ischemic heart disease. *Anesth. Analg.* 60, 802—809.

Sanders, L.D., Davies-Evans, J., Rosen, M. and Robinson, J.O. (1989) Comparison of diazepam with midazolam as I.V. sedation for outpatient gastroscopy. *Br. J. Anaesth.* 63, 726—731.

Schou-Olesen, A. and Huttel, M.S. (1978) Circulatory collapse following intravenous administration of Stesolid MR. *Ugeskr. Laeg.* 140, 2644.

Schou-Olesen, A. and Huttel, M.S. (1980) Local reactions to I.V. diazepam in three different formulations. *Br. J. Anaesth.* 52, 609—611.

Schweitzer, S.A. (1978) Chlormethiazole (Hemineurin) infusion as supplemental sedation during epidural block. *Anaesth. Intensive Care* 6, 248—250.

Scott, D.B., Beamish, D., Hudson, I.N. and Jostell, K.G. (1980) Prolonged infusion of chlormethiazole in intensive care. *Br. J. Anaesth.* 52, 541—545.

Seow, L.T., Roberts, J.G., Mather, L.E. and Cousins, M.J. (1981) Two-stage infusion of chlormethiazole for basal sedation. *Br. J. Anaesth.* 53, 1203—1210.

Short, T.G. and Galletly, D.C. (1989) Residual psychomotor effects following reversal of midazolam sedation with flumazenil. *Anaesth. Intensive Care* 17, 290—297.

Sinclair, C.J., Fagan, D. and Scott, D.B. (1985) Cardiovascular effects of chlormethiazole infusion in combination with extradural anaesthesia. *Br. J. Anaesth.* 57, 587—590.

Slogoff, S., Allen, G.W., Wessels, J.V. and Cheney, D.H. (1974) Clinical experience with subanesthetic ketamine. *Anesth. Analg.* 53, 354—358.

Stanski, D.R. and Hug, C.C. (1982) Alfentanil — a kinetically predictable narcotic analgesic. *Anesthesiology* 57, 435—438.

Sury, M.R.J. and Cole, P.V. (1988a) Nalbuphine combined with midazolam for outpatient sedation. An assessment of safety on volunteers. *Anaesthesia* 43, 281—284.

Sury, M.R.J. and Cole, P.V. (1988b) Nalbuphine combined with midazolam for outpatient sedation. An assessment in fibreoptic bronchoscopy patients. *Anaesthesia* 43, 285—288.

Thompson, G.E. and Moore, D.C. (1971) Ketamine, diazepam and Innovar, a computerised comparative study. *Anesth. Analg.* 50, 458—463.

Thorn-Alquist, A.M. (1977) Parenteral use of diazepam in an emulsion formulation. A clinical study. *Acta Anaesthesiol. Scand.* 21, 400—404.

Thornton, J.A. and Martin V.C. (1976) Flunitrazepam in dental outpatients. *Anaesthesia* 31, 297.

Tomlin, P.J. and Gjessing, J. (1978) Balanced regional analgesia-an hypothesis. *Can. Anaesth. Soc. J.* 25, 412—415.

Valtonen, M., Salonen, M., Forssell, H., Scheinin, M. and Viinamaki, O. (1989) Propofol infusion for sedation in outpatient oral surgery. A comparison with diazepam. *Anaesthesia* 44, 730—734.

Van Steenberge, A., Fanard, L. and Van der Puyl, F. (1987) Sedatives in regional anaesthesia. *Acta Anaesthesiol. Belg.* Suppl. 1, 38, 19—22.

Vindhya, P.K., Sheets, J.H., Tolia, N.H. and Tomlinson, L.J. (1987) Retrobulbar block using pentothal as a sedative for ambulatory cataract surgery. *J. Cataract Refract. Surg.* 13, 321—322.

Ward, M.E. and Rose, N.M. (1982) Out-patient sedation for oral surgery. A new technique using etomidate. *Anaesthesia* 37, 289—294.

Ward-Booth, R.P. (1986) Intravenous opiates and benzodiazepine sedation. *Br. Dent. J.* 161, 241.

White, M. and Kenny, G.N.C. (1989) Intraoperative control of propofol using a computerised infusion system. *Br. J. Anaesth.* 63, 620—621.

White, P.F., Way, W.L. and Trevor, A.J. (1982) Ketamine — its pharmacology and therapeutic uses. *Anesthesiology* 56, 119—136.

Whitwam, J.G., Al-Khudhairi, D. and McCloy, R.F. (1983) Comparison of midazolam and diazepam in doses of comparable potency during gastroscopy. *Br. J. Anaesth.* 55, 773—777.

Willatts, S.M. and Kong, K.L. (1989) Sedation Techniques. In: *Recent Advances in Anaesthesia and Analgesia* 16. Editors: R.S. Atkinson and A.P. Adams, Churchill Livingstone, Edinburgh, pp. 83—103.

Wilson, E., Mackenzie, N. and Grant, I.S. (1988) A comparison of propofol and midazolam by infusion to provide sedation in patients who receive spinal anaesthesia. *Anaesthesia* 43, Suppl. 91—94.

Wilson, E., David, A., Mackenzie, N. and Grant, I.S. (1990) Sedation during spinal anaesthesia: comparison of propofol and midazolam. *Br. J. Anaesth.* 64, 48—52.

Wilson, J., Stephen, G.W. and Scott, D.B. (1969) A study of the cardiovascular effects of chlormethiazole. *Br. J. Anaesth.* 41, 840—843.

Wise, C.C., Robinson, J.S., Heath, M.J. and Tomlin, P.J. (1969) Physiological responses to intermittent methohexitone for conservative dentistry. *Br. Med. J.* 2, 540—543.

*B. Kay (ed.) Total Intravenous Anaesthesia*



# 15

# *Intravenous anaesthesia for day-care surgery*

Jan Van Hemelrijck and Paul F. White

## INTRODUCTION

Outpatient anaesthesia has been practiced since 1842; however, it is only over the last decade that economic considerations have resulted in an explosive growth in this surgical practice. Furthermore, the patient population treated on an ambulatory basis has been extended with regard to age and physical fitness. The ability to provide safe and effective anaesthesia care with a rapid recovery and minimal side effects has become critically important to meet the demands of a busy outpatient unit. Complications and side effects which commonly delay discharge include excessive pain, prolonged emergence, dizziness and nausea and vomiting. In developing an anaesthesia treatment plan, the anaesthesiologist should consider the possible influence of the drugs and anaesthetic technique on these important factors, as well as the medical history of the individual patient.

Regional anaesthesia can offer advantages over general anaesthesia for many outpatient procedures. However, for many patients intravenous (i.v.) sedative or analgesic medications are essential adjuvants during regional anaesthesia. Uncomfortable positioning, anxiety and pain can adversely influence patient cooperation during surgery and produce deleterious haemodynamic changes, especially in the cardiac compromised. Intermittent bolus administration of i.v. sedative-hypnotic and analgesic drugs is the most widely used technique in this situation. However, in a closed claims analysis of factors contributing to unexpected cardiac arrest during regional anaesthesia, intravenous sedation was one of the factors that may have contributed to the adverse outcome (Caplan et al., 1988). Excessive doses of sedative and analgesic medication can result in delayed recovery and discharge. Use of continuous intravenous infusions of anaesthetic and analgesic drugs has been found to be associated with fewer intra-operative side effects and shorter recovery times than the traditional intermittent bolus technique (White, 1983; White et al., 1986).

Concerns regarding the recovery characteristics following different types of general anaesthesia have resulted in controversy over the choice of volatile or intravenous anaesthetic techniques for outpatient surgery. Intravenous anaesthetics are popular induction agents because of their ease of administration, rapid onset of action and high patient acceptance. In contrast, maintenance of anaesthesia has traditionally been achieved with nitrous oxide and volatile anaesthetics, while intravenous drugs (sedative-hypnotics, analgesics, muscle relaxants) had only a minor adjunctive role. In the outpatient setting, intravenous anaesthetic techniques must compete with the rapid and predictable reversibility of the volatile anaesthetics. In addition, they will have to compare favourably with respect to peri-operative side effects.

The ideal i.v. agent for outpatient anaesthesia should be non-irritating to the tissues and produce a rapid and smooth onset of action without excitatory effects or cardiocirculatory depression; it should possess both analgesic and amnesic properties, and provide excellent operative conditions; its pharmacokinetic profile should allow for a rapid and complete recovery without side effects; finally, the drug should have anti-emetic properties or at least it should not increase the incidence of postoperative nausea and vomiting. Although this ideal i.v. anaesthetic has yet to be discovered, some of the newer benzodiazepines (e.g. midazolam), sedative hypnotics (e.g. propofol), analgesics (e.g. alfentanil) and muscle relaxants (e.g. mivacurium) possess advantages over the prototypic compounds in these drug groups. Combinations of these newer i.v. drugs, with the addition of some exciting new adjuvant drugs (e.g. dexmedetomidine, esmolol, ondansetron) may result in an intravenous anaesthetic technique that compares favourably with the more traditional approaches and more closely meets the needs of the ambulatory surgery patient.

## PHARMACOLOGY OF INTRAVENOUS DRUGS USED FOR OUTPATIENT ANAESTHESIA

### Sedative-hypnotics

#### *Barbiturates*

The barbiturates used for anaesthesia (e.g. thiopentone, thiamylal and methohexitone) cause a dose-dependent depression of the central nervous system, ranging from sedation to coma. Their mechanism of action is not completely understood. The short duration of action is due to a rapid redistribution. Methohexitone clearance is 3—5 times more rapid than thiopentone, contributing to elimination half-life values of 3—5 and 10—12 h, respectively (Hudson et al., 1983). This difference in elimination half-life values may contribute to the more prolonged recovery after a thiopentone infusion as compared to a methohexitone infusion (White, 1984). When administered by repeated bolus doses, methohexitone allows for a more rapid recovery than thiopentone. It is clear that methohexitone's pharmacokinetic properties appear to be more suitable for outpatient anaesthesia than thiopentone's, especially when anaesthesia is maintained with a continuous infusion technique.

The alkaline barbiturate solutions can cause tissue irritation and pain if injected extravenously. Barbiturates produce a concentration-dependent respiratory and circulatory depression. The cardiocirculatory depression is due to both direct myocardial depression and dilatation of the venous capacitance vessels. Barbiturates also cause a coupled decrease of cerebral metabolism and blood flow, with a decrease in intracranial pressure.

The use of methohexitone causes a high incidence of excitatory effects (e.g. myoclonus, hiccups), which can be minimized by slow injection and by pretreatment with a narcotic analgesic. Although methohexitone is generally considered to be superior to thiopentone for outpatient procedures because of its shorter recovery time, or to etomidate because of its lower incidence of postoperative side effects (Cooper, 1984; White, 1984), complete recovery of fine motor skills may be as prolonged after methohexitone as after thiopentone (Korttila et al., 1975). When used for sedation (Urquhart and White, 1989) or hypnosis (White, 1984) during outpatient procedures, a carefully titrated variable-rate infusion of methohexitone can provide optimal intra-operative conditions and rapid emergence with minimal residual central nervous system impairment. Rectal methohexitone (25 mg/kg) can also be used for induction of anaesthesia in paediatric outpatients (Hannallah et al., 1985). The time to the onset of sleep is 5—10 min and correlates well with the plasma concentration of the drug (Liu et al., 1985). Sedation can also be provided by intramuscular administration of a 2—5% solution (Varner et al., 1985).

*Etomidate*

Etomidate is an imidazole-based compound, which is structurally unrelated to any other intravenous anaesthetic. Rapid redistribution is responsible for its relatively short duration of action. Recovery of psychomotor function after an induction dose of etomidate (0.2—0.4 mg/kg) is intermediate between thiopentone and methohexitone (White, 1984). The drug is rapidly metabolized to inactive metabolites by hepatic microsomal enzymes and plasma esterases. This results in a relatively short elimination half-life (2—5 h). Etomidate can be administered by an intermittent bolus or a continuous infusion technique. The major advantage of etomidate is its minimal depressant effect on the cardiovascular system. Etomidate also decreases cerebral blood flow, cerebral metabolism and intracranial pressure. This combination of properties makes it the drug of choice for patients with a compromised cerebral perfusion pressure.

Etomidate is dissolved in propylene glycol and can therefore provoke pain and occasional venous irritation when rapidly infused for induction of anaesthesia. Although it has anticonvulsant properties, etomidate can produce myoclonic movements by disinhibition of subcortical neuronal activity. The incidence of myoclonic activity can be decreased by pretreatment with an opiate analgesic (e.g.

fentanyl 1.5 μg/kg) or a benzodiazepine (e.g. midazolam 0.07 mg/kg) (Giese et al., 1985). The use of etomidate may be associated with a high incidence of nausea and vomiting (White, 1984; Kestin and Dorje, 1987). Prophylactic administration of an anti-emetic drug (e.g. droperidol 0.6—1.2 mg, metoclopramide 10—20 mg i.v.) is recommended. Etomidate causes a transient enzymatic blockade of the adrenal steroidogenesis pathway (Wagner and White, 1984; Wagner et al., 1984). This postoperative depression of adrenal steroidogenesis lasts 6—8 h after the usual induction dose. The clinical significance of this transient drug effect is unknown. Prolonged infusions of etomidate are not recommended because they can result in drug accumulation and prolonged suppression of the adrenal function.

Etomidate has been used for induction and maintenance of anaesthesia for outpatient procedures (White, 1984). Recovery is at least as rapid and perhaps more predictable than after thiopentone (Horrigan et al., 1980). Early recovery may be equivalent to recovery after methohexitone (Miller et al., 1978). An etomidate infusion has also been used to provide a stable level of sedation during regional anaesthesia, with a rapid recovery and minimal side effects, comparable to methohexitone and midazolam (Urquhart and White, 1989).

### *Ketamine*

Ketamine is an arylcyclohexylamine, which is structurally related to phencyclidine. The drug produces a so-called 'dissociative' anaesthetic state, resulting from the functional dissociation between the thalamocortical and limbic systems. Ketamine inhibits the effects of neuro-excitatory neurotransmitters such as acetylcholine and glutamate, and binds to the sigma opiate receptor. In addition, it may have some opioid-like activity at the spinal cord mu-receptor. Nevertheless, the analgesia produced by ketamine appears to be primarily related to interference with the transmission of pain signals to the higher brain centers, which are responsible for the affective-emotional component of pain perception.

The ketamine molecule contains a chiral center, producing two optical enantiomers, *S*(+) and *R*(−) ketamine. The drug is available commercially as a racemic mixture containing equal amounts of both isomers. The *S*(+) isomer is three to five times more potent than the *R*(−) isomer in terms of its anaesthetic effects, and is followed by a more rapid recovery than the racemic mixture (White et al., 1980; White et al., 1985). Both isomers produce similar degrees of psychomimetic activity and cardiocirculatory stimulation. The two enantiomers, as well as the racemic mixture, also have the same pharmacokinetic properties. Ketamine has a high hepatic clearance and a large volume of distribution, resulting in an elimination half-life of 2—3 h. The principal metabolite, norketamine, is less pharmacologically active than ketamine itself.

Ketamine has direct central nervous system (CNS) stimulating effects and causes inhibition of postganglionic reuptake of norepinephrine. These properties are responsible for producing its cardiovascular stimulating effects, namely peripheral vasoconstriction, increased heart rate and blood pressure. When the sympathetic nervous system is blocked, ketamine's direct myocardial depressant and peripheral vasodilating properties may become evident. Ketamine increases cerebral metabolism and blood flow, leading to an increase in intracranial pressure in patients with decreased cerebral compliance. The drug causes only transient respiratory depression and is able to reduce airway resistance and bronchospasm. Tracheal soiling and aspiration has been reported following induction of anaesthesia, and use of ketamine does not obviate the need for endotracheal intubation in the patient with a 'full stomach'.

Ketamine's usefulness in outpatient anaesthesia is limited primarily because of its prominent psychomimetic activity during emergence (White et al., 1982). The benzodiazepines, especially midazolam, are very effective in attenuating ketamine's emergence sequelae (Cartwright and Pringel, 1984; Toft and Romer, 1987). The use of an antisialagogue is recommended to avoid respiratory problems secondary to ketamine-induced salivary gland secretion. In paediatric patients, ketamine can be used as an intramuscular (2—6 mg/kg) or rectal (6—10 mg/kg) induction agent. For maintenance of anaesthesia, use of a continuous infusion would appear to offer advantages over the traditional intermittent bolus administration (White, 1983). However, when used as a continuous infusion with nitrous oxide after thiopentone induction for outpatient gynaecological surgery, ketamine resulted in delayed discharge and more frequent side effects compared to fentanyl (White et al., 1983). Ketamine infusion (5—25 $\mu$g/kg per min) has also been used for sedation and analgesia during local anaesthesia in the outpatient setting (White et al., 1988).

### *Propofol*

The alkylphenol, propofol (2.6-di-isopropylphenol), has a high lipid solubility, which enhances its ability to cross the blood brain barrier. In contrast to the original cremophor EL formulation, the propofol emulsion has not been associated with hypersensitivity or anaphylactic reactions. The drug has a large distribution volume and high clearance rate. Its elimination pharmacokinetics have been described by both a two- and three-compartment model. Using a two-compartment model the elimination half-life is 1—3 h. When a three-compartment model is employed, elimination from the highly perfused tissues occurs in 0.5—1 h, while the terminal elimination has been estimated to occur over 3—6 h (Cockshot, 1985; White, 1988). This long elimination half-life would increase the likelihood for drug accumulation when repeated boluses or prolonged infusions are used. Nevertheless, with careful titration, emergence from anaesthesia occurs rapidly after discontinuation of an infusion (Doze et al., 1986; Doze et al., 1988). Propofol is extensively metabolized to inactive metabolites. Since its total body clearance exceeds liver blood flow, extrahepatic elimination may occur in the lung in addition to its extensive hepatic metabolism (Cockshot, 1985). Only 30 min after intravenous administration of a bolus of propofol, less than 20% of the dose can be recovered as the unchanged compound.

Propofol can be used for induction of outpatient anaesthesia (1.5—2.5 mg/kg). Due to differences in their pharmacokinetics and pharmacodynamics (Kirckpatrick et al., 1988), older patients (>60 years of age) require lower dosages for induction (1.5—1.75 mg/kg) and maintenance (Dundee et al., 1986; Doze et al., 1988). In children, the $ED_{90}$ for induction is 2.8 mg/kg in the unpremedicated and 2 mg/kg after premedication with trimeprazine (Patel et al., 1988). A high incidence of pain on injection and a quick recovery have been reported in children (Mirakhur, 1988).

Given its pharmacokinetic and dynamic profile, continuous infusion of propofol is a rational approach to using the drug for maintenance of anaesthesia, thereby minimizing the peaks and valleys in the blood and brain concentrations. The use of a variable rate infusion allows for titration of the propofol dose to the desired clinical effect, decreasing the total dosage requirement, improving cardiocirculatory stability and providing for a rapid recovery (Doze et al., 1986; Shafer et al., 1988).

Propofol has many of the characteristics of the ideal i.v. sedative-hypnotic for outpatient anaesthesia. Its rapid onset and recovery compares favourably with the barbiturates (MacKenzie and Grant, 1985). There appears to be less residual postoperative depressant effect and psychomotor impairment, while the incidence of postoperative side effects is extremely low (Wells, 1985). The low incidence of nausea and vomiting has led to the suggestion that propofol may even possess an anti-emetic action (McCollum et al., 1988). At equipotent doses, propofol appears to be similar to the barbiturates with respect to circulatory and respiratory depression. The cardiocirculatory depression produced by propofol is characterized by a decrease in arterial pressure and cardiac index, without a significant change in heart rate (Grounds et al., 1985). The drug requires careful titration when used for patients with compromised cardiac function. Reported side effects associated with propofol administration include pain on injection and involuntary muscle movements during induction, occasional dizziness, headaches, and euphoria on emergence.

Propofol is extensively used in outpatient anaesthesia, as an induction agent, for maintenance of anaesthesia, and, in lower dosage, for sedation during procedures performed under local or regional anaesthesia. Induction with propofol resulted in faster awakening and an improved recovery profile compared to methohexitone or thiopentone and isoflurane in short outpatient procedures (Raeder and Misvaer, 1988; Doze et al., 1986, 1988). After more prolonged procedures (>2 h) these authors found no significant differences. Propofol is a valuable alternative to methohexitone when repeated short periods of unconsciousness are necessary (e.g. thermocoagulation therapy of trigeminal neuralgia) (Kytta and Rosenberg, 1988). After repeated bolus doses for induction and maintenance of anaesthesia for minor gynaecological procedures, propofol was followed by a faster early recovery than thiopentone or thiamylal (Henriksson et al., 1987; Weightman and Zacharias, 1987; Sampson et al., 1988;). In some patients minor psychomotor impairment was detected up to 3 h following propofol (Weightman and Zacharias, 1987). Repeated bolus doses of propofol during diagnostic laryngeal procedures provided for a rapid emergence without nausea, vomiting, or respiratory depression (Zelcer et al., 1989).

Alfentanil supplementation of propofol-nitrous oxide anaesthesia was more effective than fentanyl in blocking the cardiocirculatory response. Compared to isoflurane for maintenance after induction with propofol, repeated boluses of propofol resulted in more rapid initial recovery (Milligan et al., 1987). Anaesthesia with repeated doses of propofol, for dental anaesthesia in children, was also followed by a more rapid recovery than a thiopentone-isoflurane anaesthetic technique (Puttick and Rosen, 1988). Propofol induction of anaesthesia for outpatient cystoscopy resulted in fewer excitatory side effects than either methohexitone or althesin, while maintenance of anaesthesia with propofol produced less myoclonia and movement than althesin and fewer hiccups than methohexitone; however, the mean minimum systolic pressure was less with propofol than with methohexitone (Kay and Healy, 1985). In the same study, addition of a small dose of alfentanil made it possible to lower the propofol infusion rate by 60%. Both immediate recovery and return to normal activities were faster following propofol than following methohexitone anaesthesia. Induction with pethidine (meperidine) (1 mg/kg) and propofol (2—2.5 mg/kg), and maintenance with a variable rate infusion (4—12 mg/min) in combination with nitrous oxide resulted in excellent intra-operative stability and a rapid recovery following brief outpatient gynaecologic procedures (Doze et al., 1986). Recovery following propofol anaesthesia compares favourably with thiopentone-isoflurane for short outpatient anaesthesia (Doze and White, 1986; Doze et al., 1988) and resulted in better patient acceptance scores (Cork and Scipione, 1989). The early and late recovery after propofol-fentanyl-nitrous oxide anaesthesia was superior to recovery after midazolam-fentanyl-isoflurane-nitrous oxide, even when the effects of midazolam were reversed by flumazenil (Forest and Galletly, 1987). Propofol anaesthesia for microlaryngeal surgery resulted in better surgical conditions, less cardiocirculatory response and better recovery scores than etomidate anaesthesia, both supplemented with alfentanil (de Grood et al., 1987). A pre-induction dose of alfentanil (10 μg/kg) effectively obtunded cardiovascular response to bronchoscopy or oesophagoscopy performed under total intravenous anaesthesia with propofol, without affecting recovery time (Kestin et al., 1989).

An infusion of propofol (e.g. a loading bolus of 0.8 mg/kg followed by an infusion at 2—4 mg/kg per h) can produce satisfactory sedation during procedures performed under local or regional anaesthesia, and allows for a more rapid recovery of cognitive functions than midazolam (Negus and White, 1988). Although controversial, it has been alleged that postoperative anxiety scores may be higher after propofol (vs. midazolam) (Gottlieb et al., 1989). Pain at the site of infusion is a frequently occurring problem with propofol (32—37%); however, it can be prevented by injecting 2—3 ml of 1% lidocaine (Negus and White, 1988).

### *Benzodiazepines*

Benzodiazepines produce dose-dependent central nervous system depressant effects by enhancing the action of the inhibitory neurotransmittors, gamma-aminobutyric acid (GABA) and glycine. The three benzodiazepines available for parenteral use, namely diazepam, lorazepam and midazolam, possess similar anxiolytic, sedative, amnesic, hypnotic, anticonvulsant and muscle relaxant properties. In the outpatient setting, midazolam has the most suitable characteristics with regard to water-solubility, onset time, rate of metabolism and duration of action. Diazepam and lorazepam are insoluble in water and the parenteral formulations contain propylene glycol, producing pain on injection and occasionally venous irritation. The parenteral formulation of water-soluble midazolam (pH 3.5) causes minimal irritation after intravenous or intramuscular injection. At physiologic pH, midazolam has a more lipid-soluble conformation.

Diazepam has a slow and somewhat unpredictable onset of action. In contrast, midazolam's onset of action is fast, which makes the drug more titratable when used for induction of anaesthesia or for sedation during local or regional anaesthesia. Diazepam and lorazepam have a low hepatic clearance rate, resulting in eliminating half-life values of 20—40 and 10—20 h, respectively. Midazolam is more rapidily and extensively metabolized by the liver, resulting in an elimination half-life of 2—4 h (Reves et al., 1985; Persson et al., 1987). In contrast with diazepam, midazolam and lorazepam have no centrally-active metabolites. Despite a shorter terminal elimination half-life than diazepam and the absence of active metabolites, lorazepam is unsuitable for outpatient anaesthesia because of the relation between time-effect, i.e., there is a marked temporal lag between the peak blood concentration and the clinical effect of lorazepam. The plasma lorazepam concentration peaks 3 h after oral administration and recovery is prolonged after parenteral administration (Greenblatt et al., 1974).

Many patients presenting in the outpatient clinic benefit from pharmacologic intervention for relief of peri-operative anxiety, irrespective of whether the procedure will be performed under local, regional or general anaesthesia. Midazolam, 0.1 mg/kg i.m., can produce sedation, anxiolysis and amnesia without delaying discharge after brief outpatient anaesthesia (Shafer et al., 1989). Compared to intravenous sedation with diazepam, midazolam produced more effective sedation, amnesia and anxiolysis, as well as a more rapid return to normal activities (Barker et al., 1986; White et al., 1988).

The slower onset of action, the prolonged recovery times, and the high incidence of residual postoperative amnesia, make benzodiazepines less suitable for use as a primary agent for induction and maintenance of general anaesthesia in the outpatient setting (Berggren and Eriksson, 1981; White, 1984; Verna et al., 1985; Reiton et al., 1986). Furthermore, induction of anaesthesia with benzodiazepines has been characterized by marked variability in the relationship between dose and response. Nevertheless, midazolam has been successfully used in combination with nitrous oxide and alfentanil for brief outpatient procedures (Crawford et al., 1984). Use of midazolam for maintenance of anaesthesia should probably be restricted for those situations where it offers a distinct advantage over other agents (White, 1985).

Although benzodiazepines appear to have limited efficacy as primary anaesthetics, they may be most effectively used as adjuvants to other general anaesthetic agents.

Midazolam can attenuate the cardiocirculatory stimulating effects and psychomimetic emergence sequelae after ketamine. The incidence of unpleasant dreams with ketamine anaesthesia was lower when combined with midazolam, 0.07 mg/kg i.v., than with diazepam, 0.12 mg/kg (Cartwright and Pringel, 1984). The frequency of emergence reactions was lower, time to complete recovery shorter, and patient's acceptance higher when ketamine anaesthesia was supplemented with midazolam compared to diazepam supplementation for endoscopy (Toft and Romer, 1987). For outpatient plastic surgery, midazolam, 0.1—0.15 mg/kg infused over 3—5 min, followed by ketamine 0.25—0.5 mg/kg i.v., produced excellent sedation, amnesia and analgesia during injection of local anaesthetic solutions, without significant cardiovascular or respiratory depression (White et al., 1988).

Varying levels of sedation, ranging from mild to subhypnotic, are frequently desirable during local and regional anaesthesia. While mild sedation is readily achievable with oral or intramuscular benzodiazepine premedication, intravenous administration is required to achieve controllable 'deeper' levels of sedation. The effects of ageing and pre-existing disease as well as the marked interpatient variability, make careful intravenous titration mandatory. Midazolam is the benzodiazepine of choice because of short onset time and elimination half-life. It appears to be 2—4 times more potent than diazepam with respect to sedative effect and more reliably produces intra-operative amnesia (White et al., 1988). Despite shorter elimination half-life, objective measures of recovery have failed to demonstrate a more rapid return to baseline cognitive function than with diazepam (Korttila and Tarkkanen, 1985). When compared to sedation with a propofol infusion (Negus and White, 1988), or with a methohexitone or etomidate infusion (Urquhart and White, 1989), sedation with a midazolam infusion resulted in less frequent recall of intra-operative events; however, it caused more pronounced sedation and amnesia in the immediate postoperative period. Nevertheless, discharge times were similar for all sedative infusion techniques (Negus and White, 1988; Urquhart and White, 1989).

The specific benzodiazepine antagonist, flumazenil, is available for clinical use in many European countries. With this new antagonist, it is possible to readily reverse the prolonged effects of midazolam, and this might lead to an increased use of this drug combination for outpatient procedures. Nevertheless, reversal of benzodiazepine sedation should not only be effective but also safe, without cardiovascular side effects or the danger of resedation. Since the elimination half-life of the antagonist is shorter than that of midazolam (1 h vs. 2—4 h), resedation may occur after discharge from the ambulatory surgery unit. Sedation as well as anaesthesia with midazolam can be effectively reversed by flumazenil without major side effects (Ricou et al., 1986; Wolff et al., 1986; Raeder et al., 1987; Kretz and Peisdersky, 1988; Jensen et al., 1989; Philip et al., 1989; White et al., 1989). Increased restlessness and fear were noted in some patients after larger doses of flumazenil (Ricou et al., 1986; Kretz and Peisdersky, 1988; Jensen et al., 1989). Other investigators noted an increased incidence of nausea and vomiting in the immediate post-reversal period (Wolff et al., 1986).

**Analgesics**

Narcotic analgesics reduce the requirement for sedative-hypnotics and inhalational anaesthetics, thereby decreasing emergence time after outpatient procedures (Horrigan et al., 1980; White and Chang, 1984). The adjunctive use of opioid analgesics also decreases the need for postoperative analgesic medication (Epstein et al., 1975). Nevertheless, even small doses of opiods (e.g. fentanyl 1.5 μg/kg) may increase the incidence of postoperative emetic symptoms (Horrigan et al., 1980). The ideal analgesic for outpatient use would have a rapid onset and short duration of effect with minimal side effects. Although the older and more traditional opioid analgesics like morphine and meperidine have been successfully used in outpatient anaesthesia, the newer, more potent and shorter-acting fentanyl-type analgesics more closely approach the ideal analgesic and are utilized extensively in the outpatient setting.

Fentanyl remains the most widely used analgesic in outpatient anaesthesia. It has a high potency, a rapid onset time and relatively short duration of effect when given in small doses. Nevertheless, its long elimination half-life may contribute to the incidence of minor postoperative sequelae (nausea, vomiting and dizziness) (Rising et al., 1985). Fentanyl 1—3 μg/kg i.v., is an effective supplement during a barbiturate-nitrous oxide anaesthetic (Epstein et al., 1975; Goroszeniuk et al., 1977).

Sufentanil is 7—10 times more potent than fentanyl and has a more rapid onset and a slightly shorter elimination half-life. The optimal pre-induction dose of sufentanil prior to a nitrous oxide-methohexitone anaesthetic for short outpatient gynaecological procedures is 10—15 μg i.v. (White et al., 1985). Higher doses produce dose-related respiratory depression and chestwall rigidity, while increasing the frequency of postoperative nausea and vomiting. When sufentanil, 0.5—1 μg/kg, was administered in combination with thiopentone (or methohexitone) and nitrous oxide, it produced equivalent anaesthesia to isoflurane and nitrous oxide, however it resulted in a higher incidence of postoperative vomiting (Wasudev et al., 1987; Zuurmond and van Leeuwen, 1987). For outpatient dilatation and curettage, sufentanil (in combination with thiopentone and nitrous oxide) compared favourably with fentanyl, with shorter times spent in the recovery room, less requirement for postoperative analgesics and a lower incidence of nausea and vomiting (Phitayakorn et al., 1987).

Alfentanil is less potent than fentanyl (1/5 to 1/10th), but it has a more rapid onset time. Alfentanil's lower lipid solubility results in a smaller distribution volume and a shorter elimination half-life (1—2 h). Its pharmacokinetic profile should decrease the potential for accumulation and for prolonged postoperative side effects. However, some otherwise normal individuals metabolize alfentanil at an abnormally slow rate, probably due to the existence of an abnormal cytochrome P-450 isoenzyme (McDonnell et al., 1982; McDonnell et al., 1984; Henthorn et al., 1985). Disadvantages of alfentanil are related to its potential for producing emetic sequelae and chestwall rigidity (Dechene, 1985). Alfentanil can be administered by either repeated injection or continuous infusion techniques. The use of a continuous infusion allows for a more precise titration of the drug, minimizing the dosage requirement and the incidence of opioid-related side effects (White et al., 1986). When used as a part of a continuous infusion technique, a loading dose of alfentanil is necessary to achieve a therapeutic concentration rapidly (Wagner, 1974; Shand et al., 1981). Administration of a small bolus dose of alfentanil may be more effective in treating autonomic responses to transient noxious stimuli than increasing the infusion rate.

In spite of its side effect profile, alfentanil is extensively used for outpatient anaesthesia. Use of alfentanil for termination of pregnancy was followed by a higher incidence of vomiting than halothane anaesthesia (Collins et al., 1985). However, pretreatment with alfentanil effectively decreased the incidence of injection pain and myoclonia on induction with etomidate and was followed by a more rapid recovery than halothane anaesthesia (Antonios et al., 1984; Moss et al., 1987) or enflurane anaesthesia (Haley et al., 1988). Alfentanil supplementation during an etomidate-enflurane anaesthetic resulted in less myoclonic activity and better haemodynamic stability (Collin et al., 1986). When compared to fentanyl, the frequency of emetic symptoms after alfentanil has been reported to be higher (Hull and Jakobson, 1983), lower (Patrick et al., 1984), or unchanged (Cooper et al., 1983; Rosow et al., 1983; Kennedy and Ogg, 1985; White et al., 1986). However, recovery times are consistently shorter with alfentanil than with fentanyl (Kay and Venkataraman, 1983; Kallar and Keenan, 1984; White et al., 1986; Haley et al., 1988). Although late postoperative impairment of psychomotor skills has been detected (Kennedy and Ogg, 1985), other investigators have reported a more rapid return to normal activities after alfentanil (Raeder and Hole, 1986).

Nalbuphine and butorphanol are antagonist-agonist narcotics which possess an antagonist effect at the mu-receptor, a partial agonist effect at the kappa-receptor and agonist activity at the sigma-receptor. Butorphanol is at least five times more potent than morphine, has a terminal half-life of 2—4 h and duration of analgesia lasting 3—5 h (Del Pizzo, 1976). The drug has a 'ceiling effect' with respect to its respiratory depressant and analgesic actions (Nagashima et al., 1976; Stehling and Zauder, 1978; Stanley et al., 1983). Butorphanol has a low physical dependence liability, but may cause postoperative psychomimetic symptoms due to a sigma receptor activity. When used as part of a standard balanced anaesthetic for outpatient procedures, butorphanol was associated with a similar incidence of postoperative nausea and vomiting to fentanyl (Pandit et al., 1987).

Nalbuphine, another agonist-antagonist, is equipotent to morphine (Beaver and Feise, 1978); however, it has minimal abuse potential. As for butorphanol, there appears to be a ceiling effect for the analgesic efficacy of nalbuphine, which parallels the ceiling effect for its respiratory depression (Gal et al., 1982). Nalbuphine has been administered in the outpatient setting with variable results. A pre-induction dose of nalbuphine decreased the intravenous anaesthetic requirement of althesin during cystoscopy, and thereby decreased the short-term recovery times (Kay et al., 1984). In paediatric outpatients undergoing tonsillectomy, nalbuphine was as effective as morphine in providing postoperative analgesia (Krishnan et al., 1985). However, in adult outpatients, recovery was prolonged and the incidence of postoperative sedation and dysphoria was increased when nalbuphine was used as an alternative to fentanyl (Garfield et al., 1987). Although nalbuphine improved the quality of sedation when administered as an adjunct to midazolam during fibre-optic bronchoscopy, it prolonged recovery and increased the incidence of side effects (Sury and Cole, 1988). The agonist-antagonist analgesics do not appear to offer any significant advantages over fentanyl and its newer analogs in outpatient anaesthesia.

**Muscle relaxants**

Muscle relaxants play an important role as adjuvants during outpatient anaesthesia. They not only facilitate tracheal intubation, but also improve the surgical conditions for procedures requiring muscle relaxation. The short duration of most outpatient procedures necessitates the use of short-acting compounds, devoid of side effects or complications that could delay discharge after ambulatory surgery. Relaxation for longer procedures can be provided by compounds with an intermediate duration of action or by utilizing infusions of short-acting muscle relaxants.

Suxamethonium (succinylcholine) remains the most widely used relaxant for brief outpatient procedures, because of a uniquely rapid onset and short duration of effect. Unfortunately, suxamethonium has many possible side effects and complications. It can produce postoperative myalgia when not preceded by a defasciculating dose of a non-depolarizing muscle relaxant. The incidence of muscle pain is highest after short operations with early mobilization. Suxamethonium increases intraocular, intracranial and intragastric pressure. It has the potential to trigger malignant hyperthermia, and produces bradycardia with repeated bolus doses. It can provoke potassium release, and even anaphylactoid reactions have been reported in sensitized individuals. A phase II block can develop with prolonged administration. Acquired cholinesterase deficiency (e.g. during pregnancy) or the presence of atypical cholinesterase enzymes can lead to unexpectedly prolonged neuromuscular blockade. Despite all its drawbacks, there is still a place for suxamethonium during short outpatient procedures. In the absence of specific contraindications, it is most frequently administered by intravenous bolus dose (preferably preceded by a defasciculating dose of a non-depolarizing relaxant), with or without a continuous infusion (Manchicanti et al., 1985). With the availability of non-depolarizing muscle relaxants with intermediate durations of action, indications for administration of suxamethonium are continuing to decrease.

Many outpatient procedures are of sufficiently long duration to justify the use of muscle relaxants with an intermediate duration of action, namely vecuronium and atracurium (Gyasi et al., 1985; Dodgson et al., 1986). Both intermediate-acting relaxants have comparable onset times and half-life values. Atracurium may cause histamine release, while vecuronium is devoid of haemodynamic effects but has the potential for accumulation with repeated doses. Both drugs can be administered by continuous infusion; however, this technique is rarely necessary for outpatient surgery.

Mivacurium (BW B 1090U), is a rapidly metabolized derivative of atracurium, which is currently undergoing extensive clinical trials. It has a short terminal elimination half-life of 17 min as a result of its high plasma clearance rate (55 ml/kg per min) (deBros et al., 1987). Mivacurium, 0.1—0.25 mg/kg, produces excellent intubation conditions within 90—180 s, followed by surgical relaxation for 15—20 min, with spontaneous recovery occurring in 30—45 min (Savarese et al., 1988). Histamine release and a concurrent decrease in blood pressure may occur with the higher doses. Mivacurium is hydrolyzed by human cholinesterase and prolonged blockade occurs in the presence of atypical cholinesterase activity. Mivacurium can be effectively administered by continuous infusion at a rate of 6—8 $\mu$g/kg per min (Ali et al., 1988, Savarese et al., 1988). Spontaneous recovery of neuromuscular function is faster after discontinuation of an infusion of suxamethonium than of mivacurium. However, mivacurium can be used as an alternative to suxamethonium and the intermediate-acting non-depolarizing muscle relaxants in the outpatient setting (Poler, 1988).

Other newer non-depolarizing muscle relaxants with shorter durations of action than currently available relaxants are currently under investigation (Shanks, 1988). Preliminary studies in animals would suggest that the vecuronium derivatives ORG 7617 and ORG 9616 have a similar onset time and duration of action to suxamethonium. The short duration of muscle relaxant effect is due to extensive redistribution. Unfortunately, these compounds do not appear to offer the same degree of cardiocirculatory stability as vecuronium. The vecuronium derivate ORG 9991 produces muscle relaxation with an onset time of 0.7 ± 0.2 min and a duration of 10 ± 2.6 min in cats (Rodrigues et al., 1989). Animal studies with ORG 9273 and ORG 9426 would predict a shorter onset time and duration of action than vecuronium, while sharing cardiocirculatory stability (Shanks, 1988). However, a preliminary study in humans would suggest that the time course of neuromuscular block produced by ORG 9426 and vecuronium are similar (Nagashima et al., 1989).

### Intravenous adjuvants

Adjuvant drugs can be used in outpatient anaesthesia to decrease the need for i.v. anaesthetics and analgesics (e.g. beta-blockers, alpha 2-agonists), or to prevent side effects of surgery and anaesthesia. Pharmacological relief of pre-operative anxiety presents a dilemma in outpatient anaesthesia as rapid return of psychomotor function is also required. A non-sedative anxiolytic would be an ideal premedication for ambulatory patients. Beta-blockers have no sedative activity, but may be very useful for some anxious patients by alleviating the sympathetic symptoms of anxiety. They may be taken at home, so that the effect is well-established on arrival in the hospital. Timolol has been succesfully used for this purpose (MacKenzy and Bird, 1989).

Esmolol is a short-acting beta-blocker with a distribution half-life of 2 min and an elimination half-life of 9 min. Esmolol's pharmacokinetic profile makes the drug suitable for use during outpatient anaesthesia. The drug can be administered by a bolus dose followed by an infusion which is titrated to produce the desired effect (e.g. 1 mg/kg in bolus followed by an infusion of 0.25 mg/kg per min). Prolonged postoperative effects are avoided because of its rapid elimination. Esmolol has been used succesfully to prevent haemodynamic responses to intubation and to treat sinus tachycardia and hypertension (Evert et al., 1986; Liu et al., 1986; Gold et al., 1989; Newman et al., 1989; Parnass et al., 1989). Pretreatment with a combination of metoprolol and hydralazine was effective in preventing haemodynamic responses and dysrhythmias during laryngoscopy (Magnusson et al., 1986). Pretreatment with labetolol (0.45—1 mg/kg), a sympatholytic drug with mixed alpha- and beta-blocking properties, provides protection against increases in blood pressure and heart rate from induction through the recovery period (Amar et al., 1989).

The alpha-2 agonist drugs are currently under investigation as premedicants in the outpatient setting. These drugs exert a sympatholytic effect by stimulating presynaptic alpha-2 receptors, thereby inhibiting the release of norepinephrine both in the central and the peripheral sympathetic nervous systems. Clonidine, an alpha-2 agonist, has long been used for chronic hypertension. Sedation is produced as a result of its central sympatholytic activity. Clonidine potentiates halothane anaesthesia (Kaukinen and Pyykko, 1979; Bloor and Flacke, 1982), significantly decreases opioid analgesic requirements, attenuates sympathoadrenal response to painful surgical stimuli and improves intra-operative haemodynamic stability (Ghignone et al., 1986; Flacke et al., 1987; Pouttu et al., 1987; Ghignone et al., 1988), while decreasing the postoperative analgesic requirement (Segal et al., 1989).

Medetomidine is a more selective and more potent alpha 2-agonist than clonidine and will likely be of clinical use as an i.v. adjuvant in the future. It decreases halothane's anaesthetic requirement in animals through an alpha-2 effect (Segal et al., 1988; Vickery et al., 1988). As catecholamine depletion does not abolish this effect, alpha-2 receptors other than the auto-inhibitory presynaptic alpha-2 receptors must be involved, e.g. postsynaptic alpha-2 receptors in the locus ceruleus. Only the D-isomer of medetomidine is pharmacologically active. Use of dexmedetomidine for premedication causes a dose-dependent increase in the level of sedation, decreases blood pressure and plasma noradrenaline (norepinephrine) levels (Kallio et al., 1989). Intravenously administered dexmedetomidine decreases the thiopentone anaesthetic requirement during minor surgical procedures, without significant adverse effects (Aantaa et al., 1989).

Postoperative vomiting is a major cause of delayed discharge following outpatient surgery (Doze et al., 1987; Metter et al., 1987). The role of nitrous oxide as a cause of increased frequency of postoperative vomiting is still debated (Lonie and Harper, 1986; Kortilla et al., 1987; Melnick and Johnson, 1987; Muir et al., 1987). However. the use of total intravenous anaesthetic techniques would obviate the need for nitrous oxide. Prophylactic use of anti-emetic drugs can play a major role in diminishing the frequency of postoperative nausea and vomiting. In addition, adjuvants such as centrally-active anticholinergics, antihistamines, phenothiazines, butyrophenones and substituted benzamides possess varying degrees of anti-emetic activity (Pallazzo and Strunin, 1984). Many of these drugs have undesirable side effects (e.g. dysphoria, extrapyramidal myalgias), which make their routine use in outpatient anaesthesia questionable. Metoclopramide, a substituted benzamide, increases lower oesophageal sphincter tone and increases resting gastric muscle tone, while facilitating transit through oesophagus, stomach and small bowel. In addition, metoclopramide possesses peripheral cholinergic and central anti-dopaminergic effects. The latter effects are responsible for the dystonic reactions which occur following higher doses (>1 mg/kg) of the anti-emetic. The effectiveness of lower doses of metoclopramide (0.15—0.3 mg/kg) as an anti-emetic agent in outpatient anaesthesia is controversial (Korttila et al., 1979; Cohen et al., 1984; Doze et al., 1987). Metoclopramide can also be a useful adjuvant to the $H_2$-receptor blocking drugs (cimetidine, ranitidine, famitidine) for prophylaxis against acid aspiration (Rao et al:, 1984; Manchicanti et al., 1986). Finally, metoclopramide has been used as an adjuvant to droperidol for prophylaxis against postoperative nausea (Doze et al., 1987).

Droperidol is a centrally-active anti-dopaminergic compound with neuroleptic properties. Besides its prominent anti-emetic effect, it has sedative, dysphoric, extrapyramidal and hypotensive side effects. Low doses of droperidol (5—15 μg/kg) decrease the incidence of postoperative emesis in adult ambulatory patients undergoing short surgical procedures (Mortensen, 1982; Millar and Hall, 1987). Low doses are also effective in adolescents undergoing short outpatient orthopaedic procedures (Rita et al., 1981). However, low dose droperidol appears to be less effective for longer outpatient procedures in adults (Valanne and Korttila, 1985). In children scheduled for strabismus surgery droperidol, 75 μg/kg i.v., was highly effective while doses less than 50 μg/kg were only partially effective (Abramowitz et al., 1983; Hardy et al, 1985; Lerman et al., 1986). The dysphoric (psychomimetic) effects of droperidol can lead to refusal of surgery when it is used for premedication (Briggs and Ogg, 1973). Even low doses can delay emergence from anaesthesia and impair psychomotor skills in the early postoperative period (Cohen et al., 1984; O'Donovan and Shaw, 1984; Vallane and Korttila, 1985). Use of droperidol (1.25 mg) for anti-emesis prophylaxis was recently reported to increase the frequency of delayed side effects (e.g. restlessness and anxiety) after discharge from the ambulatory care unit (Melnick et al., 1989).

## CONTINUOUS INFUSION TECHNIQUES

The traditional administration of intravenous drugs by intermittent bolus injection results in a depth of anaesthesia which oscillates above and below the desired level. The high peak blood concentration which occurs after each bolus is due to rapid redistribution of the drug, followed by a rapid decrease, producing fluctuating drug levels. The magnitude of the fluctuations depends on the size of the bolus doses and the frequency of their administration. Wide variation in plasma concentration can result in haeodynamic instability due to rapid changes in the depth of anaesthesia and variable cardiovascular effects of the drugs. By more closely titrating the drug administration to the desired clinical effect, it is possible to minimize the 'peak and valley' pattern in blood concentration. By providing a narrower band of blood and brain concentrations, it might be possible to improve anaesthetic conditions, as well as decreasing side effects and recovery times (White, 1983). As intravenous drugs with shorter terminal half-life values and thus less potential for accumulation become available for clinical use, administration by continuous infusion will likely become more popular in the future. This mode of administration is a logical extension of the incremental bolus methods of intravenous drug titration, as a continuous infusion is equivalent to the sequential administration of several small bolus doses.

The newer, more rapid and shorter-acting sedative-hypnotics, analgesics and muscle relaxants are better suited pharmacologically for continuous administration techniques than the traditional agents because they can be more accurately titrated to meet the unique and changing needs of the individual patient (White, 1989). Since none of the currently available intravenous drugs can provide for a complete anaesthetic state without producing undesirable side effects and prolonged recovery times, it is usually necessary to administer a combination of drugs which provide for hypnosis, amnesia, analgesia and muscle relaxation. Selecting a combination of intravenous drugs with similar pharmacokinetics and compatible pharmacodynamic profiles should improve anaesthetic and surgical conditions.

In order to achieve a therapeutic blood level rapidly, it is necessary to administer a loading dose. To maintain the desired clinical effect, a maintenance infusion is usually necessary. Although a drug can be titrated to the desired clinical effect using the traditional intermittent bolus technique, a knowledge of basic pharmacokinetic principles may be helpful in accurately predicting the initial dosage requirements. Loading dose (LD) and the initial maintenance infusion rate (MIR) can be calculated from previously determined population pharmacokinetics.

$$\text{LD} = Cp\ (\mu\text{g/ml}) \times Vd\ (\text{ml/kg})$$
$$\text{MIR} = Cp\ (\mu\text{g/kg}) \times Cl\ (\text{ml/kg per min})$$

where: $Cp$ = plasma drug concentration,
$Vd$ = volume of distribution,
$Cl$ = clearance of the drug.

The loading dose can be administered as a bolus or as a rapid loading ('priming') infusion. The later method causes less fluctuation in drug concentration and side effects. The required plasma drug concentration depends on the desired pharmacological effect (e.g. hypnosis, sedation, analgesia, degree of muscle relaxation), the concomitant use of other drugs (with additive, potentiating, antagonistic pharmacodynamic actions, or producing pharmacokinetic interactions), the type of operation (e.g. superficial, intra-abdominal, intracranial) and the individual patient's sensitivity to the drug (e.g. age, drug history, pre-existing diseases) (Ausems et al., 1983; Shafer et al., 1988). The initial MIR must replace the amount of drug that is removed from the brain by redistribution and elimination. When redistribution assumes less importance, the MIR will decrease as it becomes dependent solely on the drug's elimination (or clearance rate) and the desired plasma concentration. Although computer programs are available that allow prediction of concentration-time profiles for intravenous anaesthetics and analgesics, their clinical usefulness is unclear given the marked pharmacokinetic and pharmacodynamic variability which exists among surgical patients (Shafer et al., 1986; Maitre et al., 1987; Maitre et al., 1988; Shafer et al., 1989). Therefore, drug administration has to be titrated to the desired clinical effect (suppressing individual responses to a given surgical stimulus). Which clinical signs are most useful in determining the optimal maintenance infusion rate during intravenous anaesthesia? Most often anaesthetists rely on somatic and autonomic signs for assessing depth of anaesthesia, and titrate intravenous infusions in a manner which is similar to the way in which we currently administer volatile anaesthetics. The most sensitive clinical signs of depth of anaesthesia appear to be changes in muscle tone and ventilatory pattern. However, if the patient has been given muscle relaxants, the anaesthesiologist must rely on signs of autonomic hyperactivity (e.g. tachycardia, hypertension, lacrimation, diaphoresis). Changes in peripheral vascular resistance may be a more reliable indicator of depth of anaesthesia than blood pressure because blood pressure also depends upon the ability of the heart to maintain cardiac output in the face of an increased afterload. Blood pressure response to surgical stimulation appears to be a less useful guide with intravenous techniques than with volatile anaesthetics (White, 1989). The heart rate response to surgical stimulation may be more useful than changes in blood pressure in determining the need for additional anaesthesia or analgesia. In the presence of drugs with highly specific cardiovascular effects (e.g. beta-blockers, calcium-antagonists, alpha-2 agonists), the signs of autonomlc hyperactivity may be partially or completely masked, decreasing their usefulness as guides for intravenous anaesthetic delivery. Autonomic activity can also be blunted by the administration of potent opioid analgesics, without assuring that this patient is unconscious. A simple, non-invasive depth of anaesthesia monitor with a predictable dose-response relationship for commonly used anaesthetic and analgesic drugs and which would reliably predict a patient's response to a given surgical stimulus would be extremely valuable with total intravenous anaesthetic techniques. Electromyographic (EMG) activity of the frontal muscles increases significantly in patients who move in response to a specific surgical stimulus; however, this event occurs late (Chang et al., 1980). Furthermore, interpretation of EMG activity is hindered by muscle relaxants. The electroencephalographic (EEG) changes depend largely on the anaesthetic drugs, although with increasing depression of central nervous frequency, a common pattern can by recognized. Univariate descriptors (e.g. spectral edge frequency, median frequency) of EEG activity appear to be of limited clinical use (Levy, 1984). In a recent study, no correlation was found between spectral edge frequency and haemodynamic response to surgical stimuli during propofol-nitrous oxide anaesthesia (White and Boyle, 1989). Although lower oesophagal contracility (LEC) monitoring was reported to correlate with autonomic responses during surgery in adults anaesthetized with volatile anaesthetics (Evans et al., 1984; Evans et al., 1987; Maccioli et al., 1988), it was less useful in children (Watcha and White, 1989). When evaluated during balanced anaesthesia (e.g. nitrous oxide-narcotic-muscle relaxant), LEC monitoring was of limited usefulness in judging depth of anaesthesia (Sessler et al., 1989; Monk et al., 1990). Finally, none of the available monitors of central nervous system function can detect intra-operative awareness under anaesthesia. The availability of a simple non-invasive depth of anaesthesia monitor would allow for more widespread use of intravenous anaesthetic techniques.

## USE OF TOTAL INTRAVENOUS TECHNIQUES IN THE OUTPATIENT SETTING

Controversy still exists over the optimal anaesthetic technique for outpatient anaesthesia. Currently available short-acting intravenous drugs have made it possible to administer an intravenous anaesthetic that can approach the commonly used inhalational techniques with respect to controllable intra-operative activity and residual postoperative side effects. Comparing intravenous narcotics-based techiques with inhalational agents, early recovery is usually more rapid with the balanced anaesthetic technique; however, the time to return to baseline cognitive and psychomotor function may actually be shorter when a volatile agent is used (Simpson et al., 1976; Rising et al., 1985; Zuurmond and van Leeuwen, 1986). Unrelated to the rate of recovery, inadequate pain relief and vomiting are two important factors that can contribute to delayed discharge from the outpatient surgery unit. While opioid compounds can contribute to a shorter stay in the recovery area as a result of their residual analgesic effect, the incidence of nausea and vomiting may be increased. Interestingly, in patients experiencing both nausea and pain in the immediate postoperative period, adequate treatment of pain resulted in resolution of nausea in 80% of the patients (Andersen and Krogh, 1976). Only 10% of the patients continued to experience nausea after adequate treatment of their acute pain symptoms.

If a continuous infusion is to be used in an optimal manner to suppress responses to surgical stimulation, the drug's maintenance infusion rate must be carefully adjusted to meet the individual patient's needs, analogous to the fashion in which the volatile anaesthetic agents are administered. Using a constant MIR which is sufficient to suppress responses to the most intense surgical stimuli will lead to excessive drug accumulation, a high incidence of postoperative side effects and prolonged recovery times. Gradually increasing signs of inadequate anaesthesia (either to 'deep' or to 'light') can be treated by making 25—50% changes in the MIR. Abrupt increases in autonomic activity should be treated with small bolus doses (equal to 10—25% of the initial loading dose) and then increasing the MIR if the stimulation is sustained (White, 1989). Alternatively, adjunctive drugs (e.g.

vasodilators, sympathetic drugs, and alpha-2-agonists) can be used to blunt the haemodynamic responses to more stressful surgical stimulation, thereby decreasing the need for analgesic and anaesthetic drugs. During the course of an operation, the MIR should be progressively decreased until early signs of inadequate anaesthesia are noted. Careful titration of intravenous drugs obviates the need to rely on antagonist drugs.

It is impossible to achieve an adequate depth of anaesthesia with one drug alone without administering a dose that produces significant cardiorespiratory changes, disturbing side effects, and delayed recovery. The use of drug combinations is a logical approach to achieve an optimal anaesthetic state for ambulatory surgery. By utilizing the minimal effective doses of different intravenous drugs with comparable pharmacokinetics and compatible pharmacodynamic profiles, the anaesthesiologist can achieve a rapid and smooth induction, maintenance and emergence from outpatient anaesthesia without untoward side effects.

Due to its favourable recovery profile, propofol is increasingly popular for maintenance of anaesthesia during ambulatory surgery. Using intermittent bolus doses of propofol (20 mg) to supplement a nitrous oxide based anaesthetic technique for superficial surgery, an average dose of 75 μg/kg per min was needed for maintenance of anaesthesia following premedication with morphine, 0.15 mg/kg and induction with propofol, 2.5 mg/kg (Uppington et al., 1985). Recovery following intermittent propofol administration was faster than following methohexitone or thiopentone (Cundy and Arunasalam, 1985; Uppington et al., 1985). Although propofol can be successfully administered with an intermittent bolus technique, a greater degree of intra-operative stability would be expected when the drug is administered by a continuous infusion technique. When preceded by a small dose of an opioid analgesic (e.g. fentanyl, 1—3 μg/kg, or alfentanil 5—10 μg/kg), anaesthesia is readily induced with propofol, 1.5—2.5 mg/kg. Induction is followed by an initial propofol infusion rate of 100—200 μg/kg per min, with 60—70% nitrous oxide. Following the redistribution phase (15—20 min), the infusion rate can be decreased to 50—150 μg/kg per min (Doze et al., 1986; White, 1988). Higher propofol infusion rates of 150—300 μg/kg per min were reported to be necessary, when propofol was used to maintain anaesthesia for outpatient surgery without the use of nitrous oxide (de Grood et al., 1985; McLeod and Boheimer, 1985). When an opioid analgesic was omitted, a propofol infusion rate of 250 μg/kg per min was necessary, in combination with nitrous oxide (MacKenzie and Grant, 1985). A small dose of alfentanil (7.5 μg/kg) lowered the propofol requirements for maintenance of anaesthesia during cystoscopy by 65% (Kay and Healy, 1985).

Alfentanil infusions can be used to provide analgesia during outpatient surgery. Depending on the type of procedure, loading doses have varied from 7.5 to 50 μg/kg. Lower doses are utilized in patients undergoing minor outpatient procedures (e.g. dilatation and curettage, cone biopsy), while higher doses are administered for more extensive procedures (e.g. mammoplasty, hand surgery). When smaller loading doses are employed, higher initial maintenance infusion rates will be required to compensate for redistribution and elimination processes. For example, the average maintenance infusion rate for brief outpatient procedures (7.7 μg/kg per min) (White et al., 1986) was higher than the rate required during longer, more stressful procedures (0.50—0.75 μg/kg per min) (Shafer et al., 1986) because the latter received a larger loading dose of the drug. When alfentanil is administered by a variable rate infusion during short surgical procedures, a small loading dose (7.5—15 μg/kg) is usually administered 2—3 min prior to induction of anaesthesia with thiopentone, methohexitone or propofol to minimize its respiratory and cardiovascular depressant effects. The alfentanil maintenance infusion, 0.25—1.0 μg/kg per min, can be varied depending on the response to surgical stimulation. In spontaneously breathing patients, changes in respiratory rate or tidal volume are early signs of a change in depth of anaesthesia. If anaesthesia becomes inadequate with a satisfactory respiratory rate of 10—16 BPM, a small dose of a rapidly acting sedative-hypnotic agent should be administered since intra-operative awareness can occur when using a nitrous oxide-narcotic technique (White et al., 1986).

## SUMMARY

The availability of a wide variety of rapid and short-acting intravenous drugs that are suited pharmacologically for use as part of a total intravenous technique has renewed interest in intravenous anaesthesia for short outpatient procedures. Advances in infusion pump technology will make the administration of intravenous drugs by continuous infusion easier in the future. Many of the newer sedative-hypnotics and muscle relaxants possess pharmacologic properties that approach the characteristics of the ideal intravenous anaesthetic for outpatient anaesthesia. Combining sedative-hypnotics, analgesics, muscle relaxants and adjunctive drugs with compatible characteristics, it has become possible to create a smooth intra-operative anaesthetic which is associated with a rapid recovery and minimal postoperative side effects. It has also become possible to achieve an acceptable degree of sedation without residual postoperative impairment in patients undergoing local or regional anaesthetic techniques.

Individualized titration of the drugs administered and knowledge of the pharmacokinetic principles upon which continuous drug administration is based is of paramount importance when using these techniques in the outpatient setting. The availability of a reliable central nervous system monitor of anaesthetic depth would facilitate the use of intravenous anaesthetic techniques. The important question regarding the use of intravenous or volatile techniques for outpatient anaesthesia is the subject of an ongoing debate. With the developement of new intravenous drugs (e.g. propofol, alfentanil, mivacurium, dexmetedomidine) and volatile anaesthetics (e.g. desflurane, sevoflurane), continued research in this field will be necessary to determine the optimal anaesthetic techniques for future patients undergoing ambulatory surgery.

# REFERENCES


Aantaa, R., Kallio, A., Kanto, J., Scheinin, H. and Scheinin, M. (1989) Dexmedetomidine reduces thiopental anesthetic requirements in man. *Anesthesiology* 71, A253.

Abramowitz, M.D., Oh, T.H., Epstein, B.S., Ruttimann, U.E. and Friendly, D.S. (1983) The antiemetic effect of droperidol following outpatient strabismus surgery in children. *Anesthesiology* 59, 579—583.

Ali, H.H., Savarese, J.J., Embree, P.B., Basta, S.J., Stout, R.G., Bottros, L.H. and Weakly, J.N. (1988) Clinical pharmacology of mivacurium bromide (BW B1090U) infusion, comparison with vecuronium and atracurium. *Br. J. Anaesth.* 61, 541—546.

Amar D., Shamoon H., Frishman, W.H., Lazar, E. and Sabama, M. (1989) Labetolol's effects on cardiovascular and sympathoadrenal responses to anesthesia and surgery. *Anesthesiology* 71, A76.

Andersen, R. and Krogh, K. (1976) Pain as a major cause of postoperative nausea. *Can. Anaesth. Soc. J.* 23, 366—369.

Antonios, W.R.A., Inglis, M.D. and Lees, N.W. (1984) Alfentanil in minor gynaecological surgery, use with etomidate and a comparison with halothane. *Anaesthesia* 39, 812—814.

Ausems, M.E., Hug, C.C., Jr, Stanski, D.R. and Burm, A.G.L. (1986) Plasma concentrations of alfentanil required to supplement nitrous oxide anesthesia for general surgery. *Anesthesiology* 65, 362—373.

Barker, I., Butchart, D.G.M., Gibson, J., Lawson, J. and MacKenzy, N. (1986) IV sedation for conservative dentistry. *Br. J. Anaesth.* 58, 371—377.

Beaver, W.T. and Feise, G.A. (1978) A comparison of the analgesic effect of intramuscular nalbuphine and morphine in patients with postoperative pain. *J. Pharmacol. Exp. Ther.* 204, 487—491.

Berggren, L. and Eriksson, I. (1981) Midazolam for induction of anesthesia in outpatients, a comparison with thiopentone. *Acta Anaesthesiol. Scand.* 25, 492—496.

Bloor, B.D. and Flacke, W.E. (1982) Reduction of halothane anesthetic requirement by clonidine, an alpha 2 adrenergic agonist. *Anesth. Analg.* 61, 741—745.

Briggs, R.M. and Ogg, M.J. (1973) Patient refusal of surgery after Innovar R/ premedication. *Plast. Reconstr. Surg.* 51, 158—161.

Caplan, R.A., Ward, R.J., Posner, K. and Cheney, F.W. (1988) Unexpected cardiac arrest during spinal anesthesia — a closed claims analysis of predisposing factors. *Anesthesiology*, 68, 5—11.

Cartwright, P.D. and Pringel, S.M. (1984) Midazolam and diazepam in ketamine anesthesia. *Anaesthesia* 39, 439—442.

Chang, T., Dworsky, W.A. and White, P.F. (1980) Continuous electromyography for monitoring depth of anesthesia. *Anesth. Analg.* 53, 315—334.

Cockshot, I.D. (1985) Propofol (Diprivan) pharmacokinetics and metabolism, an overview. *Postgrad. Med. J.* 61, 45—50.

Cohen S.E., Woods W.A. and Wyner J. (1984) Antiemetic efficacy of droperidol and metoclopramide. *Anesthesiology* 60, 67—69.

Collin, R.I.W., Drummond, G.B. and Spence, A.A. (1986) Alfentanil supplemented anaesthesia for short procedures. *Anaesthesia* 41, 477—481.

Collins, K.M., Plantevin, O.M., Whitburn, R.H. and Doyle J.P. (1985) Outpatient termination of pregnancy, halothane or alfentanil supplemented anaesthesia. *Br. J. Anaesth.* 57, 1226—1231.

Cooper, G.M. (1984) Recovery from anesthesia. *Clin. Anaesthesiol.* 2, 145—162.

Cooper, G.M., O'Connor, M., Mark, J. and Harvey, J. (1983) Effect of alfentanil and fentanyl on recovery from brief anaesthesia. *Br. J. Anaesth.* 55, 179S—182S.

Cork, R. and Scipione, P. (1989) Patients perception of propofol vs thiopental/isoflurane for outpatient anesthesia. *Anesthesiology* 71, A275.

Crawford, M.E., Carl, P., Andersen, R.S. and Mikkelsen B.O. (1984) Comparison between midazolam and thiopentone-based balanced anesthesia for day-case surgery. *Br. J. Anaesth.* 56, 165—167.

Cundy, J.M. and Arunasalam, K. (1985) Use of an emulsion formulation of propofol ('Diprivan') in intravenous anaesthesia for termination of pregnancy. A comparison with methohexitone. *Postgrad. Med. J.* 61, Suppl. 3, 129—131.

deBros, F., Basta, S.J., Ali, H.H., Wargin, W. and Welch, R. (1987) Pharmacokinetics and pharmacodynamics of BWB 1090U in healthy surgical patients receiving $N_2O/O_2$ isoflurane anesthesia. *Anesthesiology* 67, A609.

Dechene, J.-P. (1985) Alfentanil as an adjunct to thiopentone and nitrous oxide in short surgical procedures. *Can. Anaesth. Soc. J.* 32, 346—350.

de Grood, P.M.R.M., Ruys, A.H.C., van Egmond, J., Booij, L.H.D.J. and Crul, J.F. (1985) Propofol ('Diprivan') emulsion for total intravenous anaesthesia. *Postgrad. Med. J.* 61, Suppl. 3, 65—69.

de Grood, P.M.R.M., Mitsukuri, S. and Van Egmond, J. (1987) Comparison of etomidate and propofol for anaesthesia in microlaryngeal surgery. *Anaesthesia* 42, 366—372.

Del Pizzo, A. (1976) Butorphanol, a new intravenous analgesic, double-blind comparison with morphine sulfate in postoperative patients with moderate or severe pain. *Curr. Ther. Res.* 20, 221.

Dodgson, M.S., Heier, T. and Steen, P.A. (1986) Atracurium compared with suxamethonium for outpatient laparoscopy. *Br. J. Anaesth.*. 58, 405 (Suppl.).

Doze, V.A., Shafer, A. and White, P.F. (1987) Nausea and vomiting after outpatient anestheia, effectiveness of droperidol alone and in combination with metoclopramide. *Anesth. Analg.* 66, S41.

Doze, V.A., Shafer, A. and White, P.F. (1988) Propofol-nitrous oxide versus thiopental-isoflurane-nitrous oxide for general anesthesia. *Anesthesiology* 69, 63—71.

Doze, V.A., Westphal, L.M. and White, P.F. (1986) Comparison of propofol with methohexital for outpatient anesthesia. *Anesth. Analg.* 65, 1189—1195.

Doze, V.A. and White, P.F. (1986) Comparison of propofol with thiopental-isoflurane for induction and maintenance of outpatient anesthesia. *Anesthesiology* 65, A544.

Dundee, J.W., McCollum, J.S.C., Robinson, F.P. and Halliday, N.J. (1986) Elderly patients are unduly sensitive to propofol. *Anesth. Analg.* 65, S43.

Epstein, B.S., Levy, M.-L., Thein, M.N. and Coakley, C.S. (1975) Evaluation of fentanyl as an adjunct to thiopental-nitrous-oxygen anesthesia for short surgical procedures. *Anesthesiology Rev.* 2, 24—29.

Evans, J.M., Davies, W.L. and Wise, C.C. (1984) Lower esophageal contractility: a new monitor of anesthesia. *Lancet* 1, 1151—1154.

Evans, J.M., Bithell, J.F. and Vlachnikolis, I.G. (1987) Relationship between lower esophageal contractility, clinical signs and halothane concentration during general anesthesia and surgery in man. *Br. J. Anaesth.* 59, 1346—1355.

Evert, J., Harris, C., Pearson, J., Gilman, S. and Bradley, E.G. (1986) Comparison of the protective effects of esmolol and fentanyl during laryngoscopy. *Anesth. Analg.* 67S, 75.

Flacke, J.W., Bloor, B.C., Flacke, W.E., Wong, D., Dazza, S., Stead, S.W. and Laks H. (1987). Reduced narcotic requirement by clonidine with improved hemodynamic and adrenergic stability in patients undergoing coronary bypass surgery. *Anesthesiology* 67, 11—19.

Forrest, P. and Galletly, D.C. (1987) Comparison of propofol and antagonised midazolam anaesthesia for day-case surgery. *Anaesthesia Intensive Care* 15, 394—398.

Gal, T.J., DiFazio, C.A. and Moscicki, J. (1982) Analgesic and respiratory depressant activity of nalbuphine, a comparison with morphine. *Anesthesiology* 57, 367—374.

Garfield, J.M., Garfield, F.B., Philip, B.K., Earls, F. and Roaf, E. (1987) A comparison of clinical and psychological effects of fentanyl and nalbuphine in ambulatory gynecologic patients. *Anesth. Analg.* 66, 1303—1312.

Ghignone, M., Quintin, L., Duke, P.C., Kehler, C.H. and Calvillo, O. (1986) Effects of clonidine on narcotic requirements and hemodynamic response during induction of fentanyl anesthesia and endotracheal intubation. *Anesthesiology* 64, 36—42.

Ghignone, M., Noe, C., Calvillo, O. and Quintin, L. (1988) Anesthesia for ophthalmic surgery in the elderly, the effects of clonidine on intraocular pressure, perioperative hemodynamics and anesthetic requirement. *Anesthesiology* 68, 707—716.

Giese, J.L., Stockham, R.J., Stanley, T.H., Pace, N.L. and Nelissen, R.H. (1985) Etomidate versus thiopental for induction of anesthesia. *Anesth. Analg.* 64, 871—876.

Gold, M.I., Sacks, D.J., Grosnoff, D.B., Herrington, C. and Shillman, C.A. (1989) Use of esmolol during anesthesia to treat tachycardia and hypertension. *Anesth. Analg.* 68, 101—104.

Goroszeniuk, T., Whitwam, J.G. and Morgan, M. (1977) Use of methohexitone, fentanyl and nitrous oxide for short surgical procedures. *Anaesthesia* 32, 209—211.

Gottlieb, A., Schoenwald, P., Grimes-Rice, M., Khairallah, P.A., Yoon, H. and Estafanous, F.G. (1989) Sedation with propofol vs. midazolam during regional anesthesia. *Anesthesiology* 71, A755.

Greenblatt, D.J., Shader, R.I., Franke, K., MacLaughlin, D.S., Hornatz, J.S. and Allen, M.D., et al. (1979) Pharmacokinetics and bioavailabilty of intravenous, intramuscular and oral lorazepam in humans. *J. Pharmacol. Sci.* 68, 57—63.

Grounds, R.M., Twigley, A.J., Carli, F., Whitwam, J.G. and Morgan, M. (1985) The haemodynamic effects of intravenous induction, comparison of the effects of thiopentone and propofol. *Anaesthesia* 40, 735—740.

Gyasi, H.K., Naguib, M. and Adu-Gyamfi, Y. (1985) Atracurium for short surgical procedures, a comparison with succinylcholine. *Can. Anaesth. Soc. J.* 32, 613—617.

Haley, S., Edelist, G. and Urbach, G. (1988) Comparison of alfentanil, fentanyl and enflurane as supplements to general anaesthesia for outpatient gynaecologic surgery. *Can. J. Anaesth.* 35, 570—575.

Hannallah, R.S., Abramowitz, M.D., McGill, W.A. and Epstein, B.S. (1985) Rectal methohexitone induction in pediatric outpatients: physostigmine does not enhance recovery. *Can. Anaesth. Soc. J.* 32, 231—234.

Hardy, J.F., Girouard, G. and Charest, J. (1985) Nausea and vomiting after strabismus surgery in preschoolers, droperidol is not an effective antiemetic. *Can. Anaesth. Soc. J.* 32, 103—104.

Henriksson, B., Carlsson, P. and Hallen, B. (1987) Propofol vs thiopentone as anesthetic agents for short operative procedures. *Acta Anaesthesiol. Scand.* 31, 63—66.

Henthorn, T.K., Spina, E., Birgersson, C., Ericsson, O. and von Bahr, C. (1985) In vitro competitive inhibition of desipramine hydroxylation by alfentanil and fentanyl in human liver microsomes. *Anesthesiology* 63, A305.

Horrigan, R.W., Moyers, I.R., Johnson, B.H., Eger, E.I., Margolis, A. and Goldsmith, S. (1980) Etomidate vs thiopental with and without fentanyl, a comparative study of awakening in man. *Anesthesiology* 52, 362—364.

Hudson, R.J., Stanski, D.R. and Burch, P.G. (1983) Pharmacokinetics of methohexital and thiopental in surgical patients. *Anesthesiology* 59, 215—219.

Hull, C.J. and Jacobson, L. (1983) A clinical trial of alfentanil as an adjuvant for short anaesthetic procedures. *Br. J. Anaesth.* 55, 1735—1785.

Kallar, S.K. and Keenan, R.L. (1984) Evaluation and comparison of recovery time from alfentanil and fentanyl for short surgical procedures. *Anesthesiology* 61, A379.

Kallio, A., Karhuvaara, S., Scheinin, H. and Scheinin, M. (1989) Cardiovascular and sympatholytic effects of intramuscular dexedetomidine in man. *Anesthesiology* 71, A83.

Kaukinen, S. and Pyykko, K. (1979) The potentiation of halothane anesthesia by clonidine. *Acta Anaesthesiol. Scand.* 23, 107—111.

Kay, B. and Venkataraman, P. (1983) Recovery after fentanyl and alfentanil in anaesthesia for minor surgery. *Br. J. Anaesth.* 55, 169S—171S.

Kay, B., Hargreaves, J. and Healy, T.E.J. (1984) Nalbuphine and althesin anaesthesia. *Anaesthesia* 39, 666—672.

Kay, B. and Healy, T.E.J. (1985) Propofol ('Diprivan') for outpatient cystoscopy. Efficacy and recovery compared with Althesin and methohexitone. *Postgrad. Med. J.* 61, Suppl. 3, 108—114.

Kennedy, D.J. and Ogg, T.W. (1985) Alfentanyl and memory function, a comparison with fentanyl for day case termination of pregnancy. *Anaesthesia* 40, 537—540.

Kestin, I.G., Chapman, J.M. and Coates, M.B. (1989) Alfentanil used to supplement propofol infusion for esophagoscopy and bronchoscopy. *Anesthesiology* 71, A279.

Kestin, I.G. and Dorje, P. (1987) Anaesthesia for evacuation of retained products of conception. *Br. J. Anaesth.* 59, 364—369.

Kirckpatrick, T., Cockshot, I.D., Douglas, E.J. and Nimmo, W.S. (1988) Pharmacokinetics of propofol (Diprivan) in elderly patients. *Br. J. Anaesth.* 60, 146—150.

Korttila, K., Kauste, A. and Auvinen, J. (1979) Comparison of domperidone, droperidol and metoclopramide in the prevention and treatment of nausea and vomiting after balanced general anesthesia. *Anesth. Analg.* 58, 396—400.

Korttila, K., Linnoila, M., Ertama, P. and Hakkinen, S. (1975) Recovery and simulated driving after intravenous anesthesia with thiopental, methohexital or alphadione. *Anesthesiology* 43, 291—299.

Korttila, K. and Tarkkanen, J. (1985) Comparison of diazepam and midazolam for sedation during local anaesthesia for bronchoscopy. *Br. J. Anaesth.* 57, 581—586.

Kortilla, K., Hovorka, J. and Erkota, O. (1987) Omission of nitrous oxide does not decrease the incidence or severity of emetic symptoms after isoflurane anesthesia. *Anesth. Analg.* 66, S98.

Kretz, F.J. and Peisdersky, B. (1988) The effectiveness of the benzodiazepine-antagonist RO 15—1788 after the induction of anesthesia with midazolam. *Anaesthesist* 37, 24—28.

Krishnan, A., Tolhurst-Cleaver, C.L. and Kay B. (1985) Controlled comparison of nalbuphine and morphine for post-tonsillectomy pain. *Anaesthesia* 40, 1178—1181.

Kytta, J. and Rosenberg, P.H. (1988) Comparison of propofol and methohexitone anaesthesia for thermocoagulation therapy of trigeminal neuralgia. *Anaesthesia* 43, 50—53.

Laishley, R.S., O'Callaghan, A.C. and Lerman, J. (1986) Effect of dose and concentration of rectal methohexital for induction of anesthesia in children. *Can. Anaesth. Soc. J.* 33, 427—432.

Lerman, J., Eustis, S. and Smith, D.R. (1986) Effect of droperidol pretreatment on postanesthetic vomiting in children undergoing strabismus surgery. *Anesthesiology* 65, 322—325.

Levy, W.J. (1984) Intraoperative EEG patterns: implications for EEG monitoring. *Anesthesiology* 60, 430—434.

Liu, L.M.P., Gaudreault, P., Friedman, P.A., Goudzousian, N.G. and Liu, P.L. (1985) Methohexital plasma concentrations in children following rectal administration. *Anesthesiology* 62, 567—570.

Liu, P.L., Gatt, S. and Gugino, L.D. (1986) Esmolol for control of increases in heart rate and blood pressure during tracheal intubation after thiopentone and succinylcholine. *Can. Anaesth. Soc. J.* 33, 556—560.

Lonie, D.S. and Harper, N.J.N. (1986) Nitrous oxide anesthesia and vomiting. *Anaesthesia* 41, 703—707.

Maccioli, G.A., Kuni, D.R., Silvay, G., Evans, J.M., Calkins, J.M., and Kaplan, J. (1988) Response of lower esophageal contractility to changing concentrations of halothane or isoflurane: a multicentre study. *J. Clin. Monit.* 4, 247—255.

MacKenzie, N. and Grant, I.S. (1985) Propofol ('Diprivan') for continuous intravenous anaesthesia. A comparison with methohexitone. *Postgrad. Med. J.* 61, Suppl. 3, 70—75.

MacKenzie, N. and Grant, I.S. (1985) Comparison of the new emulsion formulation of propofol with methohexitone and thiopentone for induction of anaesthesia in day cases. *Br. J. Anaesth.* 57, 725—731.

Mackenzy, J.W. and Bird, J. (1989) Timolol, a non-sedative anxiolytic premedicant for day cases. *Br. Med. J.* 298, 363—365.

Magnusson, H., Ponten, J. and Sonander H.G. (1986) Methohexitone anaesthesia for microlaryngoscopy, circulatory modulation with metropolol and dihydralazine. *Br. J. Anaesth.* 58, 976—982.

Maitre, P.O., Voseh, S., Heykants, J., Thomson, D.A. and Stanski, D.R. (1987) Population pharmacokinetics of alfentanil: the average dose-plasma concentration relationship and interindividual variability in patients. *Anesthesiology* 66, 3—12.

Maitre, P.O., Ausems, M.E., Vozeh, S. and Stanski, D.R. (1988) Evaluating the accuracy of using population pharmacokinetic data to predict plasma concentrations of alfentanil. *Anesthesiology* 68, 59—67.

Manchikanti L., Grow J.B., Colliver J.A., Canella M.G. and Hadley, C.H. (1985) Atracurium pretreatment for succinylcholine induced fasciculation and postoperative myalgia. *Anesth. Analg.* 64, 1010—1014.

Manchikanti, L., Colliver, J.A., Grow, J.B., DeMeyer, R.G., Hadley, C.H. and Roush, J.R. (1986) Dose response effects of intravenous ranitidine on gastric pH and volume in outpatients. *Anesthesiology* 65, 180—185.

McCollum, J.S.C., Milligan, K.R. and Dundee, J.W. (1988) The antiemetic action of propofol. *Anaesthesia* 43, 239—243.

McDonnell, T.E., Bankowslti, R.R., Bonilla, F.A., Henthorn, T.K. and Williams, J.J. (1982) Non-uniformity of alfentanil pharmacokinetics in healty adults. *Anesthesiology* 57, A236.

McDonnell, T.E., Bartkowski, R.R. and Kahn, C. (1984) Evidence for polymorphic oxidation of alfentanil in man. *Anesthesiology* 61, A284.

McLeod, B. and Boheimer, N. (1985) Propofol ('Diprivan') infusion as main agent for day case surgery. *Postgrad. Med. J.* 61, Suppl. 3, 105—107.

Melnick, B.M. and Johnson, L.S. (1987) Effects of eliminating nitrous oxide in outpatient anesthesia. *Anesthesiology* 67, 982—984.

Melnick, B., Sawyer, R., Karambelkar, D., Phitayakorn, P., Lim Uy, N.T. and Patel, R. (1989) Delayed side effects of droperidol after ambulatory general anesthesia. *Anesth. Analg.* 69, 748—751.

Metter, S.E., Kitz, D.S., Young, M.L., Baldeck, A.M., Apfelbaum, J.L. and Lecky, J.H. (1987) Nausea and vomiting after outpatient laparascopy, incidence, impact on recovery room stay and cost. *Anesth. Analg.* 66, S116.

Millar, J.M. and Hall, P.J. (1987) Nausea and vomiting after prostaglandins in day case termination of pregnancy. *Anaesthesia* 42, 613—616.

Miller, B.M., Hendry, J.G.B. and Lees N.W. (1978) Etomidate and methohexital, a comparative clinical study in outpatient anesthesia. *Anaesthesia* 33, 450—453.

Milligan, K.R., O'Toole, D.P., Howe, J.P., Cooper, J.C. and Dundee, J.W. (1987) Recovery from outpatient anaesthesia, a comparison of incremental propofol and propofol-isoflurane. *Br. J. Anaesth.* 59, 1111—1114.

Mirakhur, R.K. (1988) Induction characteristics of propofol in children, comparison with thiopentone. *Anaesthesia* 43, 593—599.

Monk, T.G., Mills, A.K. and White, P.F. (1990) Hemodynamic, stress hormone and LEc responses during general anesthesia. *Anesth. Analg.* 70;S271.

Mortensen, P.T. (1982) Droperidol (dehydrobenzperidol), postoperative antiemetic effect when given intravenously to gynecological patients. *Acta Anaesthesiol. Scand.*. 26, 48—52.

Moss, E., Hindmarch, I., Pain, A.J. and Edmondson, R.S. (1987) Comparison of recovery after halothane or alfentanil anaesthesia for minor surgery. *Br. J. Anaesth.* 59, 970—977.

Muir, J.J., Warner, M.A., Offord, K.P., Burk, C.F., Harper, J.V. and Kunkel, S.E. (1987) Role of nitrous oxide and and other factors in postoperative nausea and vomiting, a randomized and blinded prospective study. *Anesthesiology* 66, 513—518.

Nagashima, H., Foldes, F.F. and Karamanian, A. (1976) Respiratory and circulatory effects of intravenous butorphanol and morphine. *Clin. Pharmacol. Ther.* 19, 738.

Nagashima, H., Nguyen, H.D., Kinsey, A., Rosa, M., Hollinger, I., Coldiner, P.C. and Foldes, F.F. (1989) The human dose response of ORG9426. *Anesthesiology* 71, A773.

Negus, J.B. and White, P.F. (1988) Use of sedative infusions during local and regional anesthesia. A comparison of midazolam and propofol. *Anesthesiology* 69, A711.

Newman, M.F., Leslie, J.B., Maccioli, G.A. and Reves, J.G. (1989) Determination of optimal bolus esmolol for prevention of intraoperative hypertension and tachycardia. *Anesthesiology* 71, A285.

O'Donnovan, N. and Shaw, J. (1984) Nausea and vomiting in day case dental anaesthesia. *Anaesthesia* 39, 1172—1176.

Pallazzo, M.G.A. and Strunin, L. (1984) Anaesthesia and emesis, II: Prevention and management. *Can. Anaesth. Soc. J.* 31, 407—415.

Pandit, S.K., Kothary, S.P., Pandit, U.A. and Mathai, M.K. (1987) Comparison of fentanyl and butorphanol for outpatient anaesthesia. *Can. J. Anaesth.* 34, 130—133.

Parnass, S., Rothenberg, D., Kerchberger, J. and Ivankovich, A. (1989) Single dose esmolol for prevention of hemodynamic changes of intubation in an ambulatory surgery unit. *Anesthesiology* 71, A12.

Patel, D.K., Keeling, P.A., Newman, G.B. and Radford, P. (1988) Induction dose of propofol in children. *Anaesthesia* 43, 949—956.

Patrick, M., Eager, B.M., Toft, D.F. and Sebel, P.S. (1984) Alfentanil-supplemented anaesthesia for short procedures. *Br. J. Anaesth.* 56, 861—865.

Persson, P., Nilsson, A., Hartvig, P. and Tamsen, A. (1987) Pharmacokinetics of midazolam in total intravenous anaesthesia. *Br. J. Anaesth.* 59, 548—556.

Philip, B.K., Hauch, M.A., Mallampati, S.R. and Simpson, Th. (1989) Flumazenil for reversal of sedation after midazolam-induced ambulatory general anesthesia. *Anesthesiology* 71, A301.

Phytayakorn, P., Melnick, B.M. and Vicinie, A.F. (1987) Comparison of continuous sufentanil and fentanyl infusions for outpatient anaesthesia. *Can. J. Anaesth.* 34, 242—245.

Poler, S.M., Luchtefeld, G. and White, P.F. (1988) Comparison of mivacurium (B1030U) and succinylcholine during outpatient laparoscopy. *Anesthesiology* 69, A523.

Pouttu, J., Scheinin, B. and Rosenberg, P.H. (1987) Oral premedication with clonidine, effects on stress responses during general anaesthesia. *Acta Anaesthesiol. Scand.* 31, 730—735.

Puttick, N. and Rosen, M. (1988) Propofol induction and maintenance with nitrous oxide in paediatric outpatient dental anesthesia. *Anaesthesia* 43, 646—649.

Raeder, J.C. and Hole, A. (1986) Out-patient laparascopy in general anesthesia with alfentanil and atracurium, a comparison with fentanyl and pancuronium. *Acta Anaesthesiol. Scand.* 30, 30—34.

Raeder, J.C., Hole, A. and Arnulf, V. (1987) Total intravenous anaesthesia with midazolam and flumazenil in outpatient clinics. *Acta Anaesthesiol. Scand.* 31, 634—637.

Raeder, J.C. and Misvaer, G. (1988) Comparison of propofol induction with thiopentone or methohexitone in short outpatient general anaesthesia. *Acta Anaesthesiol. Scand.* 32, 607—611.

Rao, T.L.K., Madhavareddy, S., Chinthagada, M. and El-Etr, A.A. (1984) Metoclopramide and cimetidine to reduce gastric fluid pH and volume. *Anesth. Analg.* 63, 1014—1016.

Reiton, J.A., Porter, W. and Braunstein, M. (1986) Comparison of psychomotor skills and amnesia after induction of anesthesia with midazolam or thiopental. *Anesth. Analg.* 65, 933—938.

Reves, J.G., Fragen, R.J., Vinik, H.R. and Greenblatt, D.J. (1985) Midazolam, pharmacology and uses. *Anesthesiology* 62, 310—324.

Ricou, B., Forster, A., Bruckner, A., Chastonay, P.N. and Gemperle, M. (1986) Clinical evaluation of a specific benzodiazepine antagonist (RO 15-1788) *Br. J. Anaesth.* 58, 1005—1011.

Rising, S., Dodgson, M.S. and Steen, P.A. (1985) Isoflurane vs fentanyl for outpatient laparascopy. *Acta Anaesthesiol. Scand.* 29, 251—257.

Rita, L., Goodarzi, M. and Seleny, F. (1981) Effect of low dose droperidol on postoperative vomiting in children. *Can. Anaesth. Soc. J.* 28, 259—262.

Rodrigues, R.C., Kyung, C., Caldwell, J.E., Sharna, M., Canfell, M.S. and Miller, R.D. (1989) Pharmacokinetics and neuromuscular blocking effects of ORG9991 in the cat. *Anesthesiology* 71, A775.

Rosow, C.E., Latta, W.B. and Keegan, C.R. (1983) Alfentanil and fentanyl in short surgical procedures. *Anesthesiology* 59, A345.

Sampson, I.H., Plosker, H., Cohen, M. and Kaplan, J.A. (1988) Comparison of propofol and thiamylal for induction and maintenance of anaesthesia for outpatient surgery. *Br. J. Anaesth.* 61, 707—719.

Savarese, J.J., Ali, H.H., Basta, S.J., Embree, P.B., Scott, R.P.F., Sunder, N., Weakly, J.N., Wastila, W.B. and El-Sayad, H.A. (1988) The clinical neuromuscular pharmacology of Mivacurium chloride (BW B1090U) *Anesthesiology* 68, 723—732.

Segal, I.S., Vickery, R.G., Walton, J.K., Doze, V.A. and Maze, M. (1988). Dexmedetomidine diminishes halothane anesthetic requirements in rats through a postsynaptic alpha 2 adrenergic receptor effect. *Anesthesiology* 69, 818—823.

Segal, I.S., Jarvis, D.A., Duncan, S.R., White, P.F. and Maze M. (1989) Transdermal clonidine as an adjunctive agent. *Anesth. Analg.* 68, S250.

Sessler, D.I., Stoen, R., Olofsson, C.I. and Chow, F. (1989) Lower esophageal contractility predicts movement during skin incision in patients anesthetized with halothane, but not with nitrous oxide and alfentanil. *Anesthesiology* 70, 42—46.

Shafer, A., Sung, M.-L. and White, P.F. (1986) Pharmacokinetics and pharmacodynamics of alfentanil infusions during general anesthesia. *Anesth. Analg.* 65, 1021—1028.

Shafer, A., Doze, V.A., Shafer, S.L. and White, P.F. (1988) Pharmacokinetics and pharmacodynamics of propofol infusions during general anesthesia. *Anesthesiology* 69, 348—356.

Shafer, A., White, P.F., Urquhart, M.L. and Doze, V.A. (1989) Outpatient premedication, use of midazolam and opioid analgesics. *Anesthesiology* 71, 495—501.

Shand, D.G., Desjardins, R.E., Bjornsson, T.D., Hammill, S.C. and Pritchett, E.L.C. (1981) The method of separate exponentials, a simple aid to devising intravenous drug-loading regimens. *Clin. Pharmacol. Ther.* 29, 542—547.

Shanks, C.A. (1988) What's new in skeletal muscle relaxants and their antagonists. In: *Anesthesiology Clinics of North America (June 1988). New Anesthetic Drugs.* Editors: R.J. Fragen and J.L. Benumof, W.B. Sauders Company, Philadelphia, pp. 343—344.

Simpson, J.E.P., Glynn, C.J., Cox, A.G. and Folkard, S. (1976) Comparative study of short-term recovery of mental efficiency after anaesthesia. *Br. Med. J.* 1, 1560—1562.

Stanley, T.H., Reddy, P., Gilmore, S. and Bennett, G. (1983) The cardiovascular effects of high dose butorphanol-nitrous oxide anesthesia before and during operation. *Can. Anaesth. Soc. J.* 30, 337—341.

Stehling, L.C. and Zauder, H.L. (1978) Double-blind comparison of butorphanol tartrate and meperidine hydrochloride in balanced anesthesia. *J. Int. Med. Res.* 6, 384.

Sury, M.R.J. and Cole, P.V. (1988) Nalbuphine combined with midazolam for outpatient sedation. An assessment in fiberoptic bronchoscopy patients. *Anaesthesia* 43, 285—290.

Toft, P. and Romer, U. (1987) Comparison of midazolam and diazepam to supplement total intravenous anesthesia with ketamine for endoscopy. *Can. J. Anaesth.*. 34, 466—470.

Uppington, J., Kay, N.H. and Sear, J.W. (1985) Propofol ('Diprivan') as a supplement to nitrous oxide-oxygen for maintenance of anaesthesia. *Postgrad. Med. J.* 61, Suppl. 3, 80—83.

Urquhart, M.L. and White, P.F. (1989) Comparison of sedative infusions during regional anesthesia. Methohexital, etomidate and midazolam. *Anesth. Analg.* 68, 249—254.

Valanne, J. and Korttila, K. (1985) Effect of a small dose of droperidol on nausea, vomiting and recovery after outpatient enflurane anesthesia. *Acta Anaesthesiol. Scand.* 29, 359—362.

Varner, P.D., Ebert, J.P., McKay, R.D., Nail, C.S. and Whitlock, T.M. (1985) Methohexital sedation for children undergoing CT-scan. *Anesth. Analg.* 64, 643—645.

Verma, R., Ramasubramanian, R. and Sachar, R.M. (1985) Anesthesia for termination of pregnancy, midazolam compared with methohexital. *Anesth. Analg.* 64, 792—794.

Vickery, R.G., Sheridan, B.C., Segal, I.S. and Maze, M. (1988) Anesthetic and hemodynamic effects of the stereoisomers of medetomidine, an alpha 2 adrenergic agonist in halothane anesthetized dogs. *Anesth. Analg.* 67, 611—615.

Wagner, J.G. (1974) A safe method for rapidly achieving plasma concentration plateaus. *Clin. Pharmacol. Ther.* 16, 691—700.

Wagner, R.L. and White, P.F. (1984) Etomidate inhibits adrenocortical function in surgical patients. *Anesthesiology* 61, 647—651.

Wagner, R.L., White, P.F. and Kan, P.B. (1984) Inhibition of adrenal steroidogenesis by the anesthetic etomidate. *N. Engl. J. Med.* 310, 1415—1421.

Wasudev, G., Kambam, J.R., Hazlehurst, W.M., Hill, P. and Adkins, R. (1987) Comparative study of sufentanil and isoflurane in outpatient surgery. *Anesth. Analg.* 66, S186.

Watcha, M.F. and White, P.F. (1989) Failure of lower esophageal contractility to predict patient movement in children anesthetized with halothane and nitrous oxide. *Anesthesiology* 71, 664—668.

Weightman, W.M. and Zacharias, M. (1987) Comparison of propofol and thiopentone anaesthesia (with special reference to recovery characteristics). *Anaesth. Intensive Care* 15, 389—393.

Wells, J.K.G. (1985) Comparison of ICI 35868, etomidate and methohexitone for day-case anaesthesia. *Br. J. Anaesth.* 57, 732—735.

White, P.F. (1983). Use of continuous infusion versus intermittent bolus administration of fentanyl or ketamine during outpatient anesthesia. *Anesthesiology* 59, 294—300.

White, P.F. (1984) Continuous infusion of thiopental, methohexital, or etomidate as adjuvants to nitrous oxide for outpatient anesthesia. *Anesth. Analg.* 63, 282.

White, P.F. (1985) The role of midazolam in outpatient anesthesia. *Anesthesiology Rev.* 12, 55—60.

White, P.F. (1988) Propofol, pharmacokinetics and pharmacodynamics. *Seminars in Anesthesia* Vol. VII; No. 1, Suppl. 1, 4—20.

White, P.F. (1989) Clinical uses of intravenous anesthetic and analgesic infusions. *Anesth. Analg.* 68, 161—171.

White, P.F., Ham, J., Way, W.L. and Trevor, A.J. (1980) Pharmacology of ketamine isomers in surgical patients. *Anesthesiology* 52, 231—239.

White, P.F., Way, W.L. and Trevor, A.J. (1982) Ketamine — Its pharmacology and therapeutic uses. *Anesthesiology* 56, 119—136.

White, P.F., Dworsky, W.A., Horai, Y. and Trevor, A.J. (1983) Comparison of continuous infusion of fentanyl or ketamine versus thiopental-determining the mean effective serum concentration for outpatient surgery. *Anesthesiology* 59, 564—569.

White, P.F. and Chang, T. (1984) Effect of narcotic premedication on the intravenous anesthetic requirements. *Anesthesiology* 61, A389.

White, P.F., Schuttler, J., Shafer, A., Stanski, D.R., Horai, Y. and Trevor, A.J. (1985) Comparative pharmacology of the ketamine isomers. *Br. J. Anaesth.* 57, 197—203.

White, P.F., Sung, M.-L. and Doze, V.A. (1985) Use of sufentanil in outpatient anesthesia — determining an optimal preinduction dose. *Anesthesiology* 63, A202.

White, P.F., Coe, V., Shafer, A. and Sung, M.-L. (1986) Comparison of alfentanil and fentanyl for outpatient anesthesia. *Anesthesiology* 64, 99—106.

White, P.F., Vasconez, L.O., Mathes, S.A., Way, W.L. and Wender, L.A. (1988) Comparison of midazolam and diazepam for sedation during plastic surgery. *Plast. Reconstr. Surg.* 84, 703—709.

White, P.F. and Boyle, W.A. (1989) Relationship between hemodynamic and electroencephalographic changes during general anesthesia. *Anesth. Analg.* 68, 177—181.

Wolff, J., Carl, P. and Clausen, T.G. (1986) RO 15-1788 for postoperative recovery. *Anaesthesia* 41, 1001—1007.

Zelcer, J., Tyers, M.R., White, P.F., Kennedy, J.T. and Sherman, G.P. (1989) Comparison of alfentanil and fentanyl as adjuvants to propofol and nitrous oxide anesthesia. *Anesthesiology* 71, A28.

Zuurmond, W.W.A. and van Leeuwen, L. (1987) Recovery from sufentanil anesthesia for outpatient arthroscopy, a comparison with isoflurane. *Acta Anaesthesiol. Scand.* 31, 154—156.

*B. Kay (ed.) Total Intravenous Anaesthesia*



# 16

# *Total intravenous anaesthesia for the high risk patient*

Colin S. Goodchild

## INTRODUCTION

When the reader examines the rest of this volume, it will become apparent that much is known of the effects of various intravenous anaesthetic agents on the physiology of normal patients and even those with compromised cardiovascular function. It is therefore possible, at least in theory, to predict the effect of intravenous anaesthesia on patients in the high risk categories. Much work has been performed comparing the effects of induction of anaesthesia with one agent as opposed to another. These are useful if one is able to duplicate the study conditions in clinical practice but usually this work is of limited use to an anaesthetist who wishes to design a total intravenous maintenance anaesthetic technique for a high risk case; the effects of boluses of drugs may be very different to effects of the same drugs when given by intravenous infusion under steady state anaesthetic conditions. There are a number of reasons for this.

Firstly, it is difficult to know what is the equivalent or equipotent dose of one intravenous agent compared with another. There have been a few attempts to determine the equipotent doses of intravenous anaesthetics given as bolus injections (Grounds et al., 1985) and infusions (Sear et al., 1979, 1981, 1983, 1984; Richards et al., 1988). The second problem with much of the published work on the effects of intravenous anaesthetics is that the speed of injection of a bolus is directly proportional to the magnitude of the side effects. This effect is further magnified in the elderly patient and the patient with a compromised circulation where a greater proportion of a bolus injection may be distributed to the brain (Steib et al., 1988). Finally, the concurrent use of other anaesthetic and analgesic agents may radically affect the conclusions of the study of the effects of an intravenous anaesthetic technique.

This chapters deals very briefly with the use of total intravenous anaesthesia for specific disease states, but the main subject is the use of total intravenous anaesthesia for high risk patients seen by the generalist. These are patients in whom the speed of recovery is quite important and also in whom it is important to minimise adverse respiratory and cardiovascular sequelae.

## SPECIFIC DISEASE STATES

For the rarer diseases one has to rely on isolated case reports as to the suitability of individual anaesthetic drugs. The trigger agents for malignant hyperpyrexia are well known and all of the commonly available (including the newer) intravenous anaesthetic agents have been reported to be suitable for patients susceptible to malignant hyperpyrexia (Marks et al., 1988). They allow one to avoid all the inhalational agents.

Hypertensive crises associated with anaesthesia for patients with phaeochromocytoma may be caused by the injection of drugs which lead to the release of histamine. The commonest technique used for anaesthesia for surgical removal of a phaeochromocytoma is a combination of opioids such as fentanyl with droperidol (neuroleptanaesthesia). Among the intravenous induction agents, it is usual to avoid the barbiturates because of their histamine-releasing capabilities. However, the safe use of propofol in such cases has been reported and this now opens up the possibility of using an infusion of propofol as the hypnotic part of a balanced anaesthetic technique instead of droperidol.

The avoidance of barbiturates and the use of ketamine for the induction of anaesthesia in the porphyrias is well known. Propofol infusions may be added to the list of suitable techniques for acute intermittent porphyria (Mitterschiffthaler et al., 1987).

All of the currently available intravenous anaesthetic agents have been reported as being suitable for anaesthesia for patients with myasthenia gravis. However, these patients may have compromised respiratory function postoperatively and the use of an agent which is cleared from the body very quickly may make the difference between successful management of these patients without postoperative ventilation and being faced with the difficult choice of suitable sedative agent for such patients on ventilators in intensive care. Intravenous infusions of propofol may be suitable for this application because of the rapid recovery profile. Propofol, along with other intravenous agents, has also been used successfully in myotonia, intubation being possible without the aid of muscle relaxants (Speedy, 1990).

### Epilepsy

The anticonvulsive properties of thiopentone are well known as is the occurrence of abnormal movements associated with intravenous anaesthesia with methohexitone and etomidate. The causes and origins of these abnormal movements are not known but the use of etomidate in known epileptics is discouraged. Various clinical reports have implicated the newer intravenous agent propofol in production of epileptogenic seizures (Cameron, 1987; Hopkins, 1988; Jones et al., 1988; Victory and McGee, 1988; Hodkinson et al., 1989). However, in other clinical reports it has been suggested that propofol has anticonvulsant properties (Wood et al., 1988). There are two related questions with regard to intravenous anaesthesia in known epileptics:

(i) Does the drug have intrinsic proconvulsant/anticonvulsant properties?

(ii) Does the rate of change, either up or down, in the drug concentration in the brain, affect the propensity for seizures originating from normal or epileptogenic foci?

This problem has been addressed in experiments in laboratory animals using two convulsive tests: the electroshock test which involves passing a brief electric current through the heads of mice and measuring the number in a group which have a convulsion; and, secondly, the pentylenetetrazol (PTZ) test which measures the convulsive threshold (the amount of the convulsant, pentylenetetrazol, required to make an individual animal fit (MCD of PTZ)). All known anticonvulsant drugs exhibit anticonvulsant activity in one or both of these tests. Using these tests it has been shown that equipotent sedative and anaesthetic doses of thiopentone and propofol both exhibit powerful anticonvulsant activity, thiopentone being more effective in the electroshock test and propofol being more effective in the pentylenetetrazol test (Lowson et al., 1990). The pentylenetetrazol test has also been used to measure the convulsive threshold in mice after induction of anaesthesia with thiopentone, etomidate, methohexitone and propofol. Figure 16.1 shows the MCD of PTZ (the convulsive threshold) against time, time 0 being the time at which withdrawal of the tail from a noxious stimulus occurred after induction of anaesthesia with the intravenous anaesthetic concerned. The arrow on each graph shows the time of full recovery of all animals in each group from the effects of the anaesthetic. It may be seen that all intravenous anaesthetic agents caused powerful anticonvulsant effects which extended beyond the time of full recovery from the anaesthetic. At no time during the recovery phase with any anaesthetic agent did the convulsive threshold fall below the level of control animals (shown as the horizontal dotted line). If a fall in the MCD of PTZ below control levels occurred it would indicate a proconvulsive effect of the anaesthetic during the recovery phase. This test is capable of showing a reduction of convulsive threshold demonstrated after the intravenous injection of the proconvulsant Ro 15-4513 (Lowson et al., 1990).

In several clinical reports of convulsions associated with propofol anaesthesia there was a family history of this disease and perhaps these patients are more likely to exhibit convulsions when intravenous anaesthetics are used. These convulsions are all the more likely to occur with the shorter-acting intravenous agents and when an agent is used for induction rather than maintenance by infusion because: (i) the anti-epileptic effects of methohexitone and propofol do not extend far into the recovery period when compared with thiopentone and (ii) patients on anti-epileptic medication may be forced to omit these drugs prior to surgery. It would, therefore, seem prudent when one is designing a total intravenous anaesthetic

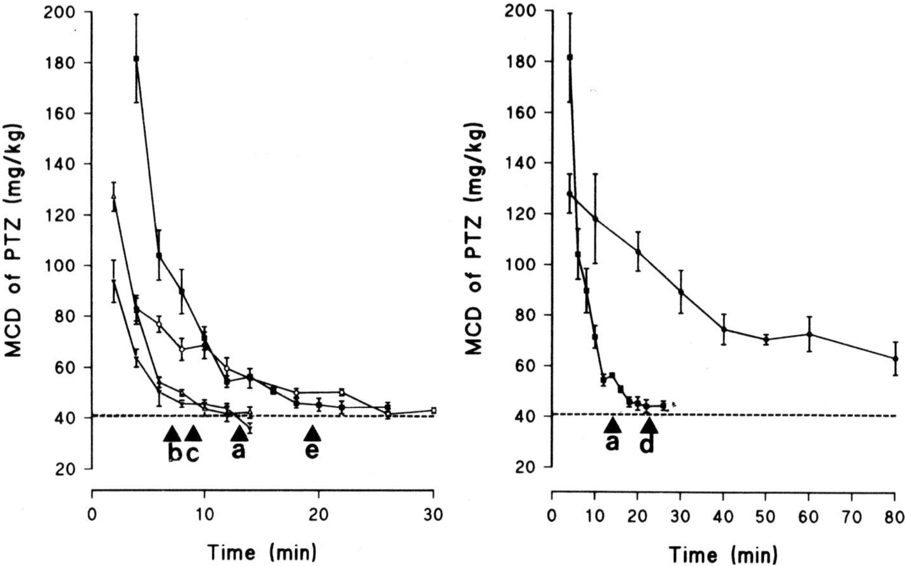


Fig. 16.1. Decrease in anticonvulsant effect (MCD of PTZ; see text) after intravenous injection of anaesthetic agents: (a) propofol 20 mg/kg, ■ ; (b) propofol 10 mg/kg, △ ; (c) methohexitone 10 mg/kg, ▲ ; (d) thiopentone 30 mg/kg, ● ; (e) etomidate 3 mg/kg, ○ . Labelled arrows show time of full recovery from anaesthesia induced with each agent. Points represent means ($n$ = 5), bars show standard error of the mean.

technique for such cases, to use thiopentone or administer an anticonvulsant prior to cessation of intravenous anaesthesia.

## SPEED OF RECOVERY

The research reporting the comparisons of speed of recovery from intravenous anaesthetic agents is of limited use to the anaesthetist who wishes to design an intravenous anaesthetic technique with a fast speed of recovery for a poor risk patient. One is particularly interested in a fast recovery of protective reflexes and respiratory and cardiovascular control. Unfortunately, the measurements of speed of recovery which have been used to compare the various intravenous anaesthetic agents are psychometric tests, e.g. time to opening of the eyes and to repeat the correct date of birth. This work, therefore, may only be used as a guide to which is the most suitable agent to use in a total intravenous anaesthetic regime in a patient for whom fast recovery of protective reflexes is regarded as important. It has been variously reported that recovery from anaesthesia with propofol is faster than or equal to recovery from thiopentone and also faster than or equal to methohexitone (Robinson et al., 1985; Herbert et al., 1985; Noble and Ogg, 1985; Valanne and Korttila, 1985; Logan et al., 1985; Grant and Mackenzie, 1985; Kirkpatrick et al., 1988; Sanders et al., 1989). When one takes into account that these were bolus injections for induction of anaesthesia and some studies used an inhalation agent and premedication, it seems that one might expect a faster recovery from total intravenous anaesthesia with propofol than with the barbiturates; this also seems to be true for the elderly who form a large part of the practice of anaesthesia in the high risk group.

## RESPIRATORY EFFECTS

The incidence of apnoea following intravenous induction of anaesthesia is well established with all agents in common usage. However, the relative incidence is difficult to assess. For instance, apnoea has been reported following intravenous propofol induction in 0—53% of cases given doses of 2 or 2.5 mg/kg (Cummings et al., 1984; Briggs and White, 1985; Bilaine and Desmonts, 1985). These were fit patients, some of whom had premedication and all of whom had rather large doses of the drug — certainly much larger and given much faster than one would wish to administer the drug to high risk groups of patients. However, one would treat all intravenous agents with caution in patients with compromised airways.

As far as anaesthesia with a total intravenous technique is concerned, rises in arterial $CO_2$ concentration have been described for thiopentone, methohexitone and propofol at depths of anaesthesia sufficient to allow surgery (Prys-Roberts et al., 1953). With all patients breathing spontaneously, they report similar elevations of $CO_2$ levels indicating a moderate degree of respiratory depression. The magnitude of this rise is of the same order as with other methods of anaesthesia. Great elevations of $CO_2$ tensions in arterial blood may follow the use of opioids in premedication or as adjuncts to intravenous anaesthesia, and these factors may become important in a poor risk patient who already has $CO_2$ retention because of pre-existing pulmonary disease. In such cases, whatever the anaesthetic technique, assisted ventilation is advisable. This would be true of the management of any anaesthetic for such a case. However, one would wish to avoid postoperative respiratory depressant effects of the drugs used and this really brings us back to the point on speed of recovery from intravenous anaesthetic drugs. Obviously, it would be desirable to include drugs which are metabolised quickly and which have the fewest respiratory effects in the postoperative period.

## CARDIOVASCULAR EFFECTS

The cardiovascular effects of various intravenous anaesthetic agents in both normal patients and those with compromised cardiovascular function have been extensively reviewed (Sear, 1989; Bovill, 1989). Whatever agent is used in the high risk patient with cardiovascular disease, the principles remain the same, i.e. to maintain the balance between myocardial oxygen demand and its supply. The avoidance of hypotension and tachycardia are keystones in the management of these patients. A related problem is the avoidance of hypertension and tachycardia associated with tracheal intubation. When deciding which drug or combinations of drugs to use in this situation one must consider first of all the effect on such a patient of inducing sleep whatever the agent used, and secondly the relative merits of different agents due to their specific effects on elements of the cardiovascular system.

The induction of sleep with any anaesthetic agent causes a centrally mediated decrease in sympathetic nervous system tone. Withdrawal of sympathetic drive from the heart produces an apparent negative inotropic effect. This is not due to a direct depressant effect of the drug on the myocardium although some anaesthetic agents also possess this property. Withdrawal of sympathetic tone from blood vessels causes a decrease in afterload and, therefore, a reduction in blood pressure. Increased peripheral perfusion causes a passive filling of peripheral veins and, therefore, an increase in capacitance and a decrease in pre-load. Further capacitance effects are caused by decreasing sympathetic tone to the capacitance vessels within the thorax and abdomen. There is, therefore, a net movement of blood away from the thorax into the periphery. This decrease in venous return tends to produce a fall in cardiac output.

All the preceding effects occur on induction of general anaesthesia, but in addition, individual anaesthetic agents possess specific properties which affect cardiovascular function. For instance, thiopentone infusions have been associated with an increase in systemic vascular resistance and also heart rate (Etsen and Li, 1955; Todd et al., 1985). Similar responses have been reported for methohexitone. By contrast, etomidate seems relatively free of these complications although small drops in blood pressure do occur when anaesthesia is induced with this agent (Colvin et al., 1979; Criado et al., 1980; Kettler and Sonntag, 1974). The hypertension and tachycardia associated with ketamine anaesthesia precludes its use from most anaesthetic practice in patients with compromised myocardial oxygen supply (Virtue et al., 1967). However, this drug does find a place in anaesthesia for hypovolaemic patients.

Benzodiazepines may also be used for the sleep element in a balanced anaesthetic technique. Midazolam has been the drug most used, usually in combination with alfentanyl or fentanyl for analgesia. This technique has been reported to produce a cardiostable anaesthetic with small decreases in blood pressure and heart rate (Nilsson et al., 1986). Similar results have also been obtained using a balanced combination of propofol and alfentanil by infusion (Schuttler et al., 1988). The effects of general anaesthetic agents on the capacitance vessels has been hitherto underestimated. Patients with compromised cardiovascular function, because of cardiac failure or hypovolaemia, may respond very badly to an anaesthetic technique which causes a relaxation of capacitance vessels. This always occurs to some extent during anaesthesia, because of reduction of sympathetic tone but some anaesthetics also exert a direct venodilator action. This has recently been shown for propofol which exerts a direct venodilator effect at anaesthetic concentrations (Goodchild and Serrao, 1989). Separation of the effects of withdrawal of sympathetic tone associated with induction and deepening of the level of anaesthesia was possible in a whole animal in which the cardiovascular system was isolated from the autonomic nervous system by bilateral vagotomy and intravenous administration of propanolol and bretylium tosylate. These results have since been confirmed in isolated portal vein and aorta (Bentley et al.,1989). Propofol exerts direct relaxant effects on both vessels, the dose response curve for relaxation of tone in the vein being significantly to the left of that for the artery.

The increase in capacitance and decrease in venous return caused by either of the mechanisms above may be counteracted very easily by either intravenous infusion of fluids or appropriate positioning of the patient; raising the legs has the advantage of improving venous return without the administration of a fluid load which may be a cause of postoperative cardiac failure when venous and arteriolar tone return to normal upon withdrawal of the anaesthetic. There is no easy answer, however, to the question of how one treats the fall in afterload associated with anaesthesia for the poor risk patient. This is particularly important in the patient with a compromised myocardium which cannot maintain reasonable perfusion pressure without a significant afterload. In such patients, a reduction of afterload is a necessary sequel to induction of general anaesthesia. The balance of evidence from the literature does not indicate that one particular intravenous anaesthetic regimen is better or worse than any other in this respect when equipotent doses are used and boluses are given at the appropriate rate for the condition of the patient. Having induced a light plane of anaesthesia with an intravenous anaesthetic regime it then remains to alter the dose according to the surgical stimulation in order to maintain a constant afterload. It may, therefore, be advantageous in this situation to use drugs which are metabolised quickly and so one may decrease the blood level of the anaesthetic relatively quickly.

## CONCLUSION

It is possible to devise total intravenous anaesthetic regimes by the addition of hypnotic or anaesthetic agents which may be given by infusions to a combination of muscle relaxant and an opioid. The use of opioids to supplement anaesthesia increases the incidence of respiratory depression in spontaneously breathing patients and hypotension, due to vasodilatation, in ventilated patients. If the hypnotic drugs are used in the same way as the inhalational agents, then good quality anaesthesia which is safe for the poor risk patient may be achieved. Instead of relying on ventilation to remove the anaesthetic drug, we must rely on metabolism. There are differences between the intravenous agents with regard to speed of elimination by metabolism from the body and these factors must be borne in mind when designing a total intravenous anaesthetic technique for the high risk patient who may have compromised hepatic and renal function. In many cases, patients have to be returned to a normal ward and even if they are admitted to intensive care good recovery of airway, cardiovascular and respiratory control will contribute to a lower incidence of morbidity and mortality in this group of patients.

## REFERENCES


Bentley, G.N., Gent, J.P. and Goodchild, C.S. (1989) Vascular effects of propofol: smooth muscle relaxation in isolated veins and arteries. *J. Pharm. Pharmacol.* 41, 797—798.

Bilaine, J. and Desmonts, J.M. (1985) Effect of premedication with atropine and hydroxyzine on induction and maintenance of anaesthesia with propofol ('Diprivan'). *Postgrad. Med. J.* 61, Suppl.3, 38—39.

Bovill, J.G. (1989) Cardiac anaesthesia. *J. Drug Dev.* 2, Suppl. 2, 111—117.

Briggs, L.P. and White, M. (1985) The effects of premedication on anaesthesia with propofol ('Diprivan'). *Postgrad. Med. J.* 61, Suppl. 3, 35—37.

Cameron, A.E. (1987) Opisthotonos again. *Anaesthesia* 42, 112—114.

Colvin, M.P., Savage, T.M., Newland, P.E., Weaver, E.J.M., Waters, A.F., Brookes, J.M. and Inniss, R. (1979) Cardiorespiratory changes following induction of anaesthesia with etomidate in patients with cardiac disease. *Br. J. Anaesth.* 51, 551—556.

Criado, A., Maseda, J., Navarro, E., Escarpa, A. and Avello, F. (1980) Induction of anaesthesia with etomidate: haemodynamic study of 36 patients. *Br. J. Anaesth.* 52, 803—806.

Cummings, G.C., Dixon, J., Kay, N.H., Windsor, J.P., Major, E., Morgan, M., Sear, J.W., Spence, A.A. and Stephenson, D.K. (1984) Dose requirements of ICI 35,868 (propofol, 'Diprivan') in a new formulation for induction of anaesthesia. *Anaesthesia* 12, 1168—1171.

Etsten, B. and Li, T.H. (1955) Haemodynamic changes during thiopental anaesthesia in humans. *J. Clin. Invest.* 34, 500—510.

Goodchild, C.S. and Serrao, J.M. (1989) Cardiovascular effects of propofol in the anaesthetised dog. *Br. J. Anaesth.* 63, 87—92.

Grant, I.S. and Mackenzie, N. (1985) Recovery following propofol ('Diprivan') anaesthesia — a review of three different anaesthetic techniques. *Postgrad. Med. J.* 61, Suppl. 3, 133—137.

Grounds, T.M., Twigley, H.A., Carli, F., Whitwam, J.G. and Morgan, M. (1985) The haemodynamics of intravenous induction. Comparison of the effects of thiopentone and propofol. *Anaesthesia* 40, 735—740.

Herbert, M., Makin, S.W., Bourke, J.B. and Hart, E.A. (1985) Recovery of mental abilities following thiopentone. *Postgrad. Med. J.* 61, Suppl. 3, 132.

Hodkinson, B.P., Frith, R.W. and Mee, E.W. (1987) Propofol and the electroencephalogram. *Lancet* ii, 1518.

Hopkins, C.S. (1988) Recurrent opisthotonos associated with anaesthesia. *Anaesthesia* 43, 904.

Jones, G.W., Boykett, M.H. and Klok, M. (1988) Propofol opisthotonos and epilepsy. *Anaesthesia* 43, 905.

Kettler, D. and Sonntag, H. (1974) Intravenous anaesthetics: coronary blood flow and myocardial oxygen consumption (with special reference to Althesin). *Acta Anaesthesiol. Belg.* 3, 384—401.

Kirkpatrick, T., Cockshott, D., Douglas, E.J. and Nimmo, W.S. (1988) Pharmacokinetics of propofol (Diprivan) in elderly patients. *Br. J. Anaesth.* 60, 146—150.

Logan, M.R., Lerack, I.D., Duggan, J. and Spence, A.A. (1985) Propofol ('Diprivan') compared with methohexitone for outpatient dental anaesthesia. *Postgrad. Med. J.* 61, Suppl. 3, 144.

Lowson, S.M., Gent, J.P. and Goodchild, C.S. (1990) The anticonvulsant properties of propofol and thiopentone: a comparison using two tests in laboratory mice. *Br. J. Anaesth.* 64, 59—63.

Marks, L.F., Edwards, J.C. and Linter, S.P.K. (1988) Propofol during cardiopulmonary bypass in a patient susceptible to malignant hyperpyrexia. *Anaesth. Intensive Care* 16, 482—485.

Mitterschiffthaler, G., Theiner, A., Hetzel, H. and Fuith, L.C. (1987) Safe use of propofol in a patient with acute intermittent porphyria. *Br. J. Anaesth.* 60, 109—111.

Nilsson, A., Tamsen, A. and Persson, P. (1986) Midazolam-fentanyl anaesthesia for major surgery. Plasma levels of midazolam during prolonged total intravenous anaesthesia. *Acta Anaesthesiol. Scand.* 30, 66—69.

Noble, J. and Ogg, T.W. (1985) The effect of propofol ('Diprivan') and methohexitone on memory after day case anaesthesia. *Postgrad. Med. J.* 61, Suppl. 3, 103—104.

Prys-Roberts, C., Davies, J.R., Calverley, R.K. and Goodman, N.W. (1983) Haemodynamic effects of infusions of diisopropylphenol (ICI 35868) during nitrous oxide anaesthesia in man. *Br. J. Anaesth.* 55, 105—110.

Richards, M.J., Skues, M.A., Jarvis, A.P. and Prys-Roberts, C. (1988) Total intravenous anaesthesia with propofol and alfentanyl: dose requirements for propofol. *Br. J. Anaesth.* 61, 510P.

Robinson, F.P., Dundee J.W. and Halliday J. (1985) Effect of age on "induction dose" of propofol. *Br. J. Anaesth.* 57, 349P.

Sanders, I.D., Isaac, P.A., Yeomans, W.A., Clyburn, P.A., Rosen, M. and Robinson, J.O. (1989) Propofol-induced anaesthesia. Double-blind comparison of recovery after anaesthesia induced by propofol or thiopentone. *Anaesthesia* 44, 200—204.

Schuttler, J., Kloos, S., Schwilden, H. and Stoeckel, H. (1988) Total intravenous anaesthesia with propofol and alfentanyl by computer-assisted infusion. *Anaesthesia* 43, (Suppl.) 2—7.

Sear, J.W. (1989) Intravenous anaesthetics. In: *Bailliere's Clinical Anaesthesiology: Anaesthesia for the Compromised Heart.* Bailliere, London, pp. 217—242.

Sear, J.W. and Prys-Roberts, C. (1979) Dose related haemodynamic effects of continuous infusion of althesin in man. *Br. J. Anaesth.* 51, 867—873.

Sear, J.W., Phillips, K.C., Andrews, C.J.H. and Prys-Roberts, C. (1983) Dose-response relationships for infusions of althesin and methohexitone. *Anaesthesia* 38, 931—936.

Sear, J.W., Prys-Roberts, C., Gray, A.J.G., Walsh, E.M., Curnow, J.S.N. and Dye, J. (1981) Infusion of minaxolone to supplement nitrous oxide anaesthesia. A comparison with althesin. *Br. J. Anaesth.* 53, 339—350.

Sear, J.W., Prys-Roberts, C. and Phillips, K.C. (1984) Age influences — the minimum infusion rate ($ED_{50}$) for continuous infusions of althesin and methohexitone. *Eur. J. Anesthesiol.* 1, 319—325.

Speedy, H. (1990) Exaggerated physiological responses to propofol in myotonic dystrophy. *Br. J. Anaesth.* 64, 110—112.

Steib, A., Freys, G., Beller, J.P., Curzola, V. and Otteni, J.C. (1988) Propofol in elderly high risk patients: a comparison of haemodynamic effects with thiopentone during induction of anaesthesia. *Anaesthesia* 43, (Suppl.) 111—114.

Todd, M.M., Drummond, J.C. and U, H.S. (1985) The haemodynamic consequences of high dose thiopental anaesthesia. *Anesth. Analg.* 64, 681—687.

Valanne, J. and Kortilla, K. (1985) Comparison of methohexitone and propofol ('Diprivan') for induction of enflurane anaesthesia in outpatients. *Postgrad. Med. J.* 61, Suppl. 3, 138—143.

Victory, R.A.P. and McGee, D. (1988) A case of convulsion after propofol. *Anaesthesia* 43, 904.

Virtue, R.W., Alanis, J.M., Mori, M., Lafargue, R.T., Vogel, J.H.K. and Metcalf, D.R. (1967) An anesthetic agent: 2-orthochlorophenyl,2-methylamin cyclohexanone HCl (CI-581). *Anesthesiology* 28, 823—833.

Wood, P.R., Browne, G.P.R. and Pugh, S. (1988) Propofol infusion for the treatment of status epilepticus. *Lancet* i, 480—481.

# Subject index